GERIATRICS *At* *Your* FINGERTIPS®

2023, 25th EDITION

GERIATRICS *At Your* FINGERTIPS®

2023, 25th EDITION

AUTHORS

David B. Reuben, MD

Keela A. Herr, PhD, RN

James T. Pacala, MD, MS

Bruce G. Pollock, MD, PhD

Jane F. Potter, MD

Todd P. Semla, MS, PharmD

Geriatrics At Your Fingertips® is published by the American Geriatrics Society as a service to healthcare providers involved in the care of older adults.

Although *Geriatrics At Your Fingertips®* is distributed by various companies in the healthcare field, it is independently prepared and published. All decisions regarding its content are solely the responsibility of the authors. Their decisions are not subject to any form of approval by other interests or organizations.

Some recommendations in this publication suggest the use of agents for purposes or in dosages other than those recommended in product labeling. Such recommendations are based on reports in peer-reviewed publications and are not based on or influenced by any material or advice from pharmaceutical or healthcare product manufacturers.

No responsibility is assumed by the authors or the American Geriatrics Society for any injury or damage to persons or property, as a matter of product liability, negligence, warranty, or otherwise, arising out of the use or application of any methods, products, instructions, or ideas contained herein. No guarantee, endorsement, or warranty of any kind, express or implied (including specifically no warrant of merchantability or of fitness for a particular purpose) is given by the Society in connection with any information contained herein. Independent verification of any diagnosis, treatment, or drug use or dosage should be obtained. No test or procedure should be performed unless, in the judgment of an independent, qualified physician, it is justified in the light of the risk involved.

Citation: Reuben DB, Herr KA, Pacala JT, et al. *Geriatrics At Your Fingertips: 2023, 25th Edition.* New York: The American Geriatrics Society; 2023.

ISSN 1553-152X
ISBN 978-1-886775-76-3

TABLE OF CONTENTS

AUTHORS

David B. Reuben, MD
Director, Multicampus Program in Geriatric Medicine and Gerontology
Chief, Division of Geriatrics
Archstone Foundation Chair
Professor of Medicine
David Geffen School of Medicine at UCLA, Los Angeles, CA

Keela A. Herr, PhD, RN
Kelting Professor in Nursing and Associate Dean for Faculty
Co-Director, Csomay Center for Gerontological Excellence
College of Nursing
The University of Iowa, Iowa City, IA

James T. Pacala, MD, MS
Professor and Head
Department of Family Medicine and Community Health
University of Minnesota Medical School, Minneapolis, MN

Bruce G. Pollock, MD, PhD, FRCPC, DFAPA
Peter and Shelagh Godsoe Chair in Late-Life Mental Health
Centre for Addiction and Mental Health
Professor of Psychiatry and Pharmacology
University of Toronto, Temerty Faculty of Medicine, Toronto, Ontario, Canada

Jane F. Potter, MD, AGSF, FACP
Professor, Internal Medicine, Geriatrics
Medical Director, Geriatrics Health Center
University of Nebraska Medical Center, Omaha, NE

Todd P. Semla, MS, PharmD
Associate Professor, Clinical
Departments of Medicine and Psychiatry & Behavioral Sciences
The Feinberg School of Medicine
Northwestern University, Chicago, IL

ABBREVIATIONS AND SYMBOLS

1,25(OH)2D	1,25-dihydroxyvitamin D
25(OH)D	25-hydroxyvitamin D
A1c	glycosylated hemoglobin
AAA	abdominal aortic aneurysm
AAOS	American Academy of Orthopaedic Surgeons
AASM	American Academy of Sleep Medicine
ABG	arterial blood gas
ABI	ankle-brachial (pressure) index
ACC	American College of Cardiology
ACEI	angiotensin-converting enzyme inhibitor
ACI	anemia of chronic inflammation
ACIP	Advisory Committee on Immunization Practices
ACP	advance care planning
ACPA	anticitrullinated peptide antibody
ACR	American College of Rheumatology
ACS	acute coronary syndrome
ACTH	adrenocorticotropic hormone
AD	Alzheimer disease
ADA	American Diabetes Association
ADLs	activities of daily living
ADR	adverse drug reaction
ADT	androgen deprivation therapy
AE	adverse event
AF	atrial fibrillation
AGS	American Geriatrics Society
AHA	American Heart Association
AHI	apnea-hypopnea index
AHRQ	Agency for Healthcare Research and Quality
AI	aromatase inhibitor
AIDS	acquired immune deficiency syndrome
AKI	acute kidney injury
ALS	amyotrophic lateral sclerosis
ALT	alanine aminotransferase
AMD	age-related macular degeneration
AML	acute myeloid leukemia
APAP	acetaminophen
ARB	angiotensin receptor blocker
ARNI	ARB-neprilysin inhibitor
AS	aortic stenosis
ASA	acetylsalicylic acid or aspirin
ASB	asymptomatic bacteriuria
ASCVD	atherosclerotic cardiovascular disease
ATA	American Thyroid Association
ATS	American Thoracic Society
AUA	American Urological Association
AUD	Alcohol Use Disorder
AV	atrioventricular
BC	Beers Criteria
BMD	bone mineral density
BMI	body mass index
BNP	brain natriuretic peptide

BP	blood pressure
BPH	benign prostatic hyperplasia
bpm	beats per minute
BUN	blood urea nitrogen
C&S	culture and sensitivity
CABG	coronary artery bypass graft
CAD	coronary artery disease
CAM	Confusion Assessment Method
CAP	community-acquired pneumonia
CBC	complete blood cell count
CBD	cannabidiol
CBT	cognitive-behavioral therapy
CCB	calcium-channel blocker
CDC	US Centers for Disease Control and Prevention
CDI	*Clostridioides difficile* infection
cfu	colony-forming unit
CHA_2DS_2–VASc	Congestive heart failure, Hypertension, Age ≥75 (doubled), Diabetes, Stroke (doubled), Vascular disease, Age 65–74, and Sex (female) (score)
$CHADS_2$	Congestive heart failure, Hypertension, Age ≥75, Diabetes, Stroke (doubled) (score)
CHD	congenital heart disease
CKD	chronic kidney disease
CLL	chronic lymphocytic leukemia
CMS	Centers for Medicare and Medicaid Services
CNS	central nervous system
COPD	chronic obstructive pulmonary disease
CPAP	continuous positive airway pressure
Cr	creatinine
CrCl	creatinine clearance
CRE	Carbapenem-resistant enterobacteriaceae
CRP	C-reactive protein
CSF	cerebrospinal fluid
CT	computed tomography
CUR	chronic urinary retention
CVD	cardiovascular disease
CW	Choosing Wisely recommendation
CXR	chest x-ray
CYP	cytochrome
D&C	dilation and curettage
D/C	discontinue
D5W	dextrose 5% in water
DASH	Dietary Approaches to Stop Hypertension
DBP	diastolic blood pressure
DBS	deep brain stimulation
DHEA	dehydroepiandrosterone
DHIC	detrusor hyperactivity with impaired contractility
DM	diabetes mellitus
DMARD	disease-modifying antirheumatic drug
DOAC	direct oral anticoagulant
DPI	dry powder inhaler
DPP-4	dipeptidyl peptidase-4
DSM-5	*Diagnostic and Statistical Manual of Mental Disorders*, 5th ed. (Arlington, VA: American Psychiatric Association; 2013)
DVT	deep-vein thrombosis
EBRT	external beam radiation therapy
ECF	extracellular fluid

ECG	electrocardiogram, electrocardiography
ECT	electroconvulsive therapy
ED	erectile dysfunction
EEG	electroencephalogram
EF	ejection fraction
eGFR	estimated glomerular filtration rate
EIA	enzyme immunoassay
EMR	electronic medical record
ENT	otolaryngologist
EPS	extrapyramidal symptoms
ESA	erythropoietin-stimulating agent
ESR	erythrocyte sedimentation rate
ESRD	end-stage renal disease
EULAR	European League Against Rheumatism
EWL	estimated weight loss
FAST	Functional Assessment Staging Tool
FDA	US Food and Drug Administration
FDG-PET	fluorodeoxyglucose-positron emission tomography
FEV_1	forced expiratory volume in 1 sec
FI	fecal incontinence
FRAX	Fracture Risk Assessment Tool
FTD	frontotemporal dementia
FVC	forced vital capacity
GAD	generalized anxiety disorder
GDS	Geriatric Depression Scale
GERD	gastroesophageal reflux disease
GFR	glomerular filtration rate
GI	gastrointestinal
GLP-1	glucagon-like peptide–1
GnRH	gonadotropin-releasing hormone
GSM	genitourinary syndrome of menopause
GU	genitourinary
Hb	hemoglobin
HDL	high-density lipoprotein
HF	heart failure
HIT	heparin-induced thrombocytopenia
HPV	human papillomavirus
HR	heart rate
HT	hormone therapy
HTN	hypertension
hx	history
IADLs	instrumental activities of daily living
IBS	irritable bowel syndrome
ICD	implantable cardiac defibrillator
ICS	inhaled corticosteroids
ICU	intensive care unit
IDSA	Infectious Diseases Society of America
Ig	immunoglobulin (eg, IgE, IgG, IgM)
IL	interleukin (eg, IL-1, IL-6)
INR	international normalized ratio
IOP	intraocular pressure
iPTH	intact parathyroid hormone
LABA	long-acting ß2 agonist
LAMA	long-acting antimuscarinic receptor antagonist
LBD	Lewy body dementia

LDL	low-density lipoprotein
L-DOPA	levodopa
LFT	liver function test
LGBT	lesbian, gay, bisexual, and transgender
LMWH	low-molecular-weight heparin
LUTS	lower urinary tract symptoms
LVEF	left ventricular ejection fraction
LVH	left ventricular hypertrophy
MAOI	monoamine oxidase inhibitor
MCI	mild cognitive impairment
MDI	metered-dose inhaler
MDS	myelodysplastic syndromes
MGUS	monoclonal gammopathy of undetermined significance
MI	myocardial infarction
MMA	methylmalonic acid
MME	morphine milligram equivalent (dose)
MMSE	Mini-Mental State Examination
MoCA	Montreal Cognitive Assessment
MRA	magnetic resonance angiography
MRI	magnetic resonance imaging
MRSA	methicillin-resistant *Staphylococcus aureus*
NCCN	National Comprehensive Cancer Network
NIH	National Institutes of Health
NIHSS	National Institutes of Health Stroke Scale
NNH	number needed to harm
NNT	number needed to treat
NPH	neutral protamine Hagedorn (insulin)
NPWT	negative-pressure wound treatment
NSAID	nonsteroidal anti-inflammatory drug
NYHA	New York Heart Association
OA	osteoarthritis
OIC	opioid-induced constipation
ORIF	open reduction and internal fixation
ORT OUD	Opioid Risk Tool (for opioid use disorder)
OSA	obstructive sleep apnea
OT	occupational therapy
PAD	peripheral arterial disease
PAH	pulmonary arterial hypertension
PAP	positive airway pressure
PCSK9	proprotein convertase subtilisin/kexin type 9
PDE5	phosphodiesterase type 5
PDT	photodynamic therapy
PE	pulmonary embolism
PET	positron emission tomography
PFT	pulmonary function test
PH	pulmonary hypertension
POLST	Physician Orders for Life-Sustaining Treatment
PPA	primary progressive aphasia
PPI	proton-pump inhibitor
PSA	prostate-specific antigen
PT	prothrombin time *or* physical therapy
PTH	parathyroid hormone
PTSD	posttraumatic stress disorder
PTT	partial thromboplastin time
PVR	postvoid residual

QTc	QT (cardiac output) corrected for heart rate
RA	rheumatoid arthritis
RBC	red blood cell(s)
RCT	randomized controlled trial
REM	rapid eye movement (sleep)
RF	rheumatoid factor
RLD	restrictive lung disease
RLS	restless legs syndrome
RR	respiratory rate
RZV	recombinant, adjuvanted zoster vaccine
SABA	short-acting $ß_2$ agonist
SAMA	short-acting antimuscarinic
SBP	systolic blood pressure
SCC	squamous cell carcinoma
SD	standard deviation
SGLT2	sodium-glucose cotransporter-2
SIADH	syndrome of inappropriate secretion of antidiuretic hormone
SMI	soft mist inhalers
SNF	skilled nursing facility
SNRI	serotonin norepinephrine-reuptake inhibitor
SPEP	serum protein electrophoresis
SSRI	selective serotonin-reuptake inhibitor
TAVR	transcatheter aortic valve replacement
TB	tuberculosis
TCA	tricyclic antidepressant
TCU	transitional care unit
TD	tardive dyskinesia
TENS	transcutaneous electrical nerve stimulation
TG	triglycerides
THC	tetrahydrocannabinol
TIA	transient ischemic attack
TIBC	total iron-binding capacity
TJR	total joint replacement
TMJ	temporomandibular joint
TNF	tumor necrosis factor
TSH	thyroid-stimulating hormone
TURP	transurethral resection of the prostate
tx	treatment(s), therapy (-ies)
U	unit(s)
UA	urinalysis
UFH	unfractionated heparin
UI	urinary incontinence
URI	upper respiratory infection
USPSTF	US Preventive Services Task Force
UTI	urinary tract infection
UV	ultraviolet
VEGF	vascular endothelial growth factor
VF	ventricular fibrillation
VT	ventricular tachycardia
VTE	venous thromboembolism
WBC	white blood cell(s)
WHO	World Health Organization

Drug Prescribing and Elimination

Drugs are listed by generic names; trade names are in *italics*. An asterisk (*) indicates that the drug is available OTC. Check marks (✓) indicate drugs preferred for treating older adults.

Formulations in text are bracketed and expressed in milligrams (mg) unless otherwise specified. Information in parentheses after dose ranges indicate the number of doses into which the daily dose can be split. Abbreviations for dosing, formulations, and route of elimination are defined below.

ac	before meals	OTC	over-the-counter
C	capsule, caplet	OU	both eyes
ChT	chewable tablet	pc	after meals
conc	concentrate	pch	patch
CR	controlled release	pk	pack, packet
crm	cream	po	by mouth
d	day(s)	pr	per rectum
DS	double strength	prn	as needed
ER	extended release	pwd	powder
F	fecal elimination	qam	every morning
fl	fluid	qhs	each bedtime
g	gram(s)	S	liquid (includes concentrate, elixir, solution, suspension, syrup, tincture)
gran	granules	SC	subcutaneous(ly)
gtt	drop(s)	sec	second(s)
h	hour(s)	shp	shampoo
hs	at bedtime	sl	sublingual
IM	intramuscular(ly)	sol	solution
inj	injectable(s)	Sp	suppository
IR	immediate release	spr	spray(s)
IT	intrathecal(ly)	SR	sustained release
IV	intravenous(ly)	sus	suspension
K	renal elimination	syr	syrup
L	hepatic elimination	T	tablet
lot	lotion	tab(s)	tablet(s)
max	maximum	tbsp	tablespoon(s)
mcg	microgram(s)	tinc	tincture
min	minute(s)	TR	timed release
mo	month(s)	tsp	teaspoon(s)
npo	nothing by mouth	wk	week(s)
NS	normal saline	XR	extended release
ODT	oral disintegrating tablet	y	year(s)
oint	ointment		
OL	off-label use		

INTRODUCTION

Since its first publication in 1998, *Geriatrics At Your Fingertips®* (GAYF) has been an important resource in the care of older patients. Through the years, the authors have continually updated material to reflect advances in medicine and added sections to increase the breadth of topics important in caring for older persons.

In this 25th edition, we have added new sections on dementia screening, non-pharmacologic approaches for problem behaviors in dementia, direct-to-consumer and OTC hearing aids, medical marijuana for chronic pain, and gambling disorder. We have made updates in every chapter including new chest pain management guidelines, updated information about drugs for weight loss, and anti-diabetic agents that have cardiac and renal benefits.

We have made some additional changes to keep GAYF small enough to be portable. In general, dosages of medications have been eliminated because these are typically readily available when electronically prescribing. Other topics (eg, prostate cancer treatment) that would likely be managed by specialists have been shortened or deleted. We have also moved some supplementary content into the digital edition only. These include a section on radiological imaging (Assessment and Approach), State Prescription Drug Monitoring Programs (Appropriate Prescribing), solitary thyroid nodule (Endocrine Disorders), a table on Deprescribing Guidance for Fall Risk Medications (Falls), MRSA (Infectious Diseases), nutrition information for lactose-free enteral and oral products (Malnutrition and Nutritional Health), and common foot disorders (Musculoskeletal Disorders).

Because information about the prevention and treatment of COVID-19 infections is rapidly emerging and may go out of date, we have kept the section on this disease short and have referred the reader to websites where the latest updates can be found.

The authors welcome feedback about GAYF's content and format. We continue to work toward creating an optimal balance between practicality, convenience, and comprehensiveness with the goal of maximizing GAYF's usefulness.

The following expert has reviewed portions of this edition:

Albert Shieh, MD

Editorial Staff

Hope Lafferty, AM, ELS, Medical Editor

Aimee Cegelka, MA, Managing Editor (print)

Laura Banks, Managing Editor (digital)

Pilar Wyman, Medical Indexer

Technical development and production of print and electronic versions:

Fry Communications, Inc.

Rhonda Liddick, Composition Manager

Jason Hughes, Technical Services Manager

Julie Stevens, Project Manager

Atmosphere Apps

Eric Poirier, Chief Executive Officer

Max Jones, Project Manager

ASSESSMENT AND APPROACH

ASSESSMENT

Table 1. Assessing Older Adults

Assessment Domain	Screening Methods	Further Assessments (if screen is positive)	See Page(s)
Medical			
Medical illnesses[1,2]	Hx, screening physical exam	Additional targeted physical exam, lab and imaging tests	see digital text
Medications[1,2]	Medications review/reconciliation	Pharmacy referral	16
Nutrition[1,2]	Inquire about weight loss (>10 lb in past 6 mo), calculate BMI	Dietary hx, malnutrition evaluation	204
Dentition	Oral exam	Dentistry referral	—
Hearing[1]	Handheld audioscope, Brief Hearing Loss Screener, whisper test	Ear exam, audiology referral	158
Vision[1]	Inquire about vision changes, Snellen chart testing	Eye exam, ophthalmology referral	126
Pain	Inquire about pain	Pain inventory	252
Urinary incontinence	Inquire if patient has lost urine >5 × in past year	UI evaluation	165
Mental			
Patient goals (ie, what matters)	Ask the patient: what brings you joy? What is most important in your life? What about your health or health care makes those things difficult?	Goal-oriented care planning	6
Cognitive status[1,2]	3-item recall, Mini-Cog	Mental status exam, dementia evaluation	2
Emotional status[1]			
Depression	PHQ-2: "Over the past month, have you often had little interest or pleasure in doing things? Over the past month, have you often been bothered by feeling down, depressed, or hopeless?"	PHQ-9 or other depression screen, in-depth interview	—
Anxiety	GAD-2: "Over the last 2 weeks, how often have you been bothered by the following problems: Feeling nervous, anxious, or on edge? Not being able to stop or control worrying?" (Scoring for each item: not at all = 0, several days = 1, more than half the days = 2, nearly every day = 3; total score of 3 or more is a positive screen)	GAD-7	47
Spiritual status	Spiritual hx	In-depth interview, chaplain or spiritual advisor referral	282

(cont.)

Table 1. Assessing Older Adults (cont.)			
Assessment Domain	**Screening Methods**	**Further Assessments (if screen is positive)**	**See Page(s)**
Physical			
Functional status[1]	ADLs, IADLs	PT/OT referral	—
Balance and gait[1]	Observe patient getting up and walking, orthostatic BP and HR, Romberg test, semitandem stand	Formal gait evaluation, measurement of gait speed, 6-min walk test	
Falls	Inquire if patient has had ≥2 falls or 1 injurious fall in past y or is afraid of falling due to balance and/or walking problem	Falls evaluation	138
Environmental			
Social, financial status[1]	Social hx, assess risk factors for mistreatment	In-depth interview, social work referral	10
Environmental hazards[1]	Inquire about living situation, home safety checklist	Home evaluation	141
Care Preferences			
Life-sustaining tx[1,2]	Inquire about preferences; complete POLST form		6

[1]Required elements of the Medicare Initial Annual Wellness Visit

[2]Required elements of Medicare Subsequent Annual Wellness Visits

Mini-Cog™ Screen for Dementia

Step 1: Three Word Registration

Look directly at person and say, "Please listen carefully. I am going to say 3 words that I want you to repeat back to me now and try to remember. The words are [select a list of words from the versions below]. Please say them with me now." If the person is unable to repeat the words after 3 attempts, move on to Step 2 (clock drawing).

The following and other word lists have been used in one or more clinical studies. For repeated administrations, use of an alternative word list is recommended.

Version 1	Version 2	Version 3	Version 4	Version 5	Version 6
Banana	Leader	Village	River	Captain	Daughter
Sunrise	Season	Kitchen	Nation	Garden	Heaven
Chair	Table	Baby	Finger	Picture	Mountain

Step 2: Clock Drawing

Say: "Next, I want you to draw a clock for me. First, put in all the numbers where they go." When that is completed, say, "Now, set the hands to 10 past 11."

Use preprinted circle (see mini-cog.com) for this exercise. Repeat instructions as needed as this is not a memory test. Move to Step 3 if the clock is not complete within 3 minutes.

Step 3: Three Word Recall

Ask the person to recall the 3 words you stated in Step 1. Say: "What were the 3 words I asked you to remember?" Record the word list version number and the person's answer.

Scoring

Word Recall: 0–3 points	1 point for each word spontaneously recalled without cueing.
Clock Draw: 0 or 2 points	Normal clock = 2 points. A normal clock has all numbers placed in the correct sequence and approximately correct position (eg, 12, 3, 6, and 9 are in anchor positions) with no missing or duplicate numbers. Hands are pointing to the 11 and 2 (11:10). Hand length is not scored. Inability or refusal to draw a clock (abnormal) = 0 points.
Total Score: 0–5 points	Total score = Word Recall score + Clock Draw score. A cut point of <3 on the Mini-Cog has been validated for dementia screening, but many individuals with clinically meaningful cognitive impairment will score higher. When greater sensitivity is desired, a cut point of <4 is recommended as it may indicate a need for further evaluation of cognitive status.

INTERPROFESSIONAL GERIATRIC TEAM CARE

- Most effective for care of frail older adults with multiple comorbidities
- Also appropriate for management of complex geriatric syndromes (eg, falls, confusion, dementia, depression, incontinence, weight loss, persistent pain, immobility)
- Common features of team care include:
  - Proactive assessment of multiple domains (**Table 1**)
  - Care coordination, usually performed by an advanced practice nurse or social worker
  - Care planning performed by team members

SITES OF CARE FOR OLDER ADULTS

Age-Friendly Health Systems

- Promoting Age-Friendly Health Systems is a nationwide initiative to transform healthcare systems for more effective and safe care of older adults (www.ihi.org/Engage/Initiatives/Age-Friendly-Health-Systems/Pages/default.aspx).
- Age-Friendly Health Systems consistently address the "4Ms" of older adult care:
  - What Matters to the patient (Goal-Oriented Care, p 6)
  - Medications (regular medication reconciliation, p 16; minimization of ADRs, p 18; use of AGS Beers Criteria, p 17)
  - Mentation (cognitive assessment, p 82; depression screening/tx, p 92; delirium prevention, p 77)
  - Mobility (promotion of physical activity, falls prevention and tx, p 136)

Telehealth—Supplementing In-Person Care and Improving Access

- Telephone visits
  - Advantages: low tech; effective for monitoring chronic conditions not requiring lab work and aided by home monitoring equipment; can be effective for nonvisual, cognitive services (eg, counseling, goal-setting, less acute behavioral health tx)
  - Barriers: nonvisual; can be difficult to add caregiver and interpreter input

- Video visits
  - Advantages: can accommodate many types of assessments; somewhat useful for assessing mobility, skin problems, and overall functioning; ability to see patient in own home setting
  - Barriers:
    - Technological: technology can be problematic; difficult to add remote caregiver and/or interpreter; optimal use requires 2-monitor setup
    - Patient-related: hearing impairment (improved with use of headphones); visual impairment (improved by magnification software); cognitive impairment (aided by involvement of caregiver); inability to follow directions (improved by examiner demonstrating maneuvers on camera)

Table 2. Sites of Care[1]

Site	Patient Needs and Services	Principal Funding Source
Home	ADL or IADL assistance Skilled nursing and/or rehabilitation services when patient can only occasionally leave the home at great effort	Medicaid in many states or private pay[2] for caregiving services Medicare Part A for nonphysician homecare services (eg, nursing, OT, PT); Part B for outpatient PT/ST/OT services independent of a home care agency[3]
Senior citizen housing	Housing	Private pay[2,4]
Assisted living, residential care, board-and-care facilities	ADL or IADL assistance, primarily with meals, housekeeping, and medication management Patient must be non–bedridden	Private pay,[2] Medicaid for some facilities
Hospital		
Acute care	Acute hospital care	Medicare Part A
Chronic care/ long-term acute care (LTAC facility)	Chronic skilled care (eg, chronic ventilator)	Medicare Part A, private pay,[2] Medicaid
Inpatient rehabilitation	Intensive interprofessional team rehabilitation	Medicare Part A
Skilled nursing facility		
Transitional care unit	Skilled nursing care and/or intensive interprofessional team rehabilitation	Medicare Part A[5]
Short stay/ Rehabilitation	Skilled nursing care and/or straight-forward rehabilitation	Medicare Part A[5]
Long-term care	ADL assistance and/or skilled nursing care	Private pay,[2] Medicaid

(cont.)

Table 2. Sites of Care[1] (cont.)		
Site	**Patient Needs and Services**	**Principal Funding Source**
Continuing care retirement communities	Variety of living arrangements ranging from independent to skilled	Private pay[2]
Hospice (home- or facility-based)	Palliative/comfort care for life expectancy <6 mo	Medicare Part A

[1] For useful information about sites of care for patients and families, see payingforseniorcare.com.

[2] May include long-term care insurance.

[3] A yearly cap of $2230 for these services can be exceeded if the therapist documents a "medically reasonable and necessary" exception.

[4] May be subsidized for older adults spending over one-third of income for rent. Some facilities may have access to a social worker or caregiving services for hire.

[5] Medicare Part A pays for 20 d after a hospital stay of ≥3 d, patient or co-insurance pays $200/d (in 2023) for days 21–100 with Part A covering the rest; patient or co-insurance pays 100% after day 100.

HOSPITAL CARE

Common Problems to Monitor

- Delirium (p 77)
- Intra- and postoperative coronary events: postoperative ECG to check
- Malnutrition (p 204)
- Pain (p 252)
- Polypharmacy: review medications daily, deprescribe as appropriate
- Pulmonary complications: minimized by frequent standing, coughing, deep breathing; early ambulation after surgery; incentive spirometry
- Rehabilitation: encourage early mobility
- Pressure injury (p 330)
- Constipation

Discharge Planning

- Ideally, all team members should participate in discharge planning, beginning early in the hospitalization.
- Site of care after discharge should be determined by patient's needs (**Table 2**).
- Influenza vaccination (if indicated) should be completed before discharge
- Evidence-based procedures for preventing hospital readmissions include:
  - A discharge coordinator (usually a specially trained nurse) who oversees appropriate patient and caregiver education regarding diagnoses and self-care, arrangement of posthospital care, medication use, and follow-up with the patient within 72 h of discharge
  - A clinical pharmacist to perform medication reconciliation at the time of discharge and within 1 wk of discharge
  - Clearly written discharge plans geared toward the patient, caregivers, and healthcare team members
- Tools for achieving effective transitions of care out of the hospital are available through the RED: Re-Engineered Discharge project (ahrq.gov/professionals/systems/hospital/red/toolkit), the Transitional Care Model (nursing.upenn.edu/ncth/transitional-care-model/), and the Care Transitions Program (caretransitions.org/#tools).

- For a safe and effective transfer from the hospital to the nursing home or TCU, the following should be completed by the time the patient arrives at the nursing home/TCU:
  - Interfacility transfer form (the medication administration record is inadequate) that includes a discharge medication list noting new and discontinued medications, discontinuation dates for short-term medications, and any dosage changes in all medications
  - Discharge summary (performed by physician) that includes the patient's baseline functional status, "red flags" for rare but potentially serious complications of conditions or tx, orders including medications, important tests for which results are pending, and needed next steps
  - Verbal provider-to-provider sign-out

SCHEDULED NURSING-HOME VISIT CHECKLIST

1. Evaluate patient for interval functional change
2. Check vital signs, weight, lab tests, consultant reports since last visit
3. Review medications, especially psychotropic drugs (correlate to active diagnoses)
4. Sign orders
5. Address nursing staff concerns
6. Write a SOAP note (subjective data, objective data, assessment, plan)
7. Revise problem list as needed
8. Review patient goals and update advance directives at least yearly
9. Update resident; update family member(s) as needed

PATIENT-CENTERED CARE AND MEDICAL DECISION-MAKING

Goal-Oriented Care—what matters to the patient

- Goals of care should be established for individual patients
- Goals of care should be based on:
  - Disease-specific care processes and outcomes (eg, A1c and retinopathy for patients with DM)—useful for healthier patients with isolated conditions.
  - Goal-oriented outcomes (an individual's goals potentially encompassing a variety of dimensions, including symptoms, functional status, social engagement, etc)—useful for patients with multiple conditions or who are frail.

Care Planning—a healthcare team process with patient and caregivers

- Elucidate patient's goal-oriented outcomes; operationalize goals to be specific, measurable, and time bound
- Identify chronic conditions and other stressors that threaten the achievement of goal-oriented outcomes
- Propose interventions and discuss possible risks and benefits of each for attaining goals
- Negotiate and implement the plan, which can address the following elements (all of which are required for chronic care management codes [see Coding in Geriatrics, p 369]):
  - Physical, mental, cognitive, psychosocial, and functional assessments
  - Preventive care services
  - Medication reconciliation and deprescribing
  - Therapeutic and psychosocial support services
  - Defined roster of healthcare team members and responsibilities of each

- ◦ Timeline for follow-up and reassessment of goal attainment
- Formal care planning is a requirement for Chronic Care Management coding (99490, 99487, 99489) and for the Cognition Assessment and Care Plan Code (99483).

Life Expectancy

- Many medical decisions are predicated on estimated life expectancy of the patient. **Table 3** shows life expectancy by age and sex.
- Life expectancy is associated with a number of factors in addition to age and sex, including health behaviors, presence of disease, nutritional status, race/ethnicity, and educational and financial status.
- Conditions commonly leading to death are frailty, cancer, organ failure (heart, lung, kidney, liver), and advanced dementia.
- Active life expectancy reflects the remaining years of disability-free existence. At age 65, active life expectancy is about 90% of total life expectancy; this percentage decreases with further aging.
- Estimated life expectancy can aid individualized medical decision-making, particularly when considering preventive tests. Tools such as ePrognosis (https://eprognosis.ucsf.edu/) can assist in estimating life expectancy. Alternatively, a clinician can judge the patient's health status as being above average (75th percentile), average (50th percentile), or below average (25th percentile) for age and sex, and then roughly determine life expectancy using **Table 3**.
- Another way to estimate individual life expectancy is by comorbidity, frailty, or both. Compared to the values in **Table 3**:
  - ◦ No comorbidity and low frailty roughly corresponds to the 75th percentile.
  - ◦ Low to medium comorbidities and low frailty roughly corresponds to the 50th percentile.
  - ◦ High comorbidities and low frailty roughly corresponds to the 25th percentile.
  - ◦ High comorbidities and high frailty will result in significantly lower life expectancy than the 25th percentile.

Table 3. Life Expectancy (y) by Age (United States)

	25th percentile		50th percentile		75th percentile	
Age	**Men**	**Women**	**Men**	**Women**	**Men**	**Women**
65	12	15	19	21	25	27
70	9	11	15	17	20	23
75	6	8	11	13	16	18
80	4	5	8	10	12	14
85	3	3	5	7	9	10
90	2	2	3	4	6	7
95	1	1	2	3	4	5

Source: Arias E and Xu J. United States Life Tables, 2019. *National Vital Statistics Reports.* 2022;70(19).

- After individual life expectancy is estimated, the period of time needed for the tx to result in a positive clinical outcome is estimated and compared with the life expectancy of the patient.
  - If estimated life expectancy is longer than the time needed to achieve a positive outcome, the tx is encouraged.
  - If estimated life expectancy is shorter than the time needed to achieve a positive outcome, the tx is discouraged.
  - If estimated life expectancy is about the same as the time needed to achieve a positive outcome, the potential risks and benefits of the tx should be discussed neutrally with the patient.

For example, the benefit of many cancer screening tests is not realized for ~10 y after detection of asymptomatic malignancies. If a patient's life expectancy is significantly less than 10 y based only on age and sex, and the patient has poor overall health status compared with age-matched peers, cancer screening would be discouraged because the likelihood of benefit from having the test is low.

INFORMED DECISION-MAKING AND PATIENT PREFERENCES FOR LIFE-SUSTAINING CARE

Healthcare providers have no ethical obligation to offer care that is judged to be futile.

Three elements are needed for a patient's choices to be legally and ethically valid:

- A capable decision maker: Capacity is for the decision being made; patient may be capable of making some but not all decisions. If a person is sufficiently impaired, a surrogate decision maker must be involved (**Figure 1**).
- Patient's voluntary participation in the decision-making process.
- Sufficient information: Patient must be sufficiently informed; items to disclose in informed consent include:
  - Diagnosis
  - Nature, risks, costs, and benefits of possible interventions
  - Alternative tx; relative benefits, risks, and costs
  - Likely results of no tx
  - Likelihood of success
  - Advice or recommendation of the clinician

Ideally, patient preferences for life-sustaining care should be established before the patient is critically ill.

- Preferences should be established for use of the following interventions and the conditions under which they would be used: cardiopulmonary resuscitation, hospitalization, IV hydration, antibiotics, artificially administered nutrition, other life-extending medical tx, and palliative/comfort care (Palliative Care, p 271).
- Patients should be encouraged to complete a living will and/or to establish a durable power of attorney for healthcare decision-making.
- Use of a POLST form can be very useful in formalizing patient preferences (polst.org).
- Providers may bill for discussions of patient preferences using the ACP CPT billing code of 99497 for initial ACP and 99498 for additional add-on of 30 min of face-to-face discussion.
- See also Physician-assisted Dying and Active Euthanasia, p 284.

Figure 1. Informed Decision-Making

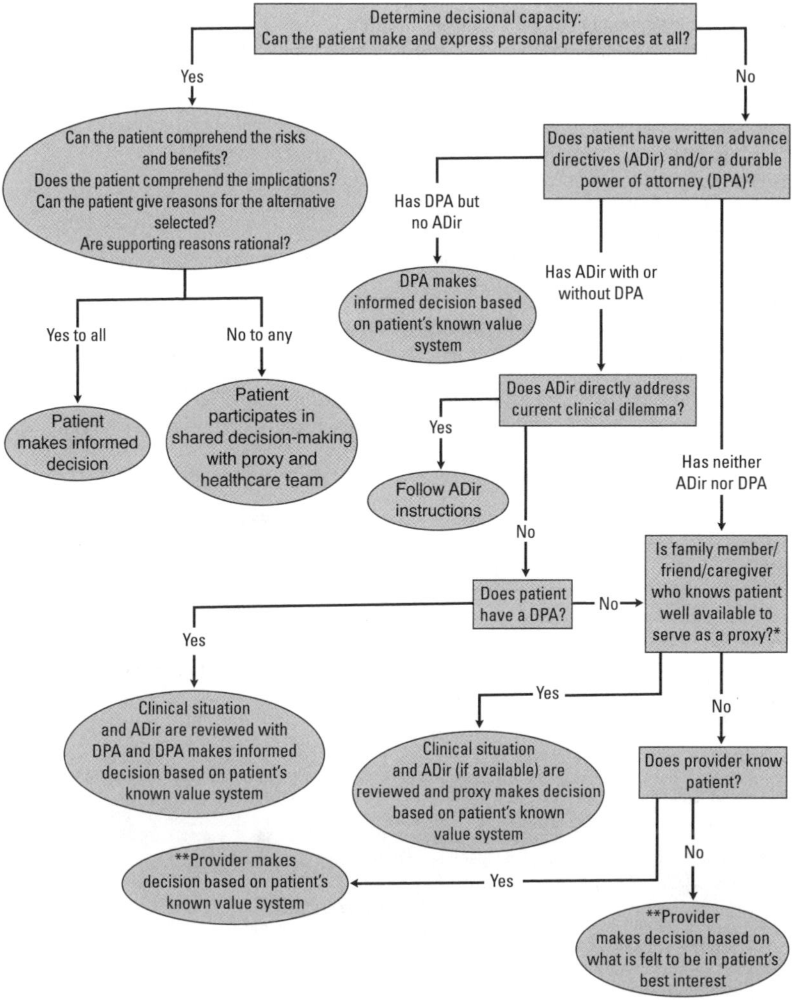

* Most states have laws specifying who should serve as proxy when no Advance Directive or Durable Power of Attorney exists. For most of these states, the specified hierarchy of decision makers is (in order): legal guardian, spouse or domestic partner, adult children, parents, adult siblings, closest living relative, close friend.

** Or court-appointed decision maker; laws vary by state.

MISTREATMENT OF OLDER ADULTS

Risk Factors for Inadequate or Abusive Caregiving

- Cognitive impairment in patient, caregiver, or both
- Dependency (financial, psychological, etc) of caregiver on elderly patient, or vice versa
- Family conflict
- Family hx of abusive behavior, alcohol or drug problems, mental illness, or developmental disability
- Financial stress
- Isolation of patient or caregiver, or both
- Depression or malnutrition in the patient
- Living arrangements inadequate for needs of the patient
- Stressful events in the family, such as death of a loved one or loss of employment

Assessment and Management

- Interview patient and caregiver separately.
- Ask patient some general screening questions, such as, "Are there any problems with family or household members that you would like to tell me about?" Follow-up a positive response with more direct questions such as those suggested in **Table 4**.
- On physical exam, look for any unusual marks, signs of injury, or conditions listed in **Table 4**.
- If mistreatment is suspected, report case to Adult Protective Services (most states have mandatory reporting laws).
- If patient is in immediate danger of harm, create and implement plan to remove patient from danger (hospital admission, court protective order, placement in safe environment, etc).

Table 4. Determining Suspicion and Clinical Signs of Possible Mistreatment of Older Adults

Abandonment
Question to Ask Patient: Is there anyone who is supposed to be helping or taking care of you?
Clinical Signs: • Evidence that patient is left alone unsafely • Evidence of sudden withdrawal of care by caregiver • Statements by patient about abandonment • Patient is dropped off (eg, in the emergency department) without contact information for the responsible party
Physical Abuse
Question to Ask Patient: Does anyone ever hit you or hurt you?
Clinical Signs: • Anxiety, nervousness, withdrawal, especially toward caregiver • Bruising, especially on face, neck, torso, genital area, soles of feet • Fractures, especially on head or face • Wounds in unusual locations or without rational explanations • Repeated emergency department visits • Repeated falls • Signs of sexual abuse • Statements by patient about physical abuse

(cont.)

Table 4. Determining Suspicion and Clinical Signs of Possible Mistreatment of Older Adults (cont.)

Exploitation

Question to Ask Patient: Is anyone taking your things or money without your permission?

Clinical Signs:

- Evidence of misuse of patient's assets
- Change in ability of patient to account for money and property or to pay for essential care
- Reports of demands for unreasonable amounts of money or goods in exchange for caregiving or services
- Unexplained loss of Social Security or pension checks
- Statements by patient about exploitation
- Requests for more frequent medication refills (possible indicator of diversion of patient's medications to others)

Neglect

Question to Ask Patient: Are you receiving enough care at home?

Clinical Signs:

- Contractures
- Dehydration
- Depression
- Diarrhea
- Fecal impaction
- Malnutrition
- Failure to respond to warning of obvious disease
- Inappropriate use of medications (may be too much or too little)
- Poor hygiene
- Pressure ulcers
- Repeated falls
- Repeated hospital admissions
- Urine burns
- Statements by patient about neglect

Psychological Abuse

Questions to Ask Patient: Does anyone scold or threaten you? Does anyone belittle or make fun of you?

Clinical Signs:

- Observed impatience, irritability, or demeaning behavior toward patient by caregiver
- Anxiety, fearfulness, ambivalence, or anger shown by patient about caregiver
- Statements by patient about psychological abuse

CROSS-CULTURAL GERIATRICS

Clinicians should remember that:

- Individuals within every ethnic group can differ widely.
- Familiarity with a patient's background is useful only if his or her preferences are linked to the cultural heritage.
- Ethnic groups differ widely in:
  - approach to decision-making (eg, involvement of family and friends)
  - disclosure of medical information (eg, cancer diagnosis)
  - end-of-life care (eg, advance directives and resuscitation preferences)

In caring for older adults of any ethnicity:

- Use the patient's preferred terminology for his or her cultural identity in conversation and in health records.
- Determine whether interpretation services are needed; if possible, use professional interpreter rather than family member. When interpreters are not available, online translation services (eg, babelfish.com or translate.google.com) or telephone translation services can be useful.
- Recognize that the patient may not conceive of illness in Western terms.
- Determine whether the patient is a refugee or survivor of violence or genocide.

- Explore early on the patient's preferences for disclosure of serious clinical findings, and reconfirm at intervals.
- Ask if the patient prefers to involve or defer to others in the decision-making process.
- Follow the patient's preferences regarding gender roles.

For further information, see the AGS *Geriatrics Cultural Navigator* (geriatricscareonline.org/ProductAbstract/Geriatrics-Cultural-Navigator/B066).

LESBIAN, GAY, BISEXUAL, TRANSGENDER, AND QUEER (LGBTQ) HEALTH

Background

- At least 1–2 million LGBTQ older adults reside in the US and grew up in a time when their behavior was criminalized and considered pathological.
- Because of discrimination many hide their sexual orientation/gender identity. Many continue to do so and may distrust healthcare providers.
- To inquire about sexual/gender identity, ask patients about past and present relationships, living situation, and sources of support to learn this information.
  - "What is your preferred name?"
  - "What are your preferred pronouns?"
  - "How do you refer to your loved ones?"
  - "Who lives with you at home?"
  - "What is your relationship status (are you single, partnered, married, open)?"
  - "Are your sexual partners women, men, or both?"
- Of LGBTQ people aged 65–75, about 50% are sexually active, as are 25% of those aged 75–85.

Medical Issues

- Provide the same basic geriatric care: syndromes, health maintenance, etc.
- Medical concerns with increased risk and or prevalence in LGBTQ patients:
  - *CVD:* especially in bisexual men but also lesbians; related to smoking, high BP, drug use; plus obesity in women; and the use of sex hormones in transgender people
  - *Anal cancer:* human papilloma virus, especially in men who have sex with men; if also HIV positive, consider screening with cytology using a PAP smear technique (*Dacron* or polyester swab moistened with water and inserted 2–3 inches into the anus, rotate 360°, fix to glass slide or place in preservative vial).
  - *Prostate cancer:* surgical and radiation tx has additional negative consequences on anal intercourse.
  - *Breast and cervical cancer:* lower prior screening rates increase risk.
  - *HIV/AIDS and other sexually transmitted infections:* older persons are less likely to use condoms and to be screened than younger persons; counsel on safe sex; evaluate for pre-exposure prophylaxis and renal function.
  - *Monkeypox:* especially in men who have sex with men
  - *Palliative care:* complicated by stigma; estrangement from family; partnerships not recognized.
  - *Advance care planning:* may need to name family of "choice" rather than biology.
  - Genital cancers in transgender people need screening based on biological sex if organs (prostate, uterus) are not removed.

Mental Health Issues

- LGBTQ persons have higher lifetime risk of depression and anxiety disorders; highest rates in transgender older adults.
- High suicide rates in young LGBTQ persons may not persist into late life.
- Important to assess for intimate partner violence.
- Better mental health results by more people (including healthcare professionals) being aware of the individual's sexual orientation.

Social and Economic Issues

- Older LGBTQ residents of long-term care facilities report higher frequency of verbal or physical harassment from other residents and staff, refused admission, or attempted discharge.
- LGBTQ older adults (especially lesbians) are more likely to live in poverty compared to heterosexual peers.
- Same-sex marriage is legal in all 50 states and recognizes federal benefits including Social Security spousal and survivor benefits, VA spousal benefits, and tax treatment of health insurance and retirement savings. However, there continues to be variability in state laws concerning adoption, transgender insurance coverage, and other relationship recognition (domestic partnerships).
  - SAGE, Advocacy & Services for LGBTQ+ Elders: sageusa.org
  - National Resource Center on LGBTQ+ Aging: lgbtagingcenter.org

COMPLETING A DEATH CERTIFICATE

- The **Cause of Death** statement in Section 32 of a Death Certificate indicates the provider's opinion, with reasonable probability, of the immediate, intermediate, and underlying causes of death and other significant contributing conditions. See below for details on completing this section.
- The **Manner of Death** statement in Section 37 indicates the provider's opinion of whether the death was natural or unnatural. Unnatural deaths will be reviewed by the coroner or medical examiner; the specific criteria for triggering a review vary by county and state.
- If a patient is on hospice care, the hospice provider usually completes the death certificate.

Immediate Cause of Death Statement (Section 32.Part I.a)

- Indicates the final disease, injury, or complication causing death (eg, aspiration pneumonia, PE, aortic rupture)
- The approximate interval between the onset of the immediate cause and death is estimated (eg, 4 wk, minutes, 1 h for the above examples).
- If the cause of death is not apparent (eg, a very elderly man without clinically apparent major illnesses is found by his daughter to have died in his sleep), some states allow the clinician to indicate "undetermined natural causes".
- Mechanistic terminal events such as asystole, electromechanical dissociation, cardiac arrest, and respiratory arrest should not be listed in this or any other cause of death section.

Intermediate/Underlying Causes of Death "Due to/Consequence of" Statement (Section 32.Part I.b–d)

- Indicates conditions and their sequence leading to the immediate cause of death, listed in reverse chronologic order.
- The last of these conditions listed is the **underlying** cause—the disease or injury that initiated the events leading to the patient's death.

- Examples:
  - A patient with osteoporosis fractures her hip, develops a DVT in the hospital, and dies of a pulmonary embolus. Pulmonary embolus would be cited as the immediate cause in Section 32.I.a, DVT would be cited as an intermediate ("due to/consequence of") cause in Section 32.I.b, hip fracture would be cited as another intermediate cause in Section 32.I.c, and osteoporosis would be entered in Section 32.I.d as the underlying cause.
  - A patient with late-state Alzheimer disease (AD) dies from apparent aspiration pneumonia. Aspiration pneumonia would be listed as the immediate cause in Section 32.I.a, and AD would be entered as the intermediate/underlying cause in Section 32.I.b.
- The approximate intervals between the onset of the intermediate/underlying causes and death is estimated.

Other Significant Conditions Leading to Death Statement (Section 32.Part II)

- Indicates conditions that likely contributed to death but did not result in underlying causes.
- Risk factors for underlying causes are often listed in this section, eg, hypertension for cerebrovascular disease (the underlying condition) leading to a massive hemorrhagic stroke (the immediate cause of death).

FRAILTY

- General definition: increased vulnerability to adverse outcomes (eg, falls, disability, delirium, failure to return to functional baseline) after exposure to a stressful event
- Frailty is associated with numerous adverse outcomes, including geriatric syndromes (falls, delirium, immobility, incontinence, dementia), poor surgical outcomes, hospitalization, and death.
- It is unknown if frailty can be arrested or reversed. Frail individuals should be strongly considered for interprofessional geriatric team care (p 3).
- Frailty models are organized around different domains:
  - Phenotypic models (eg, the phenotype Cardiovascular Health Study [CHS] scale) characterize frailty around the presence of 5 indicators:
    - weight loss (>4–5 kg or >5%/y)
    - exhaustion/fatigue (inability to walk several hundred yards or >3–4 d/wk feeling exhausted)
    - low activity (<383 kcal/wk in men or <270 kcal/wk in women)
    - weakness (low grip strength)
    - slowness (slow gait speed)
  - Cumulative deficit models (eg, the Frailty Index) classify frailty by the presence of 25 or more functional deficits, conditions, symptoms, and/or lab values, scored as the proportion of total indicators present in the patient.
  - Functional models (eg, the Clinical Frailty Scale) are based on overall functional status, primarily assessed by ADLs and IADLs.
  - Other models (eg, FRAIL scale) combine elements of functional and biologic indicators.
- Frailty indicators can be measured clinically through direct observation or self-report.
- Frailty prevalence varies widely according to scale used; ~10% of older adults are frail using either the CHS scale or the FRAIL.

MULTIMORBIDITY

- More than 50% of older adults have ≥3 chronic conditions.
- Management of patients with multimorbidity involves balancing issues of patient preferences and tx goals, prognosis, the evidence of outcomes for tx strategies of individual conditions, interactions among conditions and tx, and feasibility of tx (**Figure 2**).

Figure 2. Approach to the Evaluation and Management of the Older Adult with Multimorbidity

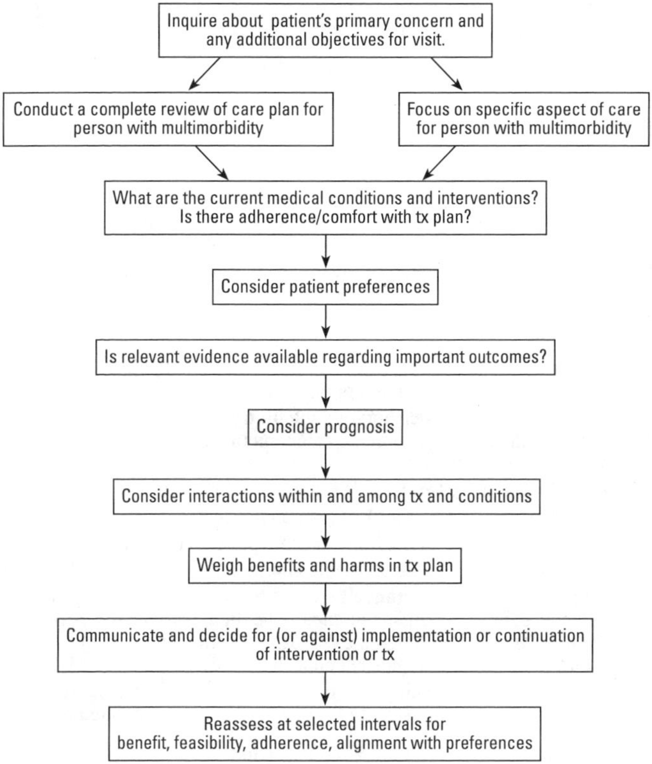

Source: AGS Expert Panel on the Care of Older Adults with Multimorbidity. *J Am Geriatr Soc* 2012;60(10):1957–1968.

APPROPRIATE PRESCRIBING, DRUG INTERACTIONS, AND ADVERSE EVENTS

HOW TO PRESCRIBE APPROPRIATELY AND REDUCE MEDICATION ERRORS

- **Obtain a complete medication history.** Ask about allergies, OTC drugs, nutritional supplements, alternative medications, alcohol, tobacco, caffeine, recreational drugs, and other prescribers.
- **Avoid prescribing before a diagnosis is made except in severe acute pain.** Consider nondrug tx.
- **Review medications regularly and before prescribing a new medication.** D/C medications that are no longer needed, ineffective, or do not have a corresponding diagnosis.
- **Know the actions, AEs, drug interactions, monitoring requirements, and toxicity profiles of prescribed meadications.** Avoid duplicative effects.
- **Consider the following for new medications:** Is the dosing regimen practical? Is the new medication affordable? Are the benefits expected to outweigh the risks?
- **Start long-term medications at a low dose and titrate dose on the basis of tolerability and response.** Use drug concentration monitoring when available.
- **Attempt to reach a therapeutic dose before switching to or adding another medication.** Use combinations cautiously: titrate each medication to a therapeutic dose before switching to a combination product.
- **Avoid using one medication to treat the AEs caused by another.**
- **Attempt to use one medication to treat 2 or more conditions.**
- **Communicate with other prescribers.** Don't assume patients do—they assume you do!
- **Avoid using drugs from the same class or with similar actions** (eg, multiple opioids).
- **Avoid confusion and know the difference between products:** Brand name products can contain different ingredients depending on their indication; *Lotrimin Ultra* crm contains butenafine, while *Lotrimin AF for Her* and *Gyne-Lotrimin* crm contain clotrimazole, and *Lotrimin AF* deodorant powder contains miconazole.
- **Adjust dose based on the patient kidney and hepatic function.** For most drugs eliminated by the kidneys, adjust dose using estimated CrCl with the Cockcroft-Gault equation:

$$\frac{\text{IBW}(140 - \text{age})\ (0.85 \text{ if female})}{(72)\ (\text{stable serum Cr})}$$

- Lab-provided eGFR can be used when eGFR is used in the drug label; most drug dose adjustments are based on CrCl.
- Both estimated CrCl and GFR values are expressed as mL/min/1.73 m^2 (BSA). For brevity, both are listed as mL/min throughout this text.
- **Use e-prescribing to reduce risk of transcription and medication errors and to check insurance coverage.**
  - Do not use ambiguous directions (eg, as directed [ud] or as needed [prn]). See ismp.org for a list of error-prone abbreviations.
  - Include the medication's purpose under indications or link to indication in the EMR.
  - Always reread prescription for errors in drug selection, strength, dosage form, quantity, and directions.
  - Always verify the patient's correct pharmacy before signing or the end of their visit.

◦ To avoid delays and server errors, send e-prescriptions at the conclusion of each patient visit, instead of in batches.
◦ Use CancelRx and other e-prescribing tools to D/C medications and stop unwanted refills.
- **Verify current prescriptions and e-prescriptions and determine whether medication refills are needed** and authorize the appropriate number
◦ Chronic, nonscheduled medications can usually be refilled up to 15 mo from the date of issue.
◦ Schedules III–V can usually be refilled up to 5 × within 6 mo from the date of issue.
◦ Schedule II medications are nonrefillable; only a 30-d supply can be prescribed at a time.
◦ A list of controlled substances by schedule can be found at www.dea.gov/drug-information/drug-scheduling.
- **Educate patient and/or caregiver about each medication.** Include the regimen, therapeutic goal, cost, and potential AEs or drug interactions. Prescribers, pharmacists, and nurses provide written instructions. Assess health literacy using the Rapid Estimate of Adult Literacy in Medicine - Short Form (REALM-SF) tool. See https://www.ahrq.gov/health-literacy/research/tools/index.html#rapid
- **Create a pill card for patients** or encourage them to create their own. See AHRQ's software program online at ahrq.gov/questions/resources/pill-card.html. For more information, see www.fda.gov/drugs/drug-safety-and-availability/ or ismp.org for a tool to create a pill card.

Medications listed as AVOID or Use with Caution in the 2023 AGS Beers Criteria® are indicated in GAYF by [BC]. Some recommendations state to AVOID the drug without exceptions or USE WITH CAUTION, and others apply only to patients with a specific disease or syndrome, or for a specific duration of use, or a specific dose below a level of kidney function (CrCl), or in combination with other drugs (drug-drug interactions [DDI]). A detailed description of the 2023 AGS Beers Criteria® including evidence tables, useful clinical tools, and patient education materials are available at the AGS website: GeriatricsCareOnline.org.

PRESCRIBING CASCADES

Definition

The prescribing of one drug to treat the adverse effects of another that can trigger additional prescribing or actions to treat adverse effects from the second drug, and so on. The adverse effects are often misinterpreted as a new medical condition. Prescribing cascades can also be categorized as intentional vs unintentional, or appropriate vs problematic.

Examples

Intentional and appropriate

- Diuretic-induced hypokalemia → potassium supplementation
- OIC → laxative use

Unintentional and problematic

- Gabapentin → peripheral edema → diuretic
- Acetylcholinesterase inhibitor → UI → anticholinergic or antimuscarinic

Preventing, Detecting, and Reversing Prescribing Cascades

- Apply the principles of appropriate prescribing (p 16).
- Apply the principles of deprescribing and discontinuing medications (pp 18–19).

DEPRESCRIBING: WHEN AND HOW TO DISCONTINUE MEDICATIONS

- Recognize opportunities to stop a medication:
  - Care transitions (ie, medication reconciliation)
  - Annual/semiannual medication review (eg, annual wellness visit)
  - Review existing medications before starting a new medication
  - Presentation or identification of a new problem or complaint
  - Palliative care or end of life
- D/C medication if:
  - Harms outweigh benefits; presence of ADRs; prescribing cascades
  - Minimal or no effectiveness or benefit
  - No indication
  - Not being taken, and adherence is not critical
  - Time to benefit > Life expectancy
  - De-escalate tx due to revised tx goals (eg, HTN, HF, DM, warfarin + ASA, DOACs + ASA)
- Plan, communicate, and coordinate:
  - Include patient, caregiver, and other healthcare providers
    - Prescribers: cancel discontinued medications in the EMR (eg, CancelRx or other available process) or by contacting the dispensing pharmacy.
    - Patients and caregivers: remove discontinued medications from the home.
  - Use motivational interviewing to link reasons to discontinue (harms) with outcomes to get patient buy-in
  - What to expect/intent
  - Instructions (eg, how to taper [if indicated])
- Monitor and follow-up:
  - Withdrawal reactions
  - Exacerbation of underlying conditions

Table 5. Examples of Medications Eligible for Deprescribing

Drug	Taper	Comments (Why, When, How)
In general, deprescribe when harms > benefits, drug no longer effective, change in goals, and lack of indication.		
Cardiovascular Agents		
Antianginal CCBs	Y	Avoid rebound CV symptoms
ASA	N	Dual antiplatelet tx >12 mo, bleeding risk, low CV risk
β blockers	Y	Avoid rebound CV symptoms
CNS antihypertensives[1]	Y	Avoid rebound HTN
Non-CNS antihypertensives	Y	When harms > benefits, frail, or >85 y; reduce daily dose 25% q3–4mo; monitor for rebound CV symptoms
Statins	N	Decrease in life expectancy, low risk of CV event, AEs

(cont.)

Table 5. Examples of Medications Eligible for Deprescribing (cont.)		
Drug	**Taper**	**Comments (Why, When, How)**
CNS Agents		
AChEIs/Memantine	Y	When of no benefit or severe end stage dementia; reduce daily dose 50% q4wk
Anticonvulsants[1]	Y	Varies by drug; monitor for seizures or return of symptoms
Antipsychotics[1]	Y	After 3 mo if for BPSD
Baclofen	Y	
Benzodiazepines[1]	Y	Reduce daily dose 12.5–25% q2wk
Dopamine agonists	Y	Lack of or inappropriate indication, AEs (falls, CNS): reduce daily dose 25% q1–4wk
Opioids[1]	Y	If for noncancer pain >100 mg MME/d; taper if dose >50 mg MME/d
Sedatives/Hypnotics[1]	Y	Reduce daily dose 12.5–25% q2wk
SSRIs/SNRIs[1]	Y	Varies by drug; reduce daily dose by 25% q1–4wk; monitor for rebound symptoms or withdrawal
Endocrine Agents		
Oral corticosteroids	Y	Dose and duration dependent
Antidiabetic agents	Y	When A1c goals change, frequent hypoglycemia: reduce daily dose q1–2wk if needed
Miscellaneous		
Allopurinol	N	Last attack >12 mo or drug-induced: uric acid <6 mg/dL and symptom free
Anti-allergy (seasonal)	Y	Off season: reduce daily dose 25–50% q1–4wk
PPIs/H2RAs	Y	Indication specific. If for GERD, consider after 4–8 wk; reduce daily dose by 50% (eg, 2×/d to 1×/d); monitor for rebound symptoms

AChEI, acetylcholinesterase inhibitor; BPSD, behavioral and psychological symptoms of dementia.

[1] Fall risk medication. Pharmacologic effects (eg, somnolence, hypotension, dizziness, impaired balance) may trigger deprescribing.

Algorithms, and other materials to help prescribers and patients decide if and how to stop a medication at:

- deprescribingresearch.org (US Deprescribing Research Network)
- www.deprescribingnetwork.ca (Canadian Deprescribing Network)
- www.nswtag.org.au/deprescribing-tools (NSW Therapeutic Advisory Group)
- www.australiandeprescribingnetwork.com.au (Australian Deprescribing Network)
- medstopper.com (based at the University of British Columbia)
- TaperMd.com (based at McMaster University, Ontario, Canada)
- www.managedhealthcareconnect.com/content/armor-a-tool-evaluate-polypharmacy-elderly-persons (ARMOR [Assess, Review, Minimize, Optimize, Reassess] tool)

MEDICATION COST SAVINGS

- Encourage patients to have a conversation with their pharmacist about possible cost-savings strategies, which may include lower-cost prescription medication plans available from the pharmacy (lower than Part D copay), OTC versions of prescription medications, use of *GoodRx* (goodrx.com) or similar services, pharmaceutical company assistance programs, or other cost-saving programs.
- Cost-saving strategies can result in a patient's medication record being incomplete at multiple pharmacies, putting the patient at risk for drug-drug interactions.

CMS GUIDANCE ON UNNECESSARY DRUGS IN THE NURSING HOME (F757)

See Appendix PP of the CMS State Operations Manual. Updated survey guidelines for antipsychotic drugs in dementia are at cms.gov/Medicare/Provider-Enrollment-and-Certification/GuidanceforLawsAndRegulations/Downloads/Appendix-PP-State-Operations-Manual.pdf

CDC GUIDANCE ON USE OF OPIOIDS FOR CHRONIC PAIN

- See complete guidance at https://www.cdc.gov/mmwr/volumes/71/rr/rr7103a1.htm.
- Tx should be individualized.

MEDICATIONS THAT SHOULD NOT BE CRUSHED

Medications that have enteric-coated (EC), sustained-release (SR), extended-release (ER), sustained-action (SA), and other long-acting oral dosage forms should not be crushed. Crushing may result in the immediate release of the entire dose and toxicity. Immediate-release (IR) tablets can be crushed and IR capsules can usually be opened for easier administration. For more information, see ismp.org or a drug's FDA label.

PHARMACOTHERAPY AND AGE-ASSOCIATED CHANGES

Table 6. Age-associated Changes in Pharmacokinetics and Pharmacodynamics

Parameter	Age Effect	Disease, Factor Effect	Prescribing Implications
Absorption	Rate and extent are usually unaffected	Achlorhydria, concurrent medications, tube feedings	Drug-drug and drug-food interactions are more likely to alter absorption
Distribution	Increase in fat:water ratio; decreased plasma protein, particularly albumin	HF, ascites, and other conditions increase body water	Fat-soluble drugs have a larger volume of distribution; highly protein-bound drugs have a greater (active) free concentration
Metabolism	Decreases in liver mass and liver blood flow decrease drug clearance; may be age-related changes in CYP2C19, while CYP3A4 and CYP2D6 are not affected	Smoking, genotype, concurrent drug tx, alcohol and caffeine intake may have more effect than aging	Lower dosages may be therapeutic
Elimination	Primarily renal; age-related decrease in GFR	Kidney impairment with acute and chronic diseases; decreased muscle mass results in less Cr production	Serum Cr not a reliable measure of kidney function; best to estimate CrCl using formula (see p 16)

(cont.)

Table 6. Age-associated Changes in Pharmacokinetics and Pharmacodynamics (cont.)			
Parameter	**Age Effect**	**Disease, Factor Effect**	**Prescribing Implications**
Pharmacodynamics	Less predictable and often altered drug response at usual or lower concentrations	Drug-drug and drug-disease interactions may alter responses	Prolonged pain relief with opioids at lower dosages; increased sedation and postural instability to benzodiazepines; altered sensitivity to β blockers

COMPLICATING FACTORS

Drug-Food or -Nutrient Interactions

Physical Interactions: Mg^{++}, Ca^{++}, Fe^{++}, Al^{++}, or zinc can lower oral absorption of levothyroxine and some quinolone antibiotics. Tube feedings decrease absorption of oral phenytoin and levothyroxine. See p 208.

Decreased Drug Effect: Warfarin and vitamin K-containing foods

Decreased Oral Intake or Appetite: Medications can alter the taste of food (dysgeusia) or decrease saliva production (xerostomia), making mastication and swallowing difficult. Medications associated with dysgeusia include allopurinol, β-lactam antibiotics, clarithromycin, and nirmatrelvir/ritonavir *(Paxlovid)*. Medications that can cause xerostomia include antihistamines, antidepressants, antipsychotics, clonidine, and diuretics.

Drug-Drug Interactions

A drug's effect can be altered, displacement from protein-binding sites, inhibition or induction of metabolic enzymes, or because 2 or more drugs have a similar pharmacologic effect. For more information, consult a drug-drug interaction text, software, or Internet resource (eg, www.fda.gov/Drugs/drug-interactions-labeling/drug-development-and-drug-interactions-table-substrates-inhibitors-and-inducers and medicine.iupui.edu/clinpharm/ddis/), and **Table 7**.

Pharmacogenomics Resources

Pharmacogenomics Knowledge Base (Pharm GKB; pharmgkb.org) provides comprehensive knowledge to clinicians and researchers about how genetic variations impact drug response.

Clinical Pharmacogenetics Implementation Consortium (CPIC; cpicpgx.org) is a useful aid for clinicians when interpreting pharmacogenetic tests. CPIC guidelines are also available at guidelines.gov.

Table 7. Potentially Clinically Important Drug-Drug Interactions That Should Be Avoided in Older Adults[BC]

Object Drug/Class	Interacting Drug/Class	Rationale	Recommendation
Renin-angiotensin system (RAS) inhibitor (ACEIs, ARBs, aliskiren) or potassium-sparing diuretics (amiloride, triamterene)	Another RAS inhibitor or potassium-sparing diuretic	Increased risk of hyperkalemia	Avoid routine use in those with CKD Stage 3a or higher.

(cont.)

Table 7. Potentially Clinically Important Drug-Drug Interactions That Should Be Avoided in Older Adults[BC] (cont.)

Object Drug/Class	Interacting Drug/Class	Rationale	Recommendation
Opioids	Benzodiazepines	Increased risk of overdose	Avoid.
	Gabapentin, pregabalin	Increased risk of severe sedative AEs, including respiratory depression and death	Avoid. Exceptions are when transitioning from opioid tx to gabapentin or pregabalin, or when using gabapentinoids to reduce opioid dose, although caution should be used in all circumstances.
Anticholinergic	Other anticholinergic	Cognitive decline, urinary retention	Avoid, minimize the number of anticholinergic drugs (**Table 35**).
CNS-active drugs	Any combination of ≥3 of these CNS-active drugs:[1] • Antidepressants (TCAs, SSRIs, and SNRIs) • Antipsychotics • Antiepileptics • Benzodiazepines and nonbenzodiazepines, benzodiazepine receptor agonists (ie, Z-drugs) • Opioids	Increased risk of falls (all) and of fracture (benzodiazepines, nonbenzodiazepines, benzodiazepine receptor agonist hypnotics)	Avoid total of ≥3 CNS-active drugs[1]; minimize number of CNS-active drugs.
Corticosteroids, oral or parenteral	NSAIDs	Peptic ulcer disease and GI bleeding	Avoid; if not possible, provide GI protection.
Lithium	ACEIs/ARBs	Lithium toxicity	Avoid, monitor lithium concentrations.
	Loop diuretics	Lithium toxicity	Avoid, monitor lithium concentrations.
	NSAIDs (including ASA)	Lithium toxicity	Avoid, monitor lithium concentrations. Extent of effect varies by NSAID.
Peripheral α-1 blockers	Loop diuretics	UI in older women	Avoid in older women, unless conditions warrant both drugs.
Warfarin	Amiodarone, Ciprofloxacin, Macrolides (excluding azithromycin), Trimethoprim-sulfamethoxazole, NSAIDs	Bleeding or increased risk of bleeding	Avoid when possible, monitor INR closely.

[1] CNS-active drugs: antiepileptics, antipsychotics, benzodiazepines, nonbenzodiazepines, benzodiazepine receptor agonist hypnotics, TCAs, SSRIs, SNRIs, and opioids.

Drug-induced Changes in Cardiac Conduction

- Intrinsic changes associated with aging in cardiac pacemaker cells and conduction system
- Increased sensitivity to drug-induced conduction disorders (eg, bradycardia and tachyarrhythmias)
- Risk increases with acute lowering of serum calcium, potassium, and magnesium
- Other causes: genetic mutations (usually younger persons); medical conditions including hypothyroidism, DM2, HF, and sepsis
- QTc prolongation exacerbated by drugs alone, drug interactions, and altered pharmacokinetics (eg, reduced kidney function)
- A comprehensive list of drugs associated with QTc prolongation or an increased risk of torsades de pointes that should be avoided by patients with congenital long QT syndrome is available at crediblemeds.org.
- If possible, do not prescribe QT-prolonging drugs to anyone with a QTc >440 millisec (women) or >420 millisec (men). Each 10 millisec increase in QTc is estimated to increase the risk of torsades de pointes by 5–7%.
- Do not allow the QTc to exceed 500 millisec during titration with these drugs as the risk of torsades de pointes is markedly increased and intervention considered necessary.

COMMONLY USED HERBAL AND ALTERNATIVE MEDICATIONS

Note: Herbal and dietary supplements are not subject to the same regulatory process by the FDA as prescription and OTC medications. Product and lot-to-lot variations can occur in composition and concentration of active ingredient(s), or be tainted with heavy metals or prescription medications (eg, sildenafil). Consumers are advised to purchase products by reputable manufacturers who follow good manufacturing procedures that contain the United States Pharmacopeia (USP) seal. For additional information on herbal and alternative medications, see NIH National Center for Complementary and Integrative Health (nccih.nih.gov).

Apoaequorin *(Prevagen)*

Common Uses: Age-associated memory complaints, MCI, brain health

AEs: Headache, dizziness, nausea, difficulty sleeping, anxiety; small number of heart and nervous system–related events

Drug Interactions: Unknown

Comments: Source is a protein derived from jellyfish. Studied in community-dwelling adults with self-reported memory concerns. Safety data in rodents only.

Black cohosh

Common uses: Vasomotor symptoms associated with menopause

AEs: Hepatotoxicity (rare); contains salicylic acid

Drug Interactions: Cardiovascular, antihypertensive, and other drugs that lower BP may lead to hypotension.

Comments: Lacks estrogenic properties. A 2012 Cochrane review concluded there was insufficient evidence to support its use for menopausal symptoms. Dose: standard 2.5% triterpene glycosides (1 mg/dose): 40–80 mg/d in divided doses; time of onset 2 wk; maximum effect at 8 wk.

Cannabis (see Substance Use Disorders)

Common Uses: Medical (pain, nausea, anxiety, sleep, other indications); recreation

AEs: Drowsiness, dizziness, ataxia, dry mouth, headache, increased appetite, derealization, hallucinations, angiogenesis

Comments: Potential lowering of CBD and THC concentrations via CYP1A2 induction (includes St John's wort) or when combined with CYP3A4 inducers, and increases of CBD and THC concentrations when combined with CYP2C9, CPY3A4 inhibitors. Concurrent use with sympathomimetics increases the risk of tachycardia.

Chondroitin/Glucosamine

Common Uses: OA, RA

AEs: Chondroitin: nausea, dyspepsia, changes in IOP; Glucosamine: anorexia, insomnia, painful and itchy skin, peripheral edema, tachycardia

Comments: Meta-analyses have reached mixed conclusions of chondroitin's effectiveness in OA of the knee. Neither the AAOS (2010) nor the ACR (2012) recommend chondroitin/ glucosamine for knee arthritis. In one trial, knee pain did not respond better to chondroitin alone or in combination with glucosamine compared with placebo in >1500 patients with OA. If patients choose a trial of chondroitin plus glucosamine, it should be glucosamine sulfate.

Cinnamon

Common Uses: DM, AD, heart disease, analgesia, and anti-inflammatory

AEs: Allergy to cinnamon or Peru balsam; cassia cinnamon contains coumarin and may increase risk of bleeding; contact dermatitis and vasomotor symptoms with large doses

Comments: May lower A1c and BP; clinical trials have concluded cinnamon does not affect factors related to DM or heart disease

Coenzyme Q_{10}

Common Uses: CVD (angina, HF, HTN), musculoskeletal disorders, periodontal diseases, DM, obesity, dementia prevention, AD, Parkinson disease; may lessen toxic effects of doxorubicin and daunorubicin; reversal of statin myopathy

AEs: Abdominal discomfort, headache, nausea, vomiting

Comments: May increase risk of bleeding; use with caution in patients with hepatic impairment, may decrease response to warfarin; may further decrease BP if taking antihypertensives or other medications that decrease BP; ubiquinol is a reduced form of coenzyme Q_{10}

Curcumin/Turmeric (Curcumin derived from turmeric; *Curcuma aromatica, C domestica, C longa*)

Common Uses: OA, pain, ulcerative colitis (enema)

AEs: Nausea, diarrhea; allergic skin reactions; increase calcium oxalate kidney stones

Comments: Drug interactions with anticoagulants, increases tacrolimus concentrations, and *C longa* potentially interacts with CYP2D6 and 3A4

Dehydroepiandrosterone (DHEA)

Common Uses: Menopausal symptoms including vaginal dryness; osteoporosis

AEs: Women: weight gain, voice changes, facial hair, headaches; Men: BPH, possible increase in hormone-sensitive tumors

Comments: Possible drug interactions with CCBs, sildenafil, carbamazepine, valproic acid/divalproex, lithium, antipsychotics, SSRIs, estrogens, and testosterone

Echinacea

Common Uses: Immune stimulant

AEs: Hepatotoxicity, allergic reactions, GI upset, rash

Drug Interactions: Immunosuppressants; reportedly inhibits CYP1A2, –3A4; induces CYP3A4 (unlikely to be clinically significant)

Comments: D/C ≥2 wk before surgery; cross-sensitivity with chrysanthemum, ragweed, daisy, and aster allergies; kidney disease; immunosuppression; mixed results regarding effectiveness to shorten duration, reduce severity, or prevent colds; should not be taken for >10 d because of concern about immunosuppression. Effect on immune response to COVID-19 is uncertain; some evidence that echinacea reduces cytokine concentrations, then may decrease cytokine storm.

Feverfew

Common Uses: Anti-inflammatory, migraine prophylaxis

AEs: Platelet inhibition, bleeding, GI upset, swelling of the lips, tongue, and oral mucosa; allergic contact dermatitis from handling fresh leaves

Drug Interactions: NSAIDs, antiplatelet agents, anticoagulants

Comments: D/C 7 d before surgery, active bleeding; cross-sensitivity with chrysanthemum and daisy; evidence lacking for either indication; minimum of 1-mo trial for migraine prophylaxis suggested

Fish Oils (*Lovaza*, omega-3 fatty acids); (see Cardiovascular and Prevention)

Common Uses: Decrease risk of CAD and CHD, hypertriglyceridemia, symptomatic tx of RA, inflammatory bowel disease, asthma, bipolar disorder, schizophrenia, memory, cognitive loss prevention, and in cases of immunosuppression

AEs: GI upset, dyspepsia, diarrhea, nausea, belching, halitosis, increased blood glucose, bleeding, increased ALT and LDL-C

Drug Interactions: Anticoagulants, antiplatelet agents, antihypertensives, cyclosporine, CYP3A4 substrates, digoxin, statins, niacin

Comments: Use with caution if allergic to seafood; monitor LFTs, TG, and LDL-C at baseline, then periodically; a 2-mo trial is adequate for hypertriglyceridemia; not proven effective for primary or secondary prevention

Flaxseed and flaxseed oil

Common Uses: RA, asthma, constipation, DM, hyperlipidemia, menopausal symptoms, prevention of stroke and CHD, BPH, laxative

AEs: Bleeding, hypoglycemia, hypotension, allergy; Flaxseed only: abdominal pain and bloating, flatulence, diarrhea

Drug Interactions: NSAIDs, antiplatelet agents, anticoagulants, insulin and hypoglycemic agents, lithium (mania)

Garlic

Common Uses: HTN, hypercholesterolemia, platelet inhibitor

AEs: Bleeding, GI upset, hypoglycemia

Drug Interactions: NSAIDs, antiplatelet agents, anticoagulants, isoniazid, NNRTIs, protease inhibitors; induction of CYP3A4 and p-glycoprotein efflux pump.

Comments: D/C 7 d before surgery; effect on lipid lowering modest and of questionable clinical value; decrease in BP if HTN, may take ≥2 mo to see effect.

Ginger

Common Uses: Antiemetic, anti-inflammatory, dyspepsia

AEs: GI upset, heartburn, diarrhea, irritation of the mouth and throat

Drug Interactions: NSAIDs, antiplatelet agents, anticoagulants

Comments: D/C 7 d before surgery

Ginkgo biloba

Common Uses: AD, memory, migraine, CVD and stroke prophylaxis

AEs: Bleeding, nausea, headache, GI upset, diarrhea, dizziness, heart palpitations; cross-allergic reactions if allergic to poison ivy, poison oak, mango rind, or cashew oil.

Drug Interactions: MAOIs (increased effect and toxicity), antiplatelet agents, anticoagulants, NSAIDs, midazolam; induces CYP2C19.

Comments: D/C 2 wk before surgery; mixed results in dementia trials; recent trials tend to have negative results

Ginseng (Panax, not American or Siberian ginseng)

Common Uses: Physical and mental performance enhancer, digestive, diuretic, immunomodulator, antineoplastic, hyperlipidemia, CNS, fatigue syndrome, and endocrine effects

AEs: HTN, tachycardia, insomnia, nausea, diarrhea, decreased appetite, confusion, depression, ED, headache, estrogenic effects (higher doses, prolonged use)

Drug Interactions: Antiplatelet agents, anticoagulants, NSAIDs, imatinib; American ginseng: hypoglycemia with hypoglycemic agents; increased warfarin clearance, decreased anticoagulant effect

Comments: D/C 7 d before surgery, kidney failure

Glucosamine (see Chondroitin)

Kava

Common Uses: Anxiety, sedative

AEs: Sedation, hepatotoxicity, GI upset, headache, dizziness, EPS, scaly skin rash, urinary retention, exacerbation of Parkinson disease, rhabdomyolysis

Drug Interactions: Anticonvulsants (increased effect), benzodiazepines, CNS depressants, L-DOPA

Comments: D/C 24 h before surgery; compared with placebo, kava has demonstrated antianxiety efficacy, but effect small and not robust

Kratom *(Mitragyna speciosa)*

Common Uses: Pain, fatigue, depression, opioid addiction

AEs: Dependence, addiction, and withdrawal potential; hyperpigmentation of the skin, constipation, nausea, vomiting, weight loss, xerostomia, loss of libido, agitation or irritability, tachycardia, drowsiness or lethargy, insomnia, confusion, HTN, and seizures

Drug Interactions: Reported to inhibit CYP3A4, -2D6, and -1A2. Concomitant use with carisoprodol, modafinil, fentanyl, diphenhydramine, morphine, O-desmethyltramadol, and others are reported to have resulted in serious and fatal adverse effects.

Comment: an unregulated herbal product

Melatonin (see Sleep Disorders)

Common Uses: Sleep disorders, insomnia, jet lag

AEs: Daytime drowsiness, headache, dizziness, enuresis, nausea, transient depression

Drug Interactions: Warfarin, ASA, clopidogrel, ticlopidine, dipyridamole (loss of hemostasis), antidiabetic agents (decreased glucose tolerance and insulin sensitivity), CNS depressants

Methylsulfonylmethane (MSM)

Common Uses: Anti-inflammatory, analgesia, OA, chronic pain, GI upset

AEs: Nausea, diarrhea, fatigue, bloating, insomnia, headache

Comments: A derivative of dimethyl sulfoxide (DMSO) that produces less odor

Red yeast rice *(Monascus purpureus,* Xue Zhi Kang, natural source of mevinolin, the active ingredient of lovastatin)

Common Uses: CHD, DM, hypercholesterolemia

AEs: Nausea, vomiting, GI upset, hepatic disorders, myopathy, rhabdomyolysis

Drug Interactions (theoretical): Cyclosporine, CYP3A4 substrates, digoxin, statins, niacin

Comments: Use with caution in patients taking other lipid-lowering agents

Rhodiola rosea *(Arctic Root,* golden root*)*

Common Uses: Energy, stamina, strength, enhanced cognitive capacity, stress, improved sexual function, mood, and anxiety

AEs: Dizziness, dry mouth

Drug Interactions: Antidiabetic drugs (hypoglycemia), antihypertensives (hypotension), moderate CYP3A4 inhibitor, immunosuppressants (may be an immunostimulant)

SAMe (S-adenosyl-methionine)

Common Uses: Depression, fibromyalgia, insomnia, OA, RA

AEs: GI distress, insomnia, dizziness, dry mouth, headache, restlessness

Drug Interactions: Antidepressants, St John's wort, NSAIDs, antiplatelet agents, anticoagulants, other drugs affecting serotonin (serotonin syndrome), antidopaminergic effects

Comments: Not effective for bipolar depression, hyperhomocysteinemia (theoretical), D/C ≥14 d before surgery

Saw palmetto

Common Uses: BPH

AEs: Headache, nausea, GI distress, erectile dysfunction, decreased libido, dizziness

Drug Interactions: Finasteride, α_1-adrenergic agonist properties in vitro may decrease efficacy; may prolong bleeding time, so use with caution with antiplatelet agents, anticoagulants, NSAIDs

Comments: Efficacy in BPH did not differ from placebo in an adequately powered, randomized clinical trial; takes 1–2 mo before any effect on BPH

St John's wort *(Hypericum perforatum)*

Common Uses: Depression, anxiety, menopausal symptoms, wound healing

AEs: Photosensitivity, hypomania, insomnia, vivid dreams, restlessness, GI upset, dry mouth, itching, fatigue, dizziness, headache; reported suicidal ideation and psychosis

Drug Interactions: Potent CYP3A4 inducer, mild CYP1A2, -2C9, -2C19 inducer, finasteride (decreased finasteride concentration and possible effectiveness), other serotonergic-acting agents

Comments: Wear sunscreen with UVA and UVB coverage; avoid in fair-skinned patients; store away from UV light; D/C 5 d before surgery; not effective in severe depression; effects reported to vary from those of conventional antidepressants, yet no more effective than placebo; evaluation of effectiveness may be complicated by product, extraction process, and composition

Valerian

Common Uses: Anxiety, insomnia

AEs: Sedation, benzodiazepine-like withdrawal, headache, GI upset, insomnia

Drug Interactions: Benzodiazepines, CNS depressants

Comments: Taper dose several weeks before surgery

ANEMIA, MYELOPROLIFERATIVE AND MYELODYSPLASTIC DISORDERS

ANEMIA

Significance

Lower Hb and mild anemia is associated with more severe disability, poorer mobility and cognition, frailty, and falls.

Evaluation

- Hematopoietic reserve capacity declines with age (eg, slower return of Hb to normal after phlebotomy); don't perform serial blood counts in clinically stable patients.[CW]
- Evaluate people aged >65 when Hb <13 g/dL in men and <12 g/dL in women.
- Evaluate if Hb falls >1 g/dL in 1 y.
- Physical exam and lab tests: BUN, Cr, ESR, CRP.
- Check WBC and peripheral blood smear; pursue suspected causes as appropriate.
- Combined deficiencies are common in older adults; reasonable to check B_{12}, folate, and iron in all cases. MCV is not reliable in combined deficiency states.
- Check reticulocyte count and reticulocyte index.
  - Reticulocyte count or index high: suspect blood loss or hemolytic anemia, p 34.
  - Reticulocyte count or index normal or low: suggests deficiency (B_{12}, folate [**Figure 3**], or iron deficiency, CKD, chronic inflammation, unexplained anemia, or MDS. [**Figure 4**]).

Figure 3. Evaluation of Hypoproliferative Anemia Due to Possible B_{12} or Folate Deficiency

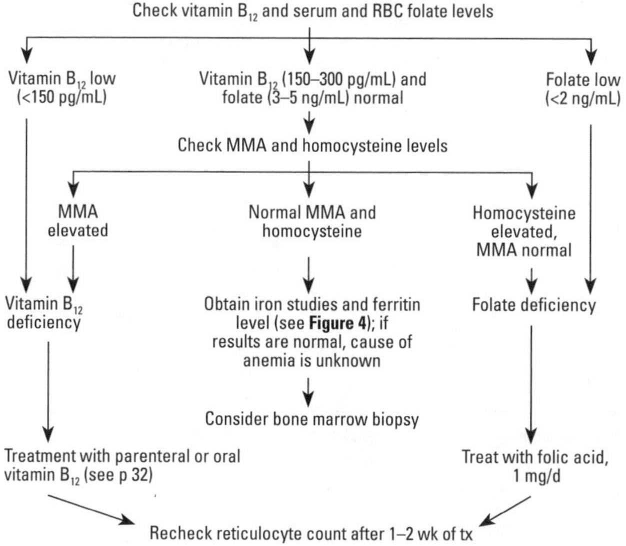

Source: Adapted from Balducci L. *J Amer Geriatr Soc* 2003; 51(3 Suppl):S2–9. Reprinted with permission.

Figure 4. Evaluation of Possible Iron Deficiency Anemia

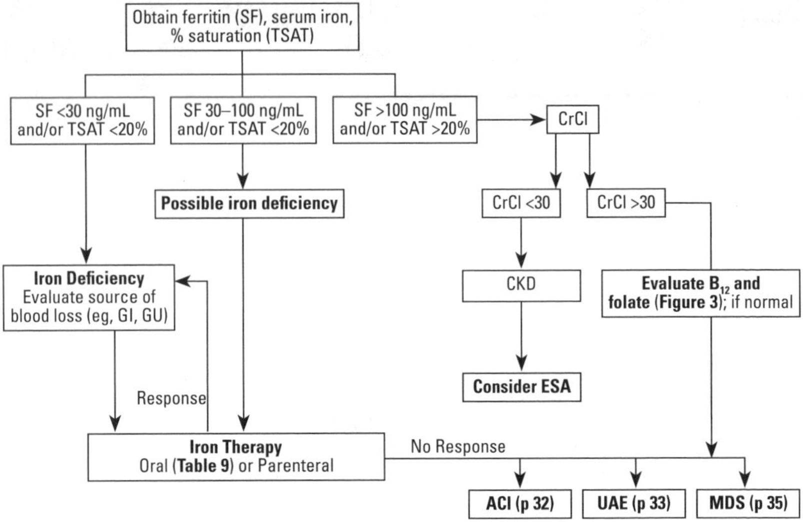

ACI, anemia of chronic inflammation; CKD, chronic kidney disease; ESA, erythropoiesis-stimulating agent; MDS, myelodysplastic syndrome; UAE, undifferentiated anemia of the elderly.

Table 8. Differentiating Anemias of Chronic Inflammation, Chronic Kidney Disease, UAE, MDS, Iron Deficiency, and Mixed ACI/Iron Deficiency

Anemia Type	Ferritin, ng/mL	TSAT, %	ESR/CRP	Other Labs	% of All Late-Life Anemias
Anemia of chronic inflammation (ACI)	>100	>20	Elevated[1]	Hb not<10; CrCl >30	6–26
Anemia of CKD	>100	>20	WNL	CrCl <30[2]	4–11
Unexplained Anemia of the Elderly (UAE)	WNL	WNL	WNL	B_{12} and folate WNL; Hb not <10	25–40
Myelodysplastic Syndrome (MDS)	WNL	WNL	WNL	Hb <10, +/- other cytopenias	?
Iron Deficiency	<30	Low	WNL	TSAT <20	15–30
Mixed Iron Deficiency and ACI	30–100	Low	Elevated	TSAT <20	?

TSAT, transferrin saturation; WNL, within normal limits; CrCl unit = mL/min.

[1] ESR >20 in men; >30 in women; or CRP >1.0 (10 mg/L)

[2] Frequency of anemia is 1% at an eGFR of 60 mL/min; 9% at an eGFR of 30 mL/min.

Iron Deficiency Anemia (Figure 4)

- Lab tests **Table 8**.
- Evaluate GI and GU source of blood loss; if not GI source, consider celiac disease (causes 11% of iron deficiency).
- Don't transfuse RBCs for iron deficiency without hemodynamic instability.[CW]
- Begin tx with oral iron using the steps outlined in **Table 9**.
- Parenteral iron (**Table 10**):
  - Use if oral iron replacement is inadequate or not tolerated.
  - Rates of anaphylaxis are low for all products, but 3–8× higher with iron dextran and ferumoxytol *(Feraheme)* than with iron sucrose *(Venofer)*.
  - IV iron is well tolerated, and premedication and test doses are unnecessary.
  - Although infusion reactions are uncommon, they are highest with iron sucrose (4.3%) and lowest with ferric carboxymaltose (1.4%), but carboxymaltose is associated with frequent (up to 70%) post-infusion incidence of hypophosphatemia; monitor for this.
  - IV iron increases risk of infection by about 1.7%, compared to oral iron.

Table 9. **Steps in Oral Iron Replacement**

	Hb, g/dL	**Oral elemental iron total replacement dose, mg**
Step 1: Estimate iron replacement dose based on Hb	>11 9–11 <9	5,000 10,000 15,000

	Preparation[1]	**No. of tabs to achieve 5000-mg elemental iron replacement**
Step 2: Select an oral iron preparation (only 10% of oral iron is absorbed)	Ferrous sulfate (elixir 2.7 mg/15 mL, 324-mg tab, 65 mg elemental iron)	75
	Ferrous gluconate (300-mg tab, 36 mg elemental iron)	140
	Ferrous fumarate (100-mg tab, 33 mg elemental iron)	150
	Iron polysaccharide (150-mg tab, 150 mg elemental iron)	33
Step 3: Decide on dosing frequency	Dosing with a single tab every other day has little difference in time to repletion compared to daily. Iron is best absorbed on an empty stomach. Assess tolerance after 1 wk (phonecall); if not tolerating, adjust dose or preparation.	
Step 4: Recheck Hb and ferritin after each 5000-mg cycle	Give additional 5000-mg cycles prn.	

[1] Tolerance to GI side effects improves, however cost increases going down the list of preparations.

Note: 1 unit packed RBCs replaces 500 mg iron, or approximately the same as is absorbed from a 5000-mg cycle of oral iron. Reticulocytosis should occur in 7–10 d. Lack of correction with replacement suggests nonadherence, malabsorption, or ongoing blood loss. H_2 blockers, antacids, and PPIs reduce absorption, and some patients will need parenteral replacement. Enterically coated preparations are less well absorbed.

Table 10. Parenteral Iron Products

Class Comments: During infusion monitor vital signs, ADRs, and injection site during and 30 min after administration; reassess need for additional iron replacement with recheck of Hb and iron studies 2–3 wk after infusions complete.

Agent (Brand)	Dose (Iron Deficiency Anemia)	Administration and Comments
Ferric carboxymaltose (*Injectafer*)	<50 kg: 15 mg/kg on day 1; repeat after >7 d (max dose 750 mg); 1500 mg/course	IV over >15 min Slow IVP: 100 mg/min
Ferric derisomaltose (*Monoferric*)	<50 mg: 20 mg/kg ×1; repeat if indicated 50 kg: 1000 mg ×1; repeat if indicated Hb <70 kg >70 kg >10 1000 mg 1500 mg <10 1500 mg 2000 mg	Infuse over 20 min
Ferric gluconate[1] (*Ferrlecit*)	CKD: 125–250 mg elemental iron/dose; repeat until hematologic or total iron requirement is met	IV: diluted over 1 h; undiluted at 12.5 mg/min per dialysis session
Ferumoxytol (*Feraheme*)	2-dose: 510 mg; repeat 3–8 d; assess 30 d after second dose. 1-dose: 1.02 g	2-dose: 15 min inf 1-dose: 30 min inf
Iron dextran complex (*INFeD*)	Total dose = 0.0442 mL (desired Hb - observed Hb) × LBW + (0.26 mL × LBW) (Max 100 mg)	IV: undiluted no faster than 50 mg/min. IM: Z-track; avoid diluting with dextran.
Iron sucrose (*Venofer*)	CKD, nondialysis: 200 mg × 5 doses within 14 d; repeat if indicated. Has been given as 500 mg on days 1 and 14.	Slow IV: undiluted over 2–5 min Diluted: <200 mg over >15 min; 300 mg over 1.5 h; 400 mg over 2.5 h; 500 mg over 3.5–4 h; assess iron status ≥48 h after last dose (rapid increase may occur).

LBW, lean body weight.

[1]OL if not on dialysis

Anemia of Chronic Inflammation (ACI; also known as anemia of chronic disease)

- Typically normocytic/normochromic and Hb about 10 g/dL
- Cause: hepcidin-induced alteration in GI iron absorption and iron trapping in macrophages.
- Most common causes in older adults:
  - Acute and chronic infection
  - Malignancy
  - Protein calorie malnutrition
  - Unidentified chronic disease
- Lab tests: see **Table 8**.
- Check erythropoietin level; if <500 mU/mL may respond to the administration of recombinant human ESAs; target level 10–11 g/dL.
- ADRs from ESA tx in ACI have not been well studied, and tx may not be reimbursed by Medicare.

Combined Iron Deficiency and Anemia of Chronic Inflammation

- Iron, TIBC, and ferritin are less reliable in the presence of inflammatory conditions (**Figure 4**).
- Anemia is often more severe than in ACI alone.
- Suspect iron deficiency if ferritin 30–100 ng/mL and/or TSAT <20%. If ferritin ≤45 ng/mL, iron deficiency is confirmed. If 45–99 ng/mL, iron deficiency is possible; either treat presumed iron deficiency and evaluate response by reticulocyte count at 2 wk or check soluble transferrin receptor (sTfR). If sTfR/log (ferritin) >2, iron deficiency is confirmed; If sTfR/log (ferritin) <1 anemia of inflammation is confirmed.

Undifferentiated (or Unexplained) Anemia of the Elderly (UAE) and Idiopathic Cytopenias of Undetermined Significance (ICUS)

- UAE is the most common type of ICUS; and most ICUS develops in old age.
- Many patients with ICUS carry 1 or more of the 40 somatic mutations associated with myeloid malignancies and a portion of these evolve into an MDS (p 35).
- Lab tests: see **Table 8**
- Additional studies: hypocellular bone marrow; erythropoietin levels low for the degree of anemia.

Anemia of Chronic Kidney Disease

- Caused by decreased erythropoietin production; check erythropoietin level, iron studies, B_{12}, and folate.
- Frequency: 1% at an eGFR of 60 mL/min; 9% at an eGFR of 30; 33–67% at eGFR of <15
- Monitor Hb annually if eGFR≥45 or 2×/y if eGFR <45
- Laboratory diagnosis: see **Table 8**
- Correct all correctable causes of anemia (iron deficiency, inflammation) before using ESAs. Keep transferrin saturation 25–50% and ferritin 200–500 ng/mL. Oral iron absorption is poor in CKD; parenteral replacement is often needed.
- Use of ESAs in anemia of CKD
  - Restoring Hb levels with ESAs decreases transfusions and fatigue but doubles stroke risk in people with DM2. Don't administer ESAs to CKD patients with Hb ≥10 g/dL without symptoms of anemia.[CW]
  - Guidelines for ESAs (kdigo.org) recommend individualized tx.
  - Use ESAs with caution (if at all) in patients with malignancy, hx of stroke, or hx of malignancy.
  - Consider ESA and iron replacement when Hb is <10 g/dL with the goal of avoiding Hb <9 g/dL and the need for transfusion. Once ESA started, follow iron studies q3mo.
  - Goal Hb is 10–11.5 using the lowest ESA dose possible. In non-DM patients, target of Hb = 11 is safe.
  - Risk of stroke and malignancy increases at Hb >12.5
  - Some patients will have improved quality of life with Hb above 11.5 g/dL and will accept the risk; do not let Hb exceed 13 g/dL.
  - Patients who do not respond to usual dosages of ESAs may be at greater risk of cardiovascular events on high ESA dosages.
  - Evaluate for antibody-mediated pure red cell aplasia in patients using ESAs for >8 wk if Hb declines 0.5–1 g/wk.

Anemia of B_{12} and Folate Deficiency **(Figure 4)**

- Lab tests: anemia or pancytopenia, macrocytosis
- Serum B_{12} 65–95% sensitivity for clinical deficiency if <200 pg/mL; deficiency is possible at <350 pg/mL; check serum MMA level to confirm deficiency.
- MMA and homocysteine normal, no deficiency; MMA and homocysteine elevated B12 deficient, possible folate deficient, MMA normal, homocysteine elevated, no B12 deficiency, consistent with folate deficiency.
- Management: Expert panels recommend parenteral replacement for severe deficiency (neurologic complications, severe anemia) and when adherence is not ensured.
  - If neurologic impairment: B_{12} 1000 mcg IM every other day for 2 wk, or until no further improvement, 1000 mcg IM q2mo for life; if no neurologic impairment, q3mo.
  - In cases of mild deficiency, RCTs support the efficacy of oral replacement; ensure there will be adherence and malabsorption is not the cause, use B_{12} 1000–2000 mcg/d po.
  - If using nonparenteral formulations, monitor MMA every 1–3 y to ensure replacement is adequate.
- Borderline folate levels 2–4 ng/mL should prompt homocysteine check. A few days of poor po intake lowers serum (but not body stores) of folate. Folate deficiency very rare except in severe malnutrition or alcoholism.
- Management: Folate 1 mg/d po for 1–4 mo or until complete hematologic recovery.

Hemolytic Anemia: not due to congenital anemia

- Hallmark is high reticulocyte count, LDH, and unconjugated bilirubin. About 2% of all anemias after age 65.
- The most common cause is autoimmune (low haptoglobin, positive direct antiglobulin) associated with CLL, medications, lymphoma, and collagen vascular disease; idiopathic, delayed transfusion reaction.
- Causes if not autoimmune: mechanical heart valve, liver disease, hypersplenism, infection.

RBC Transfusion for Anemia: Don't transfuse more units of blood than absolutely necessary.[CW] Single-unit transfusions should be the standard in stable noncardiac patients.[CW]

Acute Blood Loss

In general, withholding transfusion until Hb is 7–8 g/dL (restrictive) for people over age 65 results in equivalent outcomes (risk of bacterial infection, MI, mortality, rebleeding, pulmonary edema) compared to a more liberal transfusion for Hb <10 g/dL (liberal) transfusion policy. Exceptions are:

- Patients undergoing orthopedic procedures have better outcomes with restrictive transfusions.
- Patients with symptomatic CVD have better outcomes with liberal transfusions.

Avoid transfusions of RBC for arbitrary Hb or hematocrit thresholds and in the absence of symptoms of active coronary disease, HF, or stroke.[CW]

Chronic Anemia

- Chronic anemia due to refractory aplastic anemia, myelodysplastic syndromes, etc, will require transfusion. For these patients, the transfusion threshold is based on symptoms to generally maintain Hb >9 g/dL in men and >8 g/dL in women.

PANCYTOPENIA

Unless due to B_{12} deficiency or drug-induced, bone-marrow aspirate is indicated; causes include cancer, fibrosis, infection, myelodysplasia, splenomegaly, and aplastic anemia.

Drug-induced Pancytopenia

- Many drugs may cause this. Check the patient's complete medication list.
- Agents known to cause pancytopenia include antimicrobials, antigout, antiepileptics, antithyroid medications, cardiovascular drugs (eg, amiodarone), diuretics, and those used to treat psychiatric and rheumatologic disorders (eg, NSAIDs).

Aplastic Anemia

- Due to immune-mediated hematopoietic stem cell failure.
- Typically present with infections due to neutropenia, bleeding due to thrombocytopenia, fatigue due to anemia, or any combination of these.
- Diagnosis: hypocellular bone marrow
- Exclude MDS (see below), especially in older adults.
- Management: after age 50, horse antithymocyte globulin, cyclosporine, and eltrombopag.
- For less fit or frail, focus on relieving symptoms, improving quality of life, prolonging survival, while limiting ADRs.

Myelodysplastic Syndromes (MDS)

MDS comprise a group of hematologic malignancies characterized by clonal hematopoiesis, one or more cytopenias and abnormal cellular maturation shares clinical-pathologic features with acute myeloid leukemia (AML), but MDS has <20% blast cells.

- MDS causes risk of symptomatic anemia, infection, and bleeding; risk of transformation to AML varies by syndrome. May be responsible for a proportion of unexplained anemias (ie, UAE) and ICUS in older patients (p 33). Caused by somatic mutations in older patients.
- Suspect MDS in patients with symptoms of anemia, infections, or bleeding or bruising.

Diagnosis

The diagnosis of MDS should be considered for any older patient with unexplained cytopenia(s) or monocytosis and for those who have had UAE when Hb falls below 10 g/dL. Inspection of the peripheral blood smear and bone-marrow aspirate is a next step in evaluation. Because these alone are not diagnostic of MDS, in vitro bone-marrow progenitor cultures, trephine biopsies, flow cytometry, immunohistochemical studies, and chromosome analysis are routinely needed for diagnosis. A variety of chromosomal deletions and substitutions are diagnostic of MDS disorders.

Staging and Prognosis

- Four different classification systems are available to help estimate prognosis, but none explain most of the variability in survival.
- Classification systems stratify patients from low- to high-risk groups based on various characteristics that differ by classification system.
- In general, poorer survival occurs with a higher proportion of blast cells, complex (>3 different) karyotypes or abnormal chromosome 7, and a greater number of cell lines with cytopenias (Hb <10 g/dL, absolute neutrophils <1800/μL, platelet count <100,000/μL).
- Median survival of high-risk patients is independent of age and is under 6 mo. However, among low-risk patients, survival is substantially affected by age with mean survival for those aged <60 is about 9.4 y, >60 about 4.8 y, and >70 about 3.9 y.
- The higher the blast count, the more likely the conversion to AML; but the most common causes of death are complications of the cytopenias, not AML.

Monitoring

- Should be under the direction of a hematologist and will vary by patient age, disease stage, prognosis, and tx status.
- Monitor all patients for the development of symptomatic cytopenias (anemia, infection, bleeding) and progression to AML.

Therapy (as directed by hematology; see subspecialty sources)

Supportive Care

- **Anemia** (usually present at diagnosis) is treated with ESAs if serum erythropoietin <500 mU/mL; if no response G-CSF may be added; RBC transfusion is an alternative; transfusion threshold generally Hb <8 g/dL.
- **Iron Overload**: risk increases with 20–30 U transfused; diagnosed when serum ferritin >2500 ng/mL; the use of chelating agents improves survival for persons with low-risk MDS.
- **Infections**: are common and may be occult, respond poorly to antibiotics, and resolve slowly; bacterial skin infections are the most common; fungal disease is not uncommon. Prophylactic antibiotics are not recommended.
- In addition to influenza and pneumococcal, consider pertussis, *Shingrix,* and haemophilus influenzae B vaccines.
- Live vaccines (eg, live-attenuated flu) should **not** be given.
- Prophylactic platelet transfusions for counts <10,0000

PRIMARY MYELOPROLIFERATIVE DISORDERS

Polycythemia Vera

- A chronic myeloproliferative neoplasm characterized by clonal proliferation of myeloid cells and an elevated red blood cell mass
- Diagnosis: Hb >18.5 g/dL in men or 16.5 g/dL in women with arterial oxygen saturation >93%
- Other findings supporting diagnosis: splenomegaly, thrombocytosis and/or leukocytosis, thrombotic complications, erythromelalgia, or aquagenic pruritis
- Next step in evaluation: serum erythropoietin level (low or normal) and peripheral blood mutation screening for *JAK2* chromosome mutation in 98%; most also need bone marrow exam
- Management: phlebotomy to achieve iron deficiency and hematocrit ≤45%, and cytoreductive tx if needed.
- All patients also need ASA 40–100 mg po q12–24h; if hx of venous thrombosis, full oral anticoagulation.

Essential Thrombocytosis

- A chronic myeloproliferative neoplasm characterized by clonal proliferation of megakaryocytes
- Platelet count >450,000/μL on 2 occasions ≥1 mo apart; normal Hb, no leukocytosis or left shift
- Bone marrow showing increase in megakaryocyte lineage, enlarged mature megakaryocytes
- Presence of *JAK2, CALR,* or *MPL* mutation

- Management:
  - Is directed at preventing complications and symptoms; tx does not prolong survival or prevent progression to AML or myelofibrosis
  - Patients at intermediate risk (aged >60, no prior thrombosis, no *JAK2/MPL* mutation), use ASA 40–100 mg po q12–24h mg daily.
  - Patients at high risk (age >60 and hx of thrombosis), treat all with hydroxyurea.
    - If thrombosis was arterial, add ASA 40–100 mg po q12–24h.
    - If thrombosis was venous, give oral anticoagulant; if *JAK2/MPL*-mutated or cardiovascular risk factors, consider adding ASA 81 mg po 1×/d.
- Target platelet count on tx: 100,000–400,000/μL

Chronic Lymphocytic Leukemia (CLL)

- One of the lymphoproliferative disorders due to accumulation of functionally incompetent monoclonal B lymphocytes
- Only 30% of patients have an indolent 10- to 20-y course with the disease. Most progress more rapidly.
- Diagnosis: CBC with differential; flow cytometry of the peripheral blood for immunophenotype of circulating lymphocytes; and examination of the peripheral smear
- Don't perform baseline or surveillance CT scans in patients with asymptomatic, early stage CLL.[CW]
- Staging is based on CBC (anemia, thrombocytopenia) and physical exam (enlarged nodes, liver, or spleen); cytogenetic studies assist in prognosis and tx decisions.
- Monitoring q6- to 12-mo follow-up by hematology; treat only when CLL causes problems.
- Management/Prevention of complications:
  - Time to tx for CLL is extended in those with vitamin D sufficiency.
  - Infection: pneumococcal, influenza, *Shingrix* and other inactivated adult vaccines; **not** live vaccines; neutrophil counts 500–1000 cells/μL with signs or symptoms of infection, treat with broad-spectrum antibiotics; neutrophil count >1000 cells/μL, treat as usual adult infection as indicated.
  - Anemia in CLL is a result of hypersplenism, marrow infiltration, GI blood loss, chemotherapy, hemolytic anemia, or RBC aplasia. Tx should be directed at the underlying cause.
  - Thrombocytopenia causes include extensive tumor burden, autoimmune destruction, and hypersplenism. Tx should be directed at the underlying cause.
  - Malignancy: higher risk of nonmelanoma skin cancers; annual skin exam. Patients should undergo age- and sex-appropriate screening.

MONOCLONAL GAMMOPATHY OF UNDETERMINED SIGNIFICANCE (MGUS)

- **Definition:** Premalignant clonal plasma cell disorder with the presence of monoclonal protein <3 g/dL, <10% clonal plasma cells in bone marrow; urinary monoclonal protein <500 mg/24 h and the absence of multiple myeloma–defining events or amyloidosis (or Waldenstrom macroglobulinemia, in the case of IgM MGUS)
- **Prevalence** increases with age: 3.2% at age ≥50; 6.6% at age ≥80.

- **Evaluation:** CBC, calcium, comprehensive metabolic panel, LDH, spot urine protein, SPEP, serum immunofixation, and serum κ:λ light-chain ratio (if abnormal obtain urine electrophoresis and immunofixation).
  - If initial IgG, IgA, or IgD MGUS is <1.5 g/dL or light-chain MGUS with κ:λ normal light chains ratio, bone marrow may be deferred. Repeat lab testing at 3–6 mo and if stable; follow-up only with hx and physical exam (risk of progression 0.3–0.5%/y).
  - If IgG, IgA, or IgD MGUS ≥1.5 g/dL or any other of the risk factor (see below), obtain bone-marrow biopsy and skeletal survey, and repeat lab testing at 6 mo and annually.
  - IgM MGUS progress 1%/y to Waldenstrom macroglobulinemia, amyloidosis, or rarely myeloma. Higher risk for peripheral neuropathy (bilateral sensory and demyelinating on nerve conduction study). Even if IgM MGUS <1.5 g/dL, if there are unexplained constitutional symptoms or signs (hepatosplenomegaly, lymphadenopathy), proceed to bone-marrow biopsy, skeletal survey; echocardiography if unexplained heart disease (amyloidosis).
  - Light-chain MGUS (LC-MGUS) have increased level of the involved light chain and no monoclonal immunoglobulin heavy chain (IgG, IgA, IgD, or IgM).
    - Criteria for diagnosis of light-chain MGUS: abnormal κ:λ light chains ratio <0.26 or >1.65; increased κ if ratio >1.65 or λ if ratio <0.26; no heavy chains on immunofixation; no end-organ damage, clonal bone-marrow plasma cells <10%, urinary monoclonal protein <500 mg/24 h
- **Risk factors** for progression to myeloma: MGUS ≥1.5 g/dL, IgM MGUS, abnormal serum-free light-chain ratio (κ:λ light chains) of <0.26 or >1.65. The greater the number of factors present, the greater the risk of progression.
- Increased risk of vertebral fracture; bone turnover markers are normalized with the use of bisphosphonates and are recommended for those with osteopenia or osteoporosis.

NON-VTE INDICATIONS FOR ANTITHROMBOTIC MEDICATIONS

Table 11. Antithrombotic Medications for Selected Conditions

		Anticoagulant (Table 17)					
Indication	**Antiplatelet (Table 16)**	**VK Antagonist**	**Heparin**	**LMWH**	**Factor Xa Inhibitor**	**Direct Thrombin Inhibitor**	**Glycoprotein IIb/IIIa Inhibitor**
Atrial fibrillation without moderate to severe mitral stenosis or mechanical mitral valve	ASA	Warfarin	—	—	**Apixaban**[1] Rivaroxaban[2,4] **Edoxaban**[3,4]	Dabigatran[2]	—
Valvular disease, mechanical heart valve, TAVR[5]	ASA	**Warfarin**	—	—	—	—	—
Acute coronary syndrome	**ASA** **Clopidogrel** Prasugrel[BC] **Ticagrelor**	—	**UFH**	**Enoxaparin**[2] Dalteparin	**Fondaparinux**[2]	**Bivalirudin**	**Abciximab** **Eptifibatide** **Tirofiban**

First choice in bold text; Secondary or alternate choice in regular text; LMWH, low-molecular-weight heparin; UFH, unfractionated heparin; VK, vitamin K.

[1] Avoid in patients with CrCl <25 mL/min.[BC]

[2] Avoid in patients with CrCl <30 mL/min.[BC]

[3] Avoid in patients with CrCl <30 or >95 mL/min.[BC]

[4] Reduce dose if CrCl = 30–50 mL/min.[BC]

[5] For TAVR, if no concurrent indication for anticoagulation, low-dose ASA.

- ASA is first choice for secondary prevention of CVD and in patients with prior TIA or stroke.
- ASA or clopidogrel are first choice for patients with PAD.
- Argatroban is indicated in patients with HIT.

VTE PROPHYLAXIS, DIAGNOSIS, AND MANAGEMENT

Prophylaxis

- Prophylaxis of medical and surgical inpatients is based on patient risk factors and type of surgery.
- See **Tables 11–13** for choice of antithrombotic strategy.
- See **Tables 15** and **17** for dosages of antithrombotic medications.

DVT Diagnosis

DVT diagnosis is directed by risk score, D-dimer testing, and duplex ultrasound imaging.

- Determine risk score
  - 1 point for each of the following:
    - active cancer
    - paralysis, paresis, or plaster immobilization of lower limb

    - bedridden for 3 d or major surgery in past 12 wk
    - localized tenderness along distribution of deep venous system
    - entire leg swelling
    - calf swelling ≥3 cm over diameter of contralateral calf
    - pitting edema confined to symptomatic leg
    - collateral superficial veins
    - prior DVT
  - –2 points for alternative diagnosis as likely as DVT
- Interpret risk score and further testing
  - ≤0 points = low risk: Obtain moderately or highly sensitive D-dimer test. If negative (D-dimer in ng/mL ≤ patient age × 10), DVT is excluded. If positive, obtain ultrasound of proximal veins for diagnosis. Don't obtain imaging studies as the initial diagnostic test in patients with low pretest probability (low risk) of VTE.[CW]
  - 1–2 points = moderate risk: Obtain highly sensitive D-dimer. If negative, (D-dimer in ng/mL ≤ patient age × 10), DVT is excluded. If positive, obtain ultrasound of either proximal veins or whole leg for diagnosis.
  - ≥3 points = high risk: Obtain ultrasound of either proximal veins or whole leg. If proximal leg ultrasound is negative, repeat proximal ultrasound in 1 wk, obtain immediate highly sensitive D-dimer test, or obtain whole leg ultrasound; negative results of any of these rules out DVT.

PE Diagnosis

- Consider PE with any of the following (classic triad of dyspnea, chest pain, and hemoptysis seen in only ≤20% of cases):
  - Chest pain
  - Hemoptysis
  - Hypotension
  - Hypoxia
  - Shortness of breath
  - Syncope
  - Tachycardia
- If patient presents with shock or hypotension, obtain CT pulmonary angiography, and if positive, anticoagulate immediately with UFH and prepare for thrombolytic tx.
- If shock and hypotension are absent, calculate clinical probability of PE using clinical decision rule (**Table 14**), then follow evaluation of PE algorithm (**Figure 5**).

Table 12. DVT/PE Prophylaxis Strategies for Older Medical and Surgical Inpatients

DVT/PE Risk	Surgery Type or Medical Condition	Thromboprophylactic Options
Low	Healthy and mobile patients undergoing minor surgery Brief (<45 min) laparoscopic procedures Transurethral or other low-risk urologic procedures Joint arthroscopy Spine surgery	Aggressive early ambulation after procedure +/– intermittent pneumatic compression
Medium	Immobile (>72 h) patients Inpatients at bed rest with active malignancy, prior VTE, or sepsis Most general surgeries Open abdominopelvic surgeries Thoracic surgery Vascular surgery	Antithrombotic (**Table 13** and **Table 17**) +/– intermittent pneumatic compression
High	Acute stroke Hip or knee arthroplasty Hip, pelvic, or leg fracture Acute spinal cord injury	**Table 13**

Table 13. Antithrombotic Medications for VTE Prophylaxis

Indication	Antiplatelet (Table 16)	Anticoagulant (Table 17): VK Antagonist	Heparin	LMWH	Factor Xa Inhibitor	Direct Thrombin Inhibitor
Medical inpatients at moderate/high risk for VTE; patients with acute stroke or spinal cord injury	—	—	UFH	**Enoxaparin**[1] **Dalteparin**	**Fondaparinux**[1] Betrixaban	—
Cancer patients at moderate/high risk for VTE	—	—	—	**Enoxaparin**[1] **Dalteparin**	**Apixaban**[1] **Edoxaban**[1] Rivaroxaban[1]	
Knee or hip replacement	**ASA**	Warfarin	UFH	Enoxaparin[1] Dalteparin	**Apixaban**[1] **Fondaparinux**[1] Rivaroxaban[1]	**Dabigatran**[1] Desirudin
Hip fracture surgery	ASA	Warfarin	**UFH**	**Enoxaparin**[1] **Dalteparin**	Fondaparinux[1]	—
Non–orthopedic surgery patients at moderate/high risk of VTE	ASA	**Warfarin**	**UFH**	**Enoxaparin**[1] **Dalteparin**	Fondaparinux[1] Rivaroxaban[1]	—

First choice(s) in bold text; Secondary or alternate choice(s) in regular text; LMWH, low-molecular-weight heparin, UFH, unfractionated heparin, VK, vitamin K; VTE, venous thromboembolism (DVT/PE).

[1]Avoid or adjust dosage in patients with renal impairment; see **Table 17** for specific indications.[BC]

Figure 5. Evaluation of Suspected Pulmonary Embolism

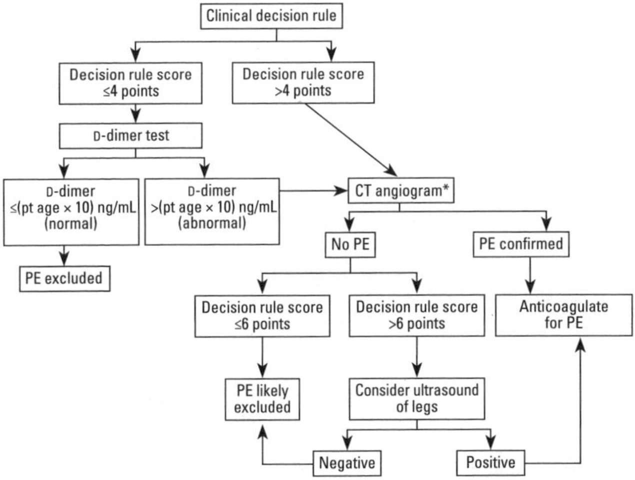

*Multidetector-row CT more sensitive than single-detector CT. Patient must be able to hold breath for 10 sec. Use ventilation perfusion scan when unable to use contrast (eg, renal dysfunction), or need to avoid ionizing radiation.

Table 14. Clinical Decision Rule for PE Probability	
Variable	**Points**
Clinical signs and symptoms of DVT (minimal leg swelling and pain with palpation of the 3 deep veins)	3
Alternative diagnosis less likely than PE	3
Heart rate >100/min	1.5
Immobilization (>3 d) or surgery in the previous 4 wk	1.5
Previous PE or DVT	1.5
Hemoptysis	1
Malignancy (receiving tx, treated in last 6 mo, or palliative)	1
	Total

Source: Wells PS et al. *Thromb Haemost* 2000;83(3):416–420. Reprinted with permission.

Management

Table 15. Antithrombotic Medications for VTE Management

		Anticoagulant (Table 17)				
Indication	**Antiplatelet (Table 16)**	**VK Antagonist**	**Heparin**	**LMWH**	**Factor Xa Inhibitor**	**Direct Thrombin Inhibitor**
Acute VTE tx	—	—	UFH	Enoxaparin[1] Dalteparin Tinzaparin	**Apixaban**[1] **Fondaparinux**[1] Rivaroxaban[1]	—
Long-term VTE tx[2]	—	Warfarin	—	Enoxaparin[1] Dalteparin Tinzaparin	**Apixaban**[1] Rivaroxaban[1] **Edoxaban**[1]	Dabigatran[1]

First choice(s) in bold text; Secondary or alternate choice(s) in regular text; LMWH, low-molecular-weight heparin; UFH, unfractionated heparin; VK, vitamin K; VTE, venous thromboembolism (DVT/PE).

[1] Avoid or adjust dosage in patients with renal impairment; see **Table 17** for specific indications.[BC]

[2] Coverage for different direct oral anticoagulants (DOACs) can vary by Medicare Part D plan.

- For acute VTE, LMWH or fondaparinux is preferred to UFH in most patients because of lower risk of hemorrhage and mortality. Reduce dosage when CrCl <30 mL/min.
- Length of long-term tx is based on cause:
  - Provoked VTE from transient cause (eg, surgery, trauma, prolonged immobility that has resolved): anticoagulate for 3 mo.
  - Unprovoked VTE: anticoagulate for at least 3 mo. Consider treating longer for patients at low bleeding risk.
  - Second unprovoked VTE: anticoagulate indefinitely.
  - The American Society of Hematology 2020 guidelines for managing VTE recommend against measuring D-dimer or using ultrasound to detect residual vein thrombosis to determine tx duration.
- If warfarin is part of a long-term anticoagulation plan, it may be started the same day as acute anticoagulant. Specific conditions may require a period of overlap when both agents should be used (eg, for DVT or PE, heparin or similar products should be used a minimum of 5 d, including 1–3 d of overlap with therapeutic INR).

- Consider low-dose ASA (100 mg/d po) after completion of long-term VTE tx (at least 3 mo of warfarin or other anticoagulant).
- Consider placement of inferior vena cava (IVC) filter in patients with PE who have an absolute contraindication to anticoagulation; filter should be removed when patient can receive anticoagulants or DVT/PE risk falls to acceptable level. IVC filters are not indicated for patients receiving anticoagulant VTE tx, VTE prophylaxis, tx of a free-floating thrombus, or preparation of the patient for thrombolysis or surgical embolectomy.
- Don't reimage DVT in the absence of a clinical change during DVT tx.[CW]
- Acute massive PE (filling defects in ≥2 lobar arteries or the equivalent by angiogram; about 5% of PE cases) associated with hypotension, severe hypoxia, or high pulmonary pressures on echocardiogram should usually be treated with thrombolytic tx within 48 h of onset.
- Submassive PE (about 20–25% of PE cases) is defined as PE with normotension and right ventricular failure; if present, thrombolytic tx should be considered. Submassive PE can be diagnosed by detection of right ventricular failure through:
  - Physical exam (eg, increased jugular venous pressure)
  - ECG (eg, right bundle branch block [RBBB] or t-wave inversions in leads V_1–V_4)
  - Elevated cardiac troponins
  - Echocardiography (eg, right ventricular hypokinesis and dilatation)
  - Chest CT showing right ventricular enlargement
- Don't perform workup for clotting disorder (order hypercoagulable testing) for patients who develop a first episode of DVT in the setting of a known cause.[CW]

ANTITHROMBOTIC MEDICATIONS

Antiplatelet Agents

Table 16. Antiplatelet Agents

Agent	Dosage	Comments (Metabolism)
Aspirin (ASA)	AF, KR, HR, HFS, SP: 75–325 mg/d po Valvular disease: 50–100 mg/d po ACS: 162–325 mg po initially, followed by 75–160 mg/d po PAD: 75–100 mg/d po	Risk of GI bleeding is dose-dependent. (L, K)
Dipyridamole/ASA	SP: 1 tab po q12h	Headache a common side effect. May decrease effectiveness of cholinesterase inhibitors. (L)
Thienopyridines	*Class effect:* increased bleeding risk when given with ASA	
Clopidogrel	ACS: 300–600 mg po initially, followed by 75 mg/d po SP, PAD: 75 mg/d po	Some patients may be poor metabolizers due to low activity of the CYP2C19 liver enzyme; unclear if testing for this enzyme activity is effective for guiding dosage; unclear if PPIs inhibit activity (L, K)
Prasugrel *(Effient)*	ACS: 60 mg po initially, followed by 10 mg/d po	Use with caution in adults aged ≥75.[BC] Consider maintenance dose of 5 mg/d in patients <60 kg (L, K)
Ticagrelor *(Brilinta)*	ACS: 180 mg po initially, followed by 90 mg po 2×/d	Should be used with ASA dosage of 75–100 mg/d po (K)

ACS, acute coronary syndrome; HFS, hip fracture surgery; HR, hip replacement; KR, knee replacement; SP, secondary stroke prevention after TIA/stroke.

Table 17. Anticoagulant Agents

Class, Agent	Dose	Comments (Metabolism)
Heparin		
Unfractionated heparin	VTE prophylaxis: 5000 U SC 2h preop and q12h postop Acute VTE tx: 5000 U/kg IV bolus followed by 15 mg/kg/h IV ACS: 60–70 U/kg (max 5000 U) IV bolus, followed by 12–15 U/kg/h IV	Bleeding, anemia, thrombocytopenia, hypertransaminasemia, urticaria (L, K)
LMWH		
Enoxaparin	KR, NOS: 30 mg SC q12h HR, HFS: 30 mg SC q12h or 40 mg SC 1×/d AS, MP: 40 mg SC 1×/d Inpatient VTE tx: 1 mg/kg SC q12h or 1.5 mg/kg SC 1×/d Outpatient DVT tx: 1 mg/kg SC q12h Unstable angina, NSTEMI: 1 mg/kg SC q12h STEMI: 30 mg IV bolus, followed by 1 mg/kg SC q12h STEMI in patients aged ≥75: 0.75 mg/kg SC q12h (no bolus)	Bleeding, anemia, hyperkalemia, hypertransaminasemia, thrombocytopenia, thrombocytosis, urticaria, angioedema[BC]; lower dose if CrCl <30 (K)
Dalteparin *(Fragmin)*	HR: 2500–5000 U SC preop, 5000 U SC 1×/d postop MP, NOS: 2500–5000 U SC preop and postop long-term VTE tx in cancer patients: 200 U/kg SC q24h × 30 d, followed by 150 U/kg SC q24g for the next 5 mo ACS: 120 IU/kg SC q12h	Same as above (K)
Tinzaparin *(Innohep)*	Acute VTE tx: 175 anti-Xa IU/kg SC 1×/d	Same as above; contraindicated in older patients with CrCl <30 (K)
Direct Factor Xa Inhibitors		*Class effect:* monitor patient at least q3mo for bleeding and side effects; follow renal function q6mo in patients aged ≥75; not recommended in patients with mechanical heart valves.[BC]
Apixaban *(Eliquis)*	AF: 5 mg po q12h HR, KR: 2.5 mg po q12h Acute VTE tx: 10 mg po q12h for 7 d, followed by 5 mg po q12h Secondary prevention of VTE recurrence: 2.5 mg po q12h	Lower dose to 2.5 mg po q12h if patient has 2 of the following: age ≥80, weight ≤60 kg, Cr ≥1.5 mg/dL (L, K)
Betrixaban *(Bevyxxa)*	MP: Initial single dose of 160 mg po, followed by 80 mg po daily for 35–42 d	Reduce dose by half if CrCl 15–29 (K)
Edoxaban *(Savaysa)*	AF: 60 mg po 1×/d VTE after patient has been treated for 5–10 d with a parenteral anticoagulant: weight ≤60 kg: 30 mg po 1×/d weight >60 kg: 60 mg po 1×/d	Reduce dose to 30 mg/d if CrCl 15–50; do not use if CrCl >95[BC] (K)

(cont.)

Table 17. Anticoagulant Agents (cont.)

Class, Agent	Dose	Comments (Metabolism)
Indirect Factor Xa Inhibitors		*Class effect:* monitor patient at least q3mo for bleeding and side effects; follow renal function q6mo in patients aged ≥75; not recommended in patients with mechanical heart valves.[BC]
Fondaparinux *(Arixtra)*	ACS: 2.5 mg SC 1×/d MP, KR, HR, NOS: 2.5 mg SC 1×/d beginning 6–8 h postop Acute VTE tx: weight <50 kg: 5 mg SC 1×/d weight 50–100 kg: 7.5 mg SC 1×/d weight >100 kg: 10 mg SC 1×/d	Lower dosage in renal impairment; contraindicated if CrCl <30[BC] (K)
Rivaroxaban *(Xarelto)*	KR, HR, NOS: 10 mg/d po, begin 6–10 h after surgery AF: 20 mg/d po with evening meal VTE: 15 mg po q12h for first 21 d, followed by 20 mg/d po	Lower dosage to 15 mg/d in AF patients with CrCl 15–50; contraindicated if CrCl <15 (L, K)
Direct Thrombin Inhibitors		
Argatroban	HIT + VTE prophylaxis or tx: 2 mcg/kg/min IV infusion	Lower dosage if hepatic impairment (L)
Bivalirudin *(Angiomax)*	ACS: 0.75 mg/kg bolus, followed by 1.75 mg/kg/h IV	(L, K)
Dabigatran *(Pradaxa)*	AF, HR[OL], KR[OL], VTE after patient has been treated for 5–10 d with a parenteral anticoagulant, secondary prevention of VTE recurrence: 150 mg po q12h	Monitor patient at least q3mo for bleeding and side effects; follow renal function q6mo in patients aged ≥75. Reduce dosage to 75 mg po q12h if CrCl = 15–30; contraindicated in patients with mechanical heart valves; use with caution in adults aged >75 or if CrCl <30[BC] (K)
Desirudin *(Iprivask)*	HR: 15 mg SC q12h starting 5–15 min before surgery	If CrCl = 31–60, starting dose is 5 mg; if CrCl <31, starting dose is 1.7 mg (K)
Glycoprotein IIb/IIIa Inhibitors		
Abciximab *(ReoPro)*	ACS: 0.25 mg/kg IV bolus, followed by 0.125 mcg/kg/min IV (max 10 mcg/min)	
Eptifibatide *(Integrilin)*	ACS: 180 mcg/kg IV bolus, followed by 2 mcg/kg/min IV	
Tirofiban *(Aggrastat)*	ACS: 0.4 mcg/kg/min IV over 30 min, followed by 0.1 mcg/kg/min	

ACS, acute coronary syndrome; AS, abdominal surgery; HFS, hip fracture surgery; HIT, heparin-induced thrombocytopenia; HR, hip replacement; KR, knee replacement; MP, medical inpatients at moderate/high risk for VTE; NA, not available; NOS, nonorthopedic surgery at moderate/high risk of VTE; [OL], off-label use; VTE, venous thromboembolism (DVT/PE). CrCl unit = mL/min.

MANAGEMENT OF BLEEDING WHILE TAKING ANTICOAGULANTS

- Major bleeding defined as bleeding at a critical site (intracranial or other CNS hemorrhage, pericardial tamponade, airway bleeding, hemothorax, abdominal bleeding, intramuscular or intra-articular bleeding), hemodynamic instability, or Hgb decrease of at least 2 g/dL.
- D/C anticoagulant, employ local bleeding control measures (pressure, packing), give volume resuscitation with IV 0.9% NaCl or Ringer's lactate.
- Use reversal agents in life-threatening bleeding due to direct oral anticoagulants:
  - Apixaban and rivaroxaban: andexanet alfa *(Andexxa)*
  - Betrixaban and edoxaban: 4-factor prothrombin complex concentrate (4F-PCC)
  - Dabigatran: idarucizumab *(Praxbind)*
- For bleeding due to warfarin, treat according to INR:
  - INR 3.6–10 without bleeding: omit next 1–2 doses and recheck INR
  - INR >10 without bleeding: omit next 1–2 doses and give Vitamin K 2.5 mg po, recheck INR
  - Any INR with major bleeding: Vitamin K 5–10 mg IV + 4F-PCC

WARFARIN THERAPY

- For anticoagulation in nonacute conditions, initiate tx by giving warfarin 2–10 mg/d po as fixed dose. The usual starting dose for patients aged >70 is 5 mg/d po, adjusted up or down depending on body size, comorbidities, and age.
- INR should be checked every 2–3 d until INR is stable. Reduce dose if INR >2.5 on day 3.
- Half-life is 31–51 h; steady state is achieved on day 5–7 of fixed dose. Genetic tests for VKORC1 (modulates sensitivity to warfarin) and CYP2C9 (modulates metabolism of warfarin) are available to help guide dosing for initiation of warfarin tx; it is unknown if their routine use significantly improves outcomes. Medicare does not cover genetic testing.
- Some drugs that **increase** INR in conjunction with warfarin (*italicized type indicates* major interaction):
  - Many antibiotics, especially fluconazole, itraconazole, ketoconazole, miconazole, ciprofloxacin, erythromycin, *moxifloxacin*, metronidazole, *sulfamethoxazole*, *trimethoprim*
  - APAP, celecoxib, *cilostazol*, *clofibrate*, *duloxetine*, *ketoprofen*, *naproxen*
- Some drugs that **decrease** INR in conjunction with warfarin: carbamazepine, dicloxacillin, nafcillin, rifampin, vitamin K
- Target INR is 2–3 for all indications except the following for which the target INR is 2.5–3.5:
  - Mechanical mitral valve (ASA 75–100 mg po 1×/d should be used in addition to warfarin)
  - Mechanical aortic valve with AF, anterior-apical STEMI, left atrial enlargement, hypercoagulable state, or low EF

SWITCHING ANTICOAGULANTS

- ***Warfarin to Direct Oral Anticoagulants*** *(DOACs):* stop warfarin and check INR daily; when INR is ≤2.5 and trending downward, start DOAC.
- ***LMWH to DOAC:*** D/C LMWH and start DOAC at time of next scheduled LMWH dose.
- ***DOAC to Warfarin*:** D/C DOAC and begin warfarin in place of the next scheduled DOAC dose. Continue warfarin and bridge with parenteral anticoagulant as indicated (**Table 106**) until INR ≥2.

ANXIETY

DIAGNOSIS

Anxiety disorders as a whole are the most common mental disorders in older adults. Panic disorder appears to be less prevalent in older adults, compared to younger adults, but phobias may be more prevalent in elders. Generalized anxiety disorder (GAD) and new-onset anxiety in older adults are often secondary to physical illness, poorer health-related quality of life, depression, or AEs of or withdrawal from medications.

DSM-5 Criteria for GAD

- Excessive anxiety and worry on more days than not for ≥6 mo, about a number of events or activities
- Difficulty controlling the worry
- The anxiety and worry are associated with 3 or more of the following symptoms:
  - restlessness or feeling keyed up or on the edge
  - muscle tension
  - being easily fatigued
  - difficulty concentrating
  - irritability
  - sleep disturbance
- Focus of anxiety and worry not confined to features of another primary psychiatric disorder; often, about routine life circumstances; may shift from one concern to another
- Anxiety, worry, or physical symptoms cause clinically significant distress or impairment in social, occupational, or other important areas of functioning
- Disturbance not due to the direct physiologic effects of a drug of abuse or a medication or to a medical condition; does not occur exclusively during a mood disorder, psychotic disorder, or a pervasive development disorder
- Generalized Anxiety Disorder 7-item scale (GAD-7) is a self-reported questionnaire for screening and measuring the severity of GAD. Research on the GAD-7 suggests that a cutoff score of 5 indicates GAD in older adults.

GAD-7 Scale

Over the last 2 weeks, how often have you been bothered by the following problems?	Not at all	Several days	Over half the days	Nearly every day
1. Feeling nervous, anxious, or on edge	0	1	2	3
2. Not being able to stop or control worrying	0	1	2	3
3. Worrying too much about different things	0	1	2	3
4. Trouble relaxing	0	1	2	3
5. Being so restless that it's hard to sit still	0	1	2	3
6. Becoming easily annoyed or irritable	0	1	2	3
7. Feeling afraid as if something awful might happen	0	1	2	3
Add the score for each column		+	+	+
Total Score *(add your column scores)* =				

If you checked off any problems, how difficult have these made it for you to do your work, take care of things at home, or get along with other people?

☐ Not difficult at all ☐ Somewhat difficult ☐ Very difficult ☐ Extremely difficult

Scoring: 0–4: minimal anxiety; 5–9: mild anxiety; 10–14: moderate anxiety; 15–21: severe anxiety

Source: Spitzer RL et al. *Arch Intern Med* 2006;116:1092–1097.

DSM-5 recognizes several other anxiety disorders or trauma- and stressor-related disorders:

- Anxiety disorder due to a general medical condition—one of the most common anxiety disorders in older adults
- Social anxiety disorder (social phobia)—another of the most common anxiety disorders in older adults
- Agoraphobia
- Obsessive-compulsive disorder (OCD)
- Panic attack
- Panic disorder
- Substance-induced anxiety disorder
- Acute stress disorder
- PTSD

DSM-5 Criteria for Panic Attack

An abrupt surge of intense fear or discomfort with ≥4 of the following (also, must peak within minutes):

- Palpitations, pounding heart, or accelerated HR
- Sweating
- Trembling or shaking
- Sensations of shortness of breath or smothering
- Feelings of choking
- Chest pain or discomfort
- Nausea or abdominal distress
- Feeling dizzy, unsteady, lightheaded, or faint
- Chills or heat sensations
- Paresthesias (numbness or tingling sensations)
- Derealization (feelings of unreality) or depersonalization (being detached from oneself)
- Fear of losing your mind or going crazy
- Fear of dying

DSM-5 Criteria for Illness Anxiety Disorder (IAD)

- The patient is preoccupied with having or acquiring a serious illness.
- The patient has no or minimal somatic symptoms.
- The patient is highly anxious about health and easily alarmed about personal health issues.
- The patient repeatedly checks health status or maladaptively avoids doctor appointments and hospitals.
- The patient has been preoccupied with illness for ≥6 mo, although the specific illness feared may change during that period.
- Symptoms are not better, accounted for by depression or another mental disorder.
- Patients who have significant somatic symptoms and are primarily concerned about the symptoms themselves are diagnosed with somatic symptom disorder.

DSM-5 Criteria for PTSD

- Exposure to actual or threatened death, serious injury, or sexual violence
- Presence of intrusion symptoms, ie, distressing memories of the event, recurrent distressing dreams related to the event, dissociative reactions (flashbacks), psychological distress or marked physiological reactions to internal or external cues that resemble an aspect of the traumatic event(s)
- Persistent avoidance of stimuli associated with the traumatic event(s)
- Negative altercations in cognitions and mood associated with the traumatic event(s) (eg, dissociative amnesia)
- Marked alterations in arousal and reactivity, ie, irritable behavior and angry outbursts, reckless or self-destructive behavior, hypervigilance, exaggerated startle response, problems with concentration, sleep disturbance
- Duration of disturbance >1 mo (if duration is 3 d to 1 mo after traumatic event, then acute stress disorder)
- Clinically significant impairment in functioning
- Not attributable to the physiological effects of substance abuse or medical condition

Differential Diagnosis

- Physical conditions producing anxiety
  - Cardiovascular: arrhythmias, angina, MI, HF
  - Endocrine: hyperthyroidism, hypoglycemia, pheochromocytoma
  - Neurologic: movement disorders, temporal lobe epilepsy, mild cognitive impairment (MCI), AD, stroke
  - Respiratory: COPD, asthma, PE
- Medications producing anxiety
  - Caffeine
  - Corticosteroids
  - Nicotine
  - Thyroid hormones: overreplacement
  - Psychotropics: antidepressants, antipsychotics, stimulants
  - Sympathomimetics: pseudoephedrine, β-agonists
- Withdrawal states: alcohol, sedatives, hypnotics, benzodiazepines, SSRIs, SNRIs
- Depression

EVALUATION

- Psychiatric hx
- Drug review: prescribed, OTC, alcohol, caffeine
- Mental status exam
- Physical exam: Focus on signs and symptoms of anxiety (eg, tachycardia, tachypnea, sweating, tremor).
- Lab tests: Consider CBC, blood glucose, TSH, B_{12}, ECG, oxygen saturation, drug and alcohol screening.

MANAGEMENT

Nonpharmacologic Interventions

- CBT may be useful for GAD, panic disorder, and PTSD; efficacy in both individual and group formats.
- In view of potential limitations (eg, availability, cost), free online CBT may be considered. See https://ecouch.com.au/.
- Graded desensitization used in panic and phobia relies on gradual exposure with learning to manage resultant anxiety.
- May be effective alone but mostly used in conjunction with pharmacotherapy.
- Requires a cognitively intact, motivated patient.
- For IAD, it is important to have a clear line of communication with other clinicians to help minimize inconsistent or conflicting messages.

Pharmacotherapy (Table 42 for dosing of antidepressants and indication of generic status)

- GAD
  - Suggested order: duloxetine, pregabalin, venlafaxine XR, escitalopram
- Panic: sertraline, escitalopram, venlafaxine XR, secondary choices include β blockers and second-generation antipsychotics
- Social phobia: sertraline, venlafaxine XR
- PTSD: sertraline
  - Avoid benzodiazepines.[CW]
  - For nightmares, prazosin may be helpful (initiate at 1 mg qhs and titrate slowly to avoid orthostatic syncope).

Alternative Agents

Buspirone

- Serotonin 1A partial agonist effective in GAD and anxiety symptoms accompanying general medical illness (although geriatric evidence is limited)
- Not effective for acute anxiety or panic disorder
- May take 2–4 wk for tx response
- Recommended starting dosage: 7.5–10 mg po q12h, up to max 60 mg/d
- No dependence, tolerance, withdrawal, or CNS depression
- Risk of serotonin syndrome with SSRIs, MAOIs, TCAs, 5-hydroxytryptamine 1 receptor agonists, ergot alkaloids, lithium, St John's wort, opioids, dextromethorphan

Pregabalin

- Although pregabalin is not FDA approved for the tx of GAD, evidence supporting its use as either single or adjunctive tx is limited, including in older adults. (Avoid concurrent use with opioids except when transitioning from opioid tx[BC]; reduce dose if CrCl <60 mL/min because of CNS AEs.[BC])
- Onset of tx response may be longer than that observed in younger adults
- Adverse effects are predominantly somnolence and dizziness
- Risk of dependence or withdrawal appears minimal but is Schedule V medication in the United States
- Current evidence does not support the use of gabapentin as an alternative to pregabalin to treat anxiety disorders

Benzodiazepines (Avoid if hx of falls or fractures, or if concurrent use with an opioid.[BC])

- Restrict use to severe GAD unresponsive to other tx[CW] (**Table 18**)
- Avoid long-acting benzodiazepines (eg, flurazepam, diazepam, chlordiazepoxide)
- Linked to cognitive impairment, falls, sedation, psychomotor impairment, delirium
- Problems: dependence, misuse (p 352), tolerance, withdrawal, more so with short-acting benzodiazepines; seizure risk with alprazolam withdrawal
- Potentially fatal if combined with alcohol or other CNS depressants
- Only short-term (60–90 d) use recommended
- Refer to deprescribing.org for suggested algorithm for mitigating benzodiazepine use
- Nonbenzodiazepine hypnotics should not be used for tx of anxiety disorders (Sleep Disorders, **Table 131**).

Table 18. Benzodiazepines for Anxiety for Older Adults

Drug	Dosage	Elimination + Half-life	Comments
Lorazepam	0.5–2 mg po in 2–3 divided doses	10–20 h	intermediate half-life drugs inactivated by direct conjugation in liver and therefore less affected by aging
Oxazepam	10–15 mg po q8–12h	3–21 h	

CARDIOVASCULAR DISEASES

PREVENTIVE CARDIOLOGY

Screening/Calculating Risk in Persons Without History of CVD (2019 ACC/AHA Guidelines)

- Assess/quantify CVD risk regularly (eg, q4–6y) in persons up to age 75 without hx of CVD by assessing traditional risk factors
  - Traditional risk factors for quantifying risk are increasing age, male sex, Black race, total cholesterol >170, HDL cholesterol <50, SBP >120, tx for high BP, DM, and current smoking
  - Additional risk factors include family hx of premature CVD, chronic inflammatory disease (RA, lupus, HIV), CKD, metabolic syndrome, elevated biomarkers (CRP, lipoprotein(a), apolipoprotein B), ABI <0.9
  - 10-y risk of CVD can be calculated using a downloadable spreadsheet available at https://tools.acc.org/ascvd-risk-estimator-plus/#!/calculate/estimate/
  - If 10-y risk of CVD is elevated (≥7.5%), patient should be considered for intensive lipid management, lifestyle alteration, and assessment and tx for obesity
  - If 10-y risk of CVD is intermediate (≥7.5% to <20%), coronary calcium scoring can help guide decisions for statin tx. In patients with coronary artery calcium scores of 0–100, statin tx is unlikely to significantly reduce CVD events.
- Don't order coronary artery calcium scoring for screening purposes on low-risk asymptomatic individuals except those with a family hx of premature CAD.[CW]
- Don't routinely order coronary CT angiography for screening asymptomatic individuals.[CW]

DYSLIPIDEMIA MANAGEMENT

Nonpharmacologic Interventions

A cholesterol-lowering diet should be considered initial tx for dyslipidemia and should be used as follows:

- The patient should be at low risk of malnutrition.
- The diet should be nutritionally adequate, with sufficient total calories, protein, calcium, iron, and vitamins, and low in saturated fats (<7% of total calories), trans-fatty acids, and cholesterol.
- The diet should be easily understood and affordable (a dietitian can be very helpful).
- Plant stanol/sterols (2 g/d), found in many fruits, vegetables, vegetable oils, nuts, seeds, cereals, and legumes, can lower LDL.
- Cholesterol-lowering margarines can lower LDL cholesterol by 10–15% (*Take Control* 1–2 tbsp/d, 45 calories/tbsp; *Benecol* 3 servings of 1.5 tsp each/d, 70 calories/tbsp).

Pharmacotherapy

- 2018 AHA/ACC/AACVPR/AAPA/ACPM/ADA/AGS/APhA/ASPC/NLA/PCNA guidelines:
  - Statins are dosed according to intensity of lipid lowering: high-intensity (usually lowers LDL ≥50%), moderate-intensity (usually lowers LDL 30–49%), and low-intensity (usually lowers LDL <30%) (**Table 20**).
  - Patients aged >75:
    - For those with CVD (prior MI, angina, ACS, coronary revascularization, stroke, TIA, or PAD), use a moderate-intensity statin; continue the same dose for patients already on a high-intensity statin.
    - The value of lowering LDL for primary prevention of CVD in patients aged >75 is uncertain.

- Patients aged 40–75:
  - For those with CVD or LDL ≥190, prescribe maximally tolerated statin tx, supplemented with ezetimibe as necessary to achieve a 50% LDL reduction.
  - For those with DM, prescribe a moderate-intensity statin unless they also have a 10-y CVD risk of ≥7.5% (risk calculator at https://static.heart.org/riskcalc/app/index.html#!/baseline-risk), in which case prescribe a high-intensity statin.
  - For those without CVD and a 10-y CVD risk of ≥7.5%, clinicians should discuss statin tx with patient to assess CVD risk factors, ADRs, and patient preferences. If statin tx is elected, prescribe a moderate- or high-intensity statin (especially if 10-y risk is >20%). The USPSTF recommends tx with a moderate-intensity statin for those without CVD and a 10-y CVD risk of ≥10% and recommends selective use of low- or moderate-intensity statins in those without CVD and a 10-y CVD risk of 7.5–10%.
  - Severe hypertriglyceridemia (fasting TG ≥500 mg/dL) and a 10-y CVD risk of ≥7.5% should be considered for statin tx as well as implementing dietary and behavioral interventions.
- Some experts are concerned that the risk calculator designates many more older adults as being eligible for primary prevention with statin tx than previous guidelines. For example, the calculator assesses a 10-y CVD risk of ≥7.5% in all men aged 63–75 and all women aged 71–75 with optimal values for other risk factors.

- Prescribing statins:
  - Statin tx is unlikely to significantly reduce CVD events in patients with coronary artery calcium scores of 0–100.
  - Check fasting lipids, measure ALT, and screen for DM before initiating tx. If ALT is normal, rechecking LFTs is unnecessary unless hyperbilirubinemia, jaundice, or clinically apparent hepatic disease occurs.
  - Statins should be taken in the evening.
  - Check fasting lipid profile 4–12 wk after statin initiation and q3–12mo thereafter to assess adherence and response (see above for expected percentage of LDL lowering by intensity).
  - About 10% of patients on statins report myalgias. Severe myopathy with creatine kinase levels >10× normal are very rare (about 1 in 10,000 cases).
  - If severe muscle pain develops after initiation, D/C statin immediately and check creatine kinase, Cr, and a UA for myoglobinuria. Most benign myalgias resolve within weeks of statin cessation.
  - Statin tx has been uncommonly associated with increases in A1c and fasting glucose.
- To further lower LDL and cardiovascular risk, add a PCSK9 inhibitor (**Table 20**) to statin tx.

Table 19. Treatment Choices for Dyslipidemia

	Type of Dyslipidemia		
Agent	**↑LDL**	**↑TG**	**↑ LDL + ↑TG + ↓HDL**
Statin	1	1	1
Fibrate		1	2
Ezetimibe	3		2, C
Niacin	2	2, C	
Bile Acid Sequestrant	2		2, C
Icosapent ethyl		2, 3, C	
Bempedioc acid	C		C
Omega-3 fatty acid		2, 3, C	
PCSK9 Inhibitor	C		C

1 = first-line tx; 2 = second-line tx; 3 = third-line tx; C = appropriate for combined tx with another agent.

Table 20. Medications for Dyslipidemia		
Class	**Medication**	**Dosage[1]**
Statin (HMG-CoA reductase inhibitor)[2]	Atorvastatin	H: 40–80 mg/d po; M: 10–20 mg/d po
	Fluvastatin	M: 40 mg po q12h or 80 mg XL/d po; L: 20–40 mg/d po
	Lovastatin[3]	M: 40 mg/d po; L: 10–20 mg/d po
	Pitavastatin *(Livalo)*	M: 2–4 mg/d po; L: 1 mg/d po
	Pravastatin	M: 40–80 mg/d po; L: 10–20 mg/d po
	ASA/pravastatin *(Pravigard PAC)*	1 tab/d po
	Rosuvastatin[4]	H: 20–40 mg/d po; M: 5–10 mg/d po
	Simvastatin	M: 20–40 mg/d po; L: 10 mg/d po
Fibrate (fibric acid derivative)	Fenofibrate[5]	48–200 mg/d po
	Fenofibrate delayed release	45–135 mg/d po
	Gemfibrozil[6]	300–600 mg po q12h
Cholesterol absorption inhibitor	Ezetimibe[7]	10 mg/d po
Nicotinic acid	Niacin[8]	100 mg po q8h to start; increase to 500–1000 mg po q8h; ER 150 mg po qhs to start, increase to 2000 mg po qhs prn
	Niacin ER[8]	500–2000 mg/d po
Bile acid sequestrant[9]	Colesevelam	Monotx: 1850 mg po q12h; combination tx: 2500–3750 mg/d po in single or divided doses
	Colestipol	5–30 g po mixed with liquid in 1 or more divided doses
Fatty acid	Icosapent ethyl	2 g po q12h with food
	Omega-3-acid ethyl esters *(Omacor, Lovaza)*	4 g/d po in single or divided doses
Adenosine triphosphate-citrate lyase (ACL) inhibitor[10]	Bempedoic acid *(Nexletol)*	180 mg/d po
Combination preparations	Ezetimibe/simvastatin combination[2] *(Vytorin)*[2,7]	10 mg/10 mg po to 10 mg/40 mg po qhs
	Lovastatin/niacin combination[2,3,8] *(Advicor)*	20 mg/500 mg po qhs to start; max dose 40 mg/2000 mg po
	Simvastatin/niacin combination[2,8] *(Simcor)*	20 mg/500 mg po qhs to start; max dose 40 mg/2000 mg po
	Bempedoic acid/ezetimibe[10] *(Nexlizet)*	180 mg/10 mg/d po

(cont.)

Table 20. Medications for Dyslipidemia (cont.)		
Class	**Medication**	**Dosage**[1]
PCSK9 inhibitor[10]	Alirocumab *(Praluent)*	75–150 mg SC q2wk
	Evolocumab *(Repatha)*	140 mg SC q2wk or 420 mg SC q1mo
ANGPTL3 inhibitor[10]	Evinacumab *(Evkeeza)*	15 mg/kg IV q1mo

H, high-intensity statin dose; M, moderate-intensity statin dose; L, low-intensity statin dose.

[1] Dosage ranges for statins are listed as high-intensity (usually lowers LDL ≥50%), moderate-intensity (usually lowers LDL 30–49%), and low-intensity (usually lowers LDL <30%)

[2] See p 51 for prescribing information.

[3] Many drug interactions warranting contraindication or dose adjustment of lovastatin; see package insert for details.

[4] Maximum dose is 10 mg/d if CrCl <30 mL/min.

[5] Measure Cr level at baseline, within 3 mo of initiating tx, and q6mo thereafter. Reduce dose if CrCl <60 mL/min; do not use if CrCl <30 mL/min.

[6] Contraindicated with concomitant statin tx.

[7] Use as monotx only in patients unable to tolerate statins, niacin, or a bile acid sequestrant (colesevelam, colestipol) and who have not reached LDL-lowering goal.

[8] Obtain baseline and q6mo LFTs, fasting blood glucose, or A1c, and uric acid. Monitor for flushing, pruritus, nausea, gastritis, ulcer. Dosage increases should be spaced 1 mo apart. ASA 325 mg po 30 min before first niacin dose of the day prevents AEs.

[9] Do not use if fasting TG >300 mg/dL. Use with caution if fasting TG is 250–299 mg/dL.

[10] Adjunctive tx for LDL lowering in patients with homozygous familial hypercholesterolemia and in patients with atherosclerotic vascular disease on maximally tolerated doses of a statin. Very expensive.

HYPERTENSION

Goal BP

- For older adults with HTN with multiple comorbidities, limited life expectancy, or both, individualize goal BP to consider tx benefits and ADRs and to reflect patient goals.
- The 2017 ACC/AHA guidelines recommend a tx goal BP of <130/80 mm Hg for most older adults, including those with CVD, DM, or CKD.
- The SPRINT study showed improved CVD outcomes, lower incidence of MCI, and lower all-cause mortality—along with increased risk of hypotension and possibly syncope—associated with an SBP tx goal of <120 mm Hg. This study had extensive exclusion criteria; about 1/3 of the general population aged ≥75 would have been eligible for the trial.

Definition

- Elevated BP: SBP 120–129 mm Hg and DBP <80 mm Hg
- HTN Stage 1: SBP 130–139 mm Hg or DBP 80–89 mm Hg
- HTN Stage 2: SBP ≥140 or DBP ≥90

The above definitions classify about 80% of person aged ≥65 as having HTN.

Evaluation and Assessment

- Measure both standing and sitting BP after 5 min of rest.

- Base diagnosis on ≥2 readings at each of ≥2 visits. After diagnosis is made, evaluate by:
  - Assessing cardiac risk factors: smoking, dyslipidemia, obesity, DM are important in older adults
  - Performing routine lab tests: CBC, UA, electrolytes, Cr, A1c, total cholesterol, HDL cholesterol, and ECG
  - Assessing end-organ damage as guided by clinical judgment: test for HF/LVH, CAD, cerebrovascular disease, nephropathy, PAD, retinopathy
  - Considering renal artery stenosis if new onset of diastolic HTN, sudden rise in BP in previously well controlled HTN, HTN despite tx with maximal dosages of 3 antihypertensive agents, or azotemia induced by ACEI/ARB tx.
    - Diagnostic tests for renal artery stenosis include renal artery duplex ultrasonography, CT angiography with and without contrast, or MRA.
    - Don't screen for renal artery stenosis in patients without resistant HTN and with normal renal function, even if known atherosclerosis present.[CW]
    - Medical tx for renal artery stenosis includes aggressive management of vascular risk factors and antihypertensive regimens that include an ACEI or ARB (monitor Cr closely).
    - Consider renal artery angioplasty, stenting, or both, for patients where medical tx has failed (refractory HTN, worsening renal function, intractable HF) or who have nonatherosclerotic disease (eg, fibromuscular dysplasia).

Aggravating Factors

- Amphetamines/stimulants
- Atypical antipsychotics (clozapine, olanzapine)
- Decongestants
- Emotional stress
- Excessive alcohol intake
- Excessive salt intake
- Lack of aerobic exercise
- Low potassium intake
- Low calcium intake
- Nicotine
- NSAIDs
- Obesity
- SNRIs
- Systemic corticosteroids

Management

- Initiate pharmacotherapy if goal BP (see above) is not attained using nonpharmacologic methods.
- Clinic-based BP measurements are usually consistent with home-based readings for BPs <140/90 mm Hg. Patients with clinic-based BP readings >140/90 mm Hg often have lower home-based readings.
- For patients with suspected "white coat" HTN, 24-h ambulatory BP monitoring (covered by Medicare if office-based BP >140/90 mm Hg) produces more reliable readings than office-based measurements.
- In noncardiac hospitalized patients, tx of incidental HTN or hypotension with new or altered doses of antihypertensives is not recommended.

Nonpharmacologic Interventions

- Adequate dietary potassium intake; goal 3500–5000 mg/d.
- Aerobic and resistance exercise: 90–150 min/wk for each.
- Diet rich in fruits, vegetables, whole grains, and low-fat dairy products; reduced intake of saturated and total fat.
- Moderation of alcohol intake: limit to 1 drink/d.
- Moderation of dietary sodium: watch for volume depletion with diuretic use. Goal: reduction of 1 g Na+/d, optimal total intake of ≤1.5 g Na+/d.
- Smoking cessation
- Weight reduction if obese: even a 10-lb weight loss can significantly lower BP.

Pharmacotherapy (**Table 21** lists commonly used antihypertensives.)

- Base tx decisions on standing BP.
- First-line drugs: a thiazide diuretic, an ACEI, an ARB, or a CCB.
- Follow-up BP measurements monthly until target BP is attained.
  - If BP is not at target, either increase the dose of the initial drug or add a second drug from the first-line list above.
  - Many patients require 2 or more drugs to achieve goal BP.
  - Other agents (eg, β blocker, vasodilators) can be added for refractory cases or when tx needs to be individualized if coexisting conditions are present (**Table 22**).
- Visits may be q3–6mo if BP is stable at target goal.

Hypertensive Emergencies and Urgencies

- Elevated BP alone without symptoms or target end-organ damage does not require emergent BP lowering.
- Emergent BP lowering is indicated with BP >180/120 ***and*** signs of new or worsening end-organ damage: hypertensive encephalopathy, intracranial hemorrhage, stroke, unstable angina, acute MI, acute left ventricular failure with pulmonary edema, aortic dissection, acute renal failure, and retinal hemorrhage, exudates, or papilledema
  - If emergent BP lowering is indicated, admit patient to ICU with immediate IV drug tx. Common agents include hydralazine, labetalol, nitroglycerin, nicardipine, and nitroprusside; choice is often based on underlying condition.
  - Emergent BP lowering goal is ≤20–25% during the first hour, then to 160/100–160/110 mm Hg for the next 2–6 h.
  - For BP management of acute ischemic stroke or intracerebral hemorrhage, see Neurologic Disorders, p 234.
- If no signs of new or worsening end-organ damage, emergent lowering is not indicated. Repeat BP measurement after 20–30 min of quiet rest and assess if patient has other nonemergent symptoms (headache, atypical chest pain, epistaxis).
  - If symptomatic, rapid oral agents can be given: clonidine (0.1–0.3 mg), labetalol (200–400 mg), captopril (25–50 mg), prazosin (5–10 mg), or nitroglycerin 2% topical oint (1–2 in). Avoid nifedipine.
  - If asymptomatic, adjust usual antihypertensives with follow-up in 1–7 d.
- When BP needs to be lowered for procedures or tx (such as β blockade before surgery, p 285):
  - Administer standard dose of a recommended antihypertensive orally (**Table 21**) or an extra dose of patient's usual antihypertensive.
  - If the patient is npo, give **low**-dose antihypertensive IV, titrating upward **slowly**. Options include β blocker (eg, labetalol 20 mg), ACEI (eg, enalaprilat at 0.625 mg over 5 min), or diuretic (eg, furosemide 10 mg).

Table 21. Commonly Prescribed Oral Antihypertensive Agents

Class, Medication	Geriatric Dosage Range, total	Comments (Metabolism, Excretion)
Diuretics		↓ potassium, sodium, magnesium levels; ↑ uric acid, calcium, cholesterol (mild), and glucose (mild) levels

(cont.)

Table 21. Commonly Prescribed Oral Antihypertensive Agents (cont.)		
Class, Medication	**Geriatric Dosage Range, total**	**Comments (Metabolism, Excretion)**
Thiazides		
✓Chlorothiazide	125–500 mg po 1×/d	
✓Chlorthalidone	12.5–25 mg po 1×/d	↑ AEs at >25 mg/d (L)
✓HCTZ	12.5–25 mg po 1×/d	↑ AEs at >25 mg/d (L)
✓Indapamide	0.625–2.5 mg po 1×/d	Less or no hypercholesterolemia (L)
✓Metolazone	2.5–5 mg po 1×/d	Monitor electrolytes carefully (L)
✓Polythiazide *(Renese)*	1–4 mg po 1×/d	
Loop diuretics		
♥Bumetanide	0.5–4 mg po 1–3×/d	Short duration of action, no hypercalcemia (K)
♥Furosemide	20–160 mg po 1–2×/d	Short duration of action, no hypercalcemia (K)
♥Torsemide	2.5–50 mg po 1–2×/d	Short duration of action, no hypercalcemia (K)
Potassium-sparing drugs		
Amiloride	2.5–10 mg po 1×/d	Avoid in patients with CrCl <30 (↑ potassium, ↓ sodium)[BC] (L, K)
Triamterene	25–100 mg po 1–2×/d	Avoid in patients with CrCl <30 (increased risk of kidney injury; ↑ potassium, ↓ sodium)[BC]; avoid in patients with CKD Stage 4 or 5.[BC] (L, K)
Aldosterone-receptor blockers[1]		
♥Eplerenone	25–100 mg po 1×/d	(L, K)
♥Spironolactone	12.5–50 mg po 1–2×/d	Gynecomastia; avoid if CrCl <30.[BC] (L, K)
Adrenergic Inhibitors		
α[1] Blockers[BC]		Avoid as antihypertensive unless patient has BPH; avoid in patients with syncope; avoid in patients with HF.
Doxazosin	1–16 mg po 1×/d	(L)
Prazosin	1–20 mg po 2–3×/d	(L)
Terazosin	1–20 mg po 1–2×/d	(L, K)
Central α[2] Agonist		
Clonidine	0.1–1.2 mg po 2–3×/d ***or*** 1 pch/wk	Sedation, dry mouth, bradycardia, withdrawal HTN. Avoid as first-line antihypertensive.[BC] Continue oral for 1–2 d when converting to patch (L, K)
β Blockers[1]		Bronchospasm, bradycardia, acute HF, may mask insulin-induced hypoglycemia; less effective for reducing HTN-related endpoints in older vs younger patients; lipid solubility is a risk factor for delirium

(cont.)

Table 21. Commonly Prescribed Oral Antihypertensive Agents (cont.)		
Class, Medication	**Geriatric Dosage Range, total**	**Comments (Metabolism, Excretion)**
Acebutolol	200–800 mg po 1×/d	β1, low lipid solubility, intrinsic sympathomimetic activity (L, K)
Atenolol	12.5–100 mg po 1×/d	β1, low lipid solubility (K)
Betaxolol	5–20 mg po 1×/d	β1, low lipid solubility (L, K)
♥Bisoprolol	2.5–10 mg po 1×/d	β1, low lipid solubility (L, K)
Metoprolol tartrate (IR)	25–400 mg po 2×/d	β1, moderate lipid solubility (L)
♥Metoprolol succinate (SR)	50–400 mg po 1×/d	β1, moderate lipid solubility (L)
Nadolol	20–160 mg po 1×/d	β1, β2, low lipid solubility (K)
♥Nebivolol *(Bystolic)*	2.5–40 mg po 1×/d	β1, low lipid solubility (L, K)
Pindolol	5–40 mg po 2×/d	β1, β2, moderate lipid solubility, intrinsic sympathomimetic activity (K)
Propranolol	20–160 mg po 2×/d	β1, β2, high lipid solubility (L)
Long-acting	60–180 mg po 1×/d	β1, β2, high lipid solubility (L)
Timolol	10–40 mg po 2×/d	β1, β2, low to moderate lipid solubility (L, K)
Combined α and β Blockers[1]		Postural hypotension, bronchospasm
♥Carvedilol	3.125–25 mg po 2×/d	β1, β2, high lipid solubility (L)
♥Extended-release *(Coreg CR)*	10–80 mg po 1×/d	Multiply regular daily dose of carvedilol by 1.6 to convert to CR dose; do not take within 2 h of alcohol ingestion
Labetalol	100–600 mg po 2×/d	β1, β2, moderate lipid solubility (L, K)
Direct Vasodilators		Headaches, fluid retention, tachycardia
♥Hydralazine	25–100 mg po 2–4×/d	Lupus syndrome; used in combination with isosorbide dinitrate for HF in Black pts (L, K)
Minoxidil	2.5–50 mg po 1×/d	Hirsutism (K)
Calcium Antagonists		
Nondihydropyridines		Conduction defects, worsening of systolic dysfunction,[BC] gingival hyperplasia
✓Diltiazem SR	120–360 mg/d po 1×/d	Nausea, headache (L)
✓Verapamil SR	120–360 mg po 1–2×/d	Constipation, bradycardia (L)
Dihydropyridines		Ankle edema, flushing, headache, gingival hypertrophy
✓Amlodipine	2.5–10 mg po 1×/d	(L)
✓Felodipine	2.5–20 mg po 1×/d	(L)
✓Isradipine SR	2.5–10 mg po 1×/d	(L)

(cont.)

Table 21. Commonly Prescribed Oral Antihypertensive Agents (cont.)		
Class, Medication	Geriatric Dosage Range, total	Comments (Metabolism, Excretion)
✓Nicardipine SR	30–120 mg/d po	(L)
✓Nifedipine SR	30–60 mg po 1×/d	(L)
✓Nisoldipine	10–40 mg po 1×/d	(L)
ACEIs[BC,1]		Cough (common), angioedema (rare), hyperkalemia, rash, loss of taste, leukopenia
✓♥Benazepril	2.5–40 mg po 1–2×/d	(L, K)
✓♥Captopril	12.5–150 mg po 2–3×/d	(L, K)
✓♥Enalapril	2.5–40 mg po 1–2×/d	(L, K)
✓♥Fosinopril	5–40 mg po 1–2×/d	(L, K)
✓♥Lisinopril	2.5–40 mg po 1×/d	(K)
✓Moexipril	3.75–30 mg po 1×/d	(L, K)
✓♥Perindopril	4–8 mg po 1–2×/d	(L, K)
✓♥Quinapril	5–40 mg po 1×/d	(L, K)
✓♥Ramipril	1.25–20 mg po 1×/d	(L, K)
✓♥Trandolapril	1–4 mg po 1×/d	(L, K)
Angiotensin II Receptor Blockers (ARBs)[BC,1]		Angioedema (very rare), hyperkalemia
✓Azilsartan *(Edarbi)*	20–80 mg po 1×/d	(L, K)
✓♥Candesartan	4–32 mg po 1×/d	(K)
✓Irbesartan	75–300 mg po 1×/d	(L)
✓♥Losartan	12.5–100 mg po 1–2×/d	(L, K)
✓Olmesartan	20–40 mg po 1×/d	Severe GI symptoms (rare) (L, K)
✓Telmisartan	20–80 mg po 1×/d	(L)
✓♥Valsartan	40–320 mg po 1×/d	(L, K)
Renin Inhibitor[BC]		
Aliskiren	150–300 mg po 1×/d	Monitor electrolytes in patients with renal disease; contraindicated in patients with DM who are also taking an ACEI or ARB

✓ = preferred for treating older adults; ♥ = useful in managing HFrEF

[1]See **Table 25** for target dosages in managing HF.

Note: Listing of AEs is not exhaustive, and AEs are for the drug class except when noted for individual drugs.

Table 22. Choosing Antihypertensive Therapy on the Basis of Coexisting Conditions

Condition	Appropriate for Use	Avoid or Contraindicated
Angina	β, CA	
Atrial tachycardia and fibrillation	β, NDCA	
Bronchospasm/COPD		β, αβ, L
CKD	AA, ACEI[1], ARB[1]	
DM	ACEI, ARB, β, T[2]	T[1]
Dyslipidemia		β, T[3]
Essential tremor	B[4]	
Gout		L, T
HFrEF	AA, ACEI, ARB, β, αβ, L	NDCA
Hyperthyroidism	β	
MI	β, AA, ACEI, ARB	CA
Osteoporosis	T	
Prostatism (BPH)	α	
Urge UI	CA	L, T

AA, aldosterone antagonist; α, α blocker; β, β blocker; αβ, combined α and β blocker; CA, calcium antagonist; L, loop diuretic; NDCA, nondihydropyridine calcium antagonist; T, thiazide diuretic.

[1] Use with great caution in renovascular disease.

[2] Low-dose diuretics probably beneficial in DM2; high-dose diuretics relatively contraindicated in DM1 and DM2.

[3] Low-dose diuretics have a minimal effect on lipids.

[4] Long-acting propranolol is used for tremor.

PULMONARY ARTERIAL HYPERTENSION (PAH)

Evaluation and Assessment

- Pulmonary hypertension (PH) is defined by a pulmonary artery pressure >20 mm Hg on right heart catheterization. PAH is one of 5 subtypes of PH, further defined by a pulmonary artery wedge pressure of >15 mm Hg and a pulmonary vascular resistance of ≥3 Wood units.
- PAH can be primary (unexplained) or secondary to underlying conditions.
- Almost all cases in older adults are secondary, most commonly associated with chronic pulmonary (eg, COPD, interstitial lung disease, OSA) or cardiac disease (eg, HF, mitral valvular disease), or pulmonary emboli.
- Early symptoms are often nonspecific and include dyspnea on exertion, fatigue, and vague chest discomfort.
- Late symptoms include severe dyspnea on exertion, cyanosis, syncope, chest pain, HF, arrhythmias.
- Physical exam findings relate to manifestations of the associated conditions mentioned above.
- Diagnostic tests:
  - ECG may show right-axis deviation, right atrial and ventricular hypertrophy, T-wave changes
  - CXR may show large right ventricle, dilated pulmonary arteries

- Echocardiography estimates pulmonary arterial pressure and evaluates possible valvular disease
- Right heart catheterization is gold standard
- Additional tests (eg, PFTs, sleep study) may clarify severity of coexisting conditions.

Management

- Correct or optimize underlying conditions.
- Supplemental oxygen for chronic hypoxemia
- Diuretics for volume overload from HF
- Avoid CCBs unless they have been shown to be of benefit from a right heart catheterization vasodilator challenge study.
- Other agents have been studied mainly in primary PAH and are of uncertain effectiveness and safety in secondary PAH:
  - Warfarin (p 46)
  - Prostacyclins: epoprostenol *(Flolan)* by continuous IV infusion, treprostinil *(Remodulin)* by continuous SC infusion, treprostinil or iloprost *(Ventavis)* by inhalation, or selexipag *(Uptravi)* 200–1600 mcg po q12h
  - Endothelial receptor antagonists: ambrisentan 5–10 mg/d po; bosentan 62.5 mg po q12h × 4 wk, then 125 mg po q12h; macitentan *(Opsumit)* 10 mg/d po
  - Guanylate cyclase stimulator: riociguat *(Adempas)*, 0.5 mg po q8h, increase dose gradually to maximum of 2.5 mg po q8h
  - PDE5 inhibitors: sildenafil 20–25 mg po q8h, tadalafil 40 mg/d po

CORONARY ARTERY DISEASE

Evaluation of Chest Pain (2021 AHA/ACC/ASE/CHEST/SAEM/SCCT/SCMR Guidelines)

- Chest pain should be characterized as cardiac, possible cardiac, and noncardiac upon assessment.
- See **Table 23** to determine the likelihood of cardiac pain.

Table 23. Symptoms Associated with Cardiac Pain Due to Ischemia or Angina

Symptom Parameter	Probability of Pain Due to Ischemia or Angina	
	High	**Low**
Location	Retrosternal	Right-sided or localized to a very limited area
Quality	Pain, discomfort, heaviness, tightness, pressure, constriction, squeezing, or gripping	Tearing, ripping, or burning
Time course	Gradually builds over a few minutes	Very short duration (seconds)
Antecedents	Physical exercise or emotional distress	Altered or positional change

- Differential diagnosis of chest pain includes ischemia or angina (**Table 24**), ACS (persistent ischemic pain at rest or with minimal exertion), aortic dissection (sudden onset of ripping chest pain with radiation to back), PE, pericardial disease, esophageal rupture or spasm, pneumothorax, chest wall pain.
- Women are at greater risk for underdiagnosis. Women are more likely to report accompanying symptoms of nausea, fatigue, and shortness of breath than men.

- Acute chest pain that is not clearly noncardiac in origin should be immediately evaluated in the emergency department. An EKG should be performed within 10 min of presentation.
- Subacute or stable chest pain in an outpatient setting should be evaluated with physical exam and EKG. Diagnostic testing for CAD (see next section) is based on individual characteristics. Pretest probability score instruments can help assess the likelihood of cardiac pain, but often overestimate the probability of CAD and can lead to overtesting.

Diagnostic Tests for CAD

- Cardiac catheterization is the gold standard; cardiac CT angiography is a less invasive, but less accurate, alternative.
- Stress testing: the heart is stressed either through exercise (treadmill, stationary bicycle) or, if the patient cannot exercise or the ECG is markedly abnormal, with pharmacologic agents (dipyridamole, adenosine, dobutamine). Exercise stress tests can be performed with or without cardiac imaging, while pharmacologic stress tests always include imaging. Imaging can be accomplished by echocardiography, single-photon-emission computed tomography (SPECT), or nuclear medicine (thallium stress test, sestamibi, technetium Tc 99m tetrofosmin).
- Don't perform stress cardiac imaging or advanced noninvasive imaging in the initial evaluation of patients without cardiac symptoms unless high-risk markers are present.[CW]
- Don't use coronary artery calcium scoring for patients with known CAD (including stents and bypass grafts).[CW]
- Don't obtain screening exercise ECG testing in individuals who are asymptomatic and at low risk for coronary disease.[CW]

Acute Coronary Syndrome (ACS)

- ACS encompasses diagnoses of ST segment MI (STEMI), non-ST segment MI (NSTEMI), and unstable angina.
- Type 1 MI represents plaque rupture (traditional heart attack) while Type 2 MI is caused by a mismatch between myocardial supply and demand caused by conditions like coronary spasm, hypotension or shock, severe HTN, and severe anemia.
- Suspect ACS with anginal chest pain or anginal equivalent on no or minimal exertion: arm, jaw, or abdominal pain (with or without nausea); acute functional decline; delirium; shortness of breath; syncope; unexplained fall.
- Diagnosis is based on symptoms along with cardiac serum markers and ECG findings:
    - STEMI (30% of ACS): elevated serum markers, elevated ST segments
    - NSTEMI (70% of ACS): elevated serum markers, depressed ST segments and/or inverted T-waves
    - Unstable angina: nonelevated serum markers, normal or depressed ST segments, normal or inverted T-waves
- Measuring cardiac serum markers:
    - Most protocols call for checking troponins T or I at presentation and 2 h later.
    - Among patients at low risk for MI evaluated in the emergency department for chest pain, a single negative enzyme measurement is likely sufficient to rule out MI.
    - For higher-risk patients (older adults with hx suspicious for MI, ECG changes, multiple CAD risk factors), a single negative enzyme measurement, particularly within 6 h of symptom onset, does not exclude MI; 2 negative measurements exclude MI.
    - Sensitivity of troponins is improved with the use of sensitive or ultrasensitive assays.
    - Troponins are not useful to detect reinfarction within first wk of an MI. CK-MB is the preferred marker for early reinfarction.
    - Both CK-MB and cardiac troponins can have false-positive results due to subclinical ischemic myocardial injury or nonischemic myocardial injury.

- Troponin levels can be transiently or persistently minimally elevated by many non-ACS causes:
  - type 2 MI
  - severe HTN
  - tachyarrhythmias
  - coronary spasm
  - HF
  - viral myocarditis
  - endocarditis
  - myocarditis
  - pericarditis
  - malignancy
  - cancer chemotherapy
  - trauma
  - PE
  - sepsis
  - renal failure
  - stroke
- Evaluation of elevated troponins (hx, physical exam, assessment of renal function, ECG, echocardiography) should focus on finding and treating the underlying cause.
- Elevated troponin in the face of normal CK-MB indicates increased risk of MI in the ensuing 5 y.

Initial Hospital Management of ACS (presentation to 48 h)

Follow institutional protocol.

- Unless contraindicated, all post-MI patients should take ASA, a β blocker, an ACEI, and a statin (high-intensity dose for patients aged <75, medium-intensity dose for patients aged ≥75; see Dyslipidemia Management, p 51).
- Consider tapering and then stopping β blocker tx after 1–3 y in patients with normal LVEF and without angina or signs of ischemia.
- Dual antiplatelet therapy (DAPT): in addition to ASA, give clopidogrel or ticagrelor (**Table 16**) for 3–6 mo in patients receiving stents, on medical tx, or undergoing CABG. Consider continuing DAPT beyond 6 mo if bleeding risk is low and there have been no significant bleeding events. Prasugrel (**Table 16**) can be given as an alternative to clopidogrel. Prasugrel should be considered only in patients aged <75 without hx of TIA or stroke.[BC] ASA dosage in DAPT should be 75–100 mg/d po. Recent trials suggest that after 12 mo of DAPT, continuing clopidogrel or ticagrelor might be more effective than ASA monotx.
- Angina management:
  - If β blockers are contraindicated, use long-acting nitrates or long-acting CCBs for chronic angina.
  - For refractory chronic angina despite tx with β blocker, CCB, or nitrates, consider adding ranolazine *(Ranexa)* 500–1000 mg po q12h; contraindicated in patients with QT prolongation or on QT-prolonging drugs, with hepatic impairment, or on CYP3A inhibitors, including diltiazem (p 58).
  - Use sl or spr nitroglycerin for acute angina.
- Treat HTN (p 54).
- Treat DM; see p 115 for target goals. Consider prescribing canagliflozin, dapagliflozin or empagliflozin (**Table 50**) for patients with DM, because these agents produce better cardiac outcomes in patients with CVD.
- Weight reduction in obese individuals; initial tx goal is 5–10% reduction with ultimate goal of BMI <25 kg/m^2 (p 210)
- Aerobic exercise 30–60 min/d, at least intermediate intensity (eg, brisk walking).
- Smoking cessation.
- Encourage adopting DASH (Dietary Approaches to Stop Hypertension) or Mediterranean diet.
- Consider omega-3 polyunsaturated fatty acid supplements (mixed data on effectiveness for reducing outcomes).

- Consider placement of ICD (p 76) in patients with LVEF ≤30% at least 40 d after MI or 3 mo after CABG.
- Don't perform routine annual stress testing after coronary artery revascularization.[CW]
- Avoid NSAIDs other than ASA.

HEART FAILURE (HF; 2022 AHA/ACC/HFSA GUIDELINES)

Evaluation and Assessment

- All patients initially presenting with overt HF should have an echocardiogram to evaluate left ventricular function.
  - EF ≤40% indicates systolic dysfunction and a diagnosis of HF with reduced EF (HFrEF)
  - EF ≤40% that improves to EF >40% on subsequent measurement classification is referred to as HFimpEF
  - EF ≥50% indicates diastolic dysfunction and a diagnosis of HF with preserved EF (HFpEF)
  - EF of 41–49% is a midrange classification (sometimes indicated as HFmrEF) but patients usually resemble those with HFpEF
  - Echocardiography can also evaluate cardiac dyssynchrony (**Table 24**) in patients with a wide QRS complex on ECG.
  - Echocardiography with tissue doppler imaging may be helpful in diagnosing diastolic dysfunction.

Table 24. Heart Failure Staging and Management

Clinical Profile	ACC/AHA Staging	NYHA Staging	Management
Asymptomatic but at high risk of developing HF (eg, HTN, DM, CAD present)	Stage A	—	RFR, E, SGLT2 inhibitor for patients with DM
Asymptomatic with structural disease: LVH, low EF, prior MI, or valvular disease	Stage B	Class I	RFR, E, ACEI (or ARB if unable to tolerate ACEI), β, ICD in selected patients
Normal EF; current or prior symptoms (HFpEF)	Stage C	Class I–IV	RFR, drug tx for symptomatic HF (pp 65–66), control of ventricular rate
Low EF[1]; currently asymptomatic but with hx of symptoms	Stage C	Class I	RFR, E, DW, SR, ACEI (or ARB if unable to tolerate ACEI), β
Low EF[1]; patient comfortable at rest but symptomatic on normal physical activity	Stage C	Class II	Class II–IV: RFR, E, DW, SR, drug tx for symptomatic HF (pp 65–66), consider biventricular pacing if cardiac dyssynchrony is present, consider placement of ICD if LVEF ≤35% (p 76)
Low EF[1]; patient comfortable at rest but symptomatic on slight physical activity	Stage C	Class III	
Low EF[1]; patient symptomatic at rest	Stage C	Class IV	
Refractory symptoms at rest in hospitalized patient requiring specialized interventions (eg, transplant) or hospice care	Stage D	Class IV	Decide on care preference; above measures or hospice as appropriate

RFR, cardiac risk factor reduction; E, exercise (regular walking or cycling); β, β blocker, DW, measurement of daily weight; SR, salt restriction (≤3 g/d if severe HF).

[1] Low EF = EF ≤40%

- Other routine initial assessment: orthostatic BPs, height, weight, BMI calculation, ECG, CXR, CBC, UA, electrolytes, calcium, magnesium, Cr, BUN, lipid profile, fasting glucose, LFTs, TSH, functional status.

- Measuring plasma brain natriuretic peptide (BNP) or N-terminal prohormone brain natriuretic peptide (NT-proBNP) can aid in diagnosis of HF in patients presenting with acute dyspnea.
  - BNP and NT-proBNP levels increase with age.
  - In dyspneic patients aged >70:
    - HF very unlikely (likelihood ratio negative = 0.1) if BNP <125 pg/mL or if NT-proBNP <300 pg/mL)
    - HF very likely (likelihood ratio positive = 6) if BNP >500 pg/mL or if NT-proBNP >1200 pg/mL in those aged 65–74 and >1800 pg/mL in those aged 75 and older
  - Other conditions causing increased BNP or NT-proBNP levels include ACS, heart muscle disease, valvular disease, pericardial disease, AF, anemia, impaired renal function, pulmonary disease, pulmonary HTN, OSA, critical illness, severe burns, and sepsis.
- Optional: Radionuclide ventriculography, which measures EF more precisely, evaluates right ventricular function better, and costs more than echocardiography.
- If HF is accompanied by angina or signs of ischemia, coronary angiography should be strongly considered.
- Consider coronary angiography if HF presents with atypical chest pain or in patients who have known or suspected CAD.
- Consider stress testing if HF presents in patients at high risk (ie, numerous risk factors) for CAD.
- Drugs to be avoided in patients with HF:
  - Thiazolidinediones[BC] **(Table 50)**, NSAIDs, and COX-2 inhibitors[BC]
  - Dronedarone and most antiarrhythmic agents (amiodarone preferred if necessary)
  - Nondihydropyridine CCBs in patients with HFrEF[BC]
- Use metformin with caution.
- Cilostazol is contraindicated in decompensated HF.[BC]

Drug Therapy for Symptomatic HFpEF

- For acute HFpEF with volume overload, loop diuretics and vasodilation with nitroglycerin are indicated. Parenteral nitroglycerin can cause hypotension in HFpEF patients without elevated BP, so use it cautiously if BP is normal or low.
- For HFpEF without volume overload, tx focuses on control of HTN (goal SBP <130 mm Hg), rate control, especially in patients with AF, and avoidance of digoxin.
- A combination ARB-neprilysin inhibitor (ARNI; sacubitril/valsartan [*Entresto*]) is approved for HFpEF tx based on a trial that suggested benefit in participants with EFs down to 45%.

Drug Therapy for Symptomatic HFrEF (AHA Stage C and D, NYHA Class II–IV)

For information on drug dosages and AEs not listed below, see **Table 21**. Efficacy of different medications may vary significantly across racial and ethnic groups; eg, Black people may require higher doses of ACEIs and β blockers and may benefit from isosorbide dinitrate combined with hydralazine tx.

- Diuretics if volume overload. In patients with normal renal function, IV furosemide is ~2× as potent as furosemide po. The IV and oral potencies of bumetanide and torsemide are about equal, and these 2 agents have a shorter half-life than furosemide. In refractory acute decompensated HF, consider continuous infusion of loop diuretics, supplemented by metolazone.

- ARB, ACEI, or combination ARB-neprilysin inhibitor (ARNI; sacubitril/valsartan [*Entresto*]) to target doses (**Table 25**). Use ARNI for NYHA Class II and III patients; if ARNI is not tolerated, can use ACEI or ARB. ARNI is contraindicated in patients with hx of angioedema. ARBs can improve HFrEF outcomes in older adults, while ACEIs improve outcomes in subjects aged <75 but not in those aged >75.
- In NYHA Class II and III patients taking ACEI or ARB who are chronically symptomatic, replacing ACEI or ARB with ARNI can be beneficial.
- β blocker (bisoprolol, carvedilol, metoprolol succinate) to target dose (**Table 25**) after volume status is stabilized

Table 25. **Target Dosages of Medications for HFrEF**

Agent	Starting Dosage	Target Dosage
ACEIs[BC,1]		
Benazepril	2.5 mg/d po	40 mg/d po
Captopril	6.25 mg po q8h	50 mg po q8h
Enalapril	2.5 mg po q12h	10–20 mg po q12h
Fosinopril	5 mg/d po	40 mg/d po
Lisinopril	2.5 mg/d po	20–40 mg/d po
Perindopril	2 mg/d po	8–16 mg/d po
Quinapril	5 mg po q12h	20 mg po q12h
Ramipril	1.25 mg/d po	10 mg/d po
Trandolapril	1 mg/d po	4 mg/d po
Angiotensin II Receptor Blockers (ARBs)[BC,1]		
Candesartan	4 mg/d po	32 mg/d po
Losartan	12.5 mg/d po	100 mg/d po
Valsartan	20 mg po q12h	160 mg po q12h
Angiotensin Receptor-Neprilysin Inhibitor (ARNI)[BC]		
Sacubitril/Valsartan	24/26 mg po q12h	97/103 mg po q12h
β Blockers		
Bisoprolol	1.25 mg/d po	10 mg/d po
Carvedilol	3.125 mg po q12h	25-50 mg po q12h
Carvedilol ER	10 mg/d po	80 mg/d po
Metoprolol XR	12.5–25 mg/d po	200 mg/d po
Mineralocorticoid Receptor Antagonists		
Spironolactone	12.5 mg/d po	25–50 mg/d po
Eplerenone	25 mg/d po	50 mg/d po

(cont.)

Table 25. Target Dosages of Medications for HFrEF (cont.)		
Agent	**Starting Dosage**	**Target Dosage**
SGLT2 Inhibitors		
Canagliflozin	100 mg/d po	100 mg/d po
Dapagliflozin	5 mg/d po	10 mg/d po
Empagliflozin	10 mg/d po	10 mg/d po

[1] Check Cr and electrolytes 1–2 wk after initiating tx. Titrate to target dosage by gradually increasing or doubling the dose q2wk as tolerated.

- Adding an mineralocorticoid receptor antagonist to target dose (**Table 25**) can reduce mortality in patients with NYHA Class II–IV failure. Monitor serum potassium carefully and avoid these medications if Cr >2.5 mg/dL in men or >2 mg/dL in women, or serum $K^+ \geq 5.0$ mEq/L.
- SGLT2 inhibitor to target dose (p 119, **Table 50**) for all patients with DM and those without DM but at high risk of developing HF (ACC/AHA Stage A). Also effective for all patients with symptomatic chronic HFrEF to reduce HF hospitalization and mortality.
- Adding a combination of isosorbide dinitrate and hydralazine (**Table 21**; also available as a single preparation: *BiDil* 1–2 tabs po q8h) can help patients, particularly Black patients, with persistent symptoms. Use vasodilators with caution in patients with hx of syncope.
- For patients with EF ≤35%, with stable symptoms, and in sinus rhythm with HR ≥70 who are taking maximally tolerated doses of β blockers or intolerant to β blockers, consider adding ivabradine *(Corlanor)* to reduce risk of hospitalization for HF.
- For high-risk patients with worsening HF despite the above-listed tx, consider adding vericiguat *(Verquvo)* to reduce HF hospitalization and CVD death.
- Consider low-dose digoxin; 0.0625–0.125 mg/d po (target serum levels 0.5–0.8 mg/dL) if HF is not controlled on diuretics and ACEIs, with or without an aldosterone antagonist. Avoid doses >0.125 mg/d.[BC] Digoxin may be less effective and even harmful in women and has been associated with increased mortality in patients with AF.
  - Monitor digoxin concentration with concomitant administration of many other medications.
    - The following **increase** digoxin concentration or effect, or both: amiodarone, diltiazem, erythromycin, esmolol, ibuprofen, spironolactone, tetracycline, verapamil
    - The following **decrease** digoxin concentration or effect, or both: aminosalicylic acid, antacids, antineoplastics, cholestyramine, colestipol, kaolin pectin, metoclopramide, psyllium, sulfasalazine, St John's wort
- Consider adding omega-3 polyunsaturated fatty acid supplements as adjunctive tx for symptomatic patients.
- Correct iron deficiency, for patients with or without anemia, using IV iron (**Table 9**).
- Concomitant HTN should be treated with goal SBP <130 mm Hg.
- Class I antiarrhythmics are not indicated.

LEG EDEMA

Differential

- Acute (<72 h) unilateral: DVT (by far most common and must be ruled out), ruptured Baker's cyst, ruptured medial head of the gastrocnemius
- Acute bilateral: acute worsening of HF, renal disease

- Chronic unilateral: venous insufficiency, secondary lymphedema (from tumor, radiation tx, surgery), cellulitis (warmth, erythema that does not resolve on raising leg), reflex sympathetic dystrophy
- Chronic bilateral: venous insufficiency (most common of all causes), HF, pulmonary HTN, drugs (see below), idiopathic edema, obesity, renal disease, liver disease, primary lymphedema, secondary lymphedema (from tumor, radiation tx, surgery)
- Drugs commonly causing edema include:
  - Antihypertensives: CCBs, β blockers, clonidine, hydralazine
  - Hormones: corticosteroids, sex hormones
  - NSAIDs

Evaluation

- History: duration and location of edema; overnight improvement (less likely in lymphedema), presence of pain (more likely in DVT, reflex sympathetic dystrophy); medication review; hx of heart, kidney, or liver disease; hx of cancer and/or radiation tx; sleep apnea (increases likelihood of pulmonary HTN)
- Physical exam: BMI; location of edema; tenderness (more likely in DVT); skin changes; signs of heart, kidney, or liver disease; pelvic exam if suspect pelvic tumor

Table 26. Distinguishing Lymphedema from Venous Edema

Type	Characteristics	Location	Causes	Management
Lymphedema	Pitting minimal or absent; skin is tense and thickened, with pink discoloration often accompanied by cellulitis or lymphangitis	Any extremity, commonly asymmetric	Cancer or cancer tx, infection, surgery, radiation tx	Compression, weight control, complex decompression PT (covered by Medicare)
Venous edema	Edema is soft and pitting; worse throughout course of day; skin is thickened with dark ruddy discoloration; prone to ulceration	Feet and legs, commonly symmetric	Venous insufficiency, HF, hypoalbuminemia	See below

Treatment of Venous Edema

- Venous insufficiency: leg elevation, skin care (daily mild soap and moisturizers), and compression stockings worn during the day (**Table 27**).
  - Below-the-knee stockings are usually sufficient. Above-the-knee stockings are appropriate for more extensive edema and for patients with orthostatic hypotension.
  - ABI measurement should precede use of compression stockings.
  - Compression stockings are not covered under traditional Medicare Part B unless an ulcer is present. Other insurance plans may cover them and require a doctor's prescription for coverage (although a prescription is not required to obtain them).
  - Antiembolism stockings (eg, T.E.D.™) are not designed for managing venous insufficiency.
  - Intermittent pneumatic compression pumps can be tried for recalcitrant edema.
  - Compression wraps can be used in patients who have difficulty donning compression stockings.
  - Diuretics should be used only for short-term tx of severe cases; chronic use can lead to intravascular dehydration and electrolyte imbalances.

Stocking Class (Compression Grade)	Pressure Delivered, mm Hg	Indications	Appropriate ABI Range
1 (mild)	10–20	Mild edema Varicose veins	>0.5[1]
2 (moderate–firm)	20–30	Moderate edema Pigmentation	>0.8
3 (firm–extra firm)	30–50	Severe edema Lymphedema	>0.8

Table 27. Prescribing Compression Stockings

[1] Use with great caution in patients with ABI of 0.5–0.8.

- See **Table 15** and p 42 for DVT tx.
- See pp 340–341 for management of venous stasis ulcers.
- Other tx should be directed at the underlying cause.

ATRIAL FIBRILLATION (AF)

Evaluation and Assessment

Causes

- Cardiac disease: cardiac surgery, cardiomyopathy, HF, hypertensive heart disease, ischemic disease, pericarditis, valvular disease
- Noncardiac disease: alcoholism, chronic pulmonary disease, infections, pulmonary emboli, thyrotoxicosis

Standard testing: ECG, CBC, electrolytes, Cr, BUN, TSH, echocardiogram

Management (2019 ACC/AHA Guidelines)

- Correct precipitating cause.
- Weight loss in overweight and obese patients and CVD risk factor reduction
- Patients presenting with AF and hypotension, severe angina, or advanced HF should be strongly considered for acute direct-current cardioversion.
- For acute management of AF with rapid ventricular response in patients who do not receive or respond to cardioversion, ventricular rate should be acutely lowered with one or more of the following medications:
  - β blockers (eg, metoprolol) 2.5–5 mg IV bolus over 2 min; may repeat twice
  - Diltiazem 0.25 mg/kg IV over 2 min
  - Verapamil 0.075–0.15 mg/kg IV over 2 min
- Long-term management of AF can be achieved through rate control or rhythm control.

Rate Control

- For patients with minimal symptoms or in whom sinus rhythm cannot be easily achieved, rate control (target <110 bpm in asymptomatic patients with normal EF, <80 bpm for symptomatic patients or reduced EF) plus antithrombotic tx is the preferred tx strategy.
  - In patients without left ventricular dysfunction or without HFrEF, rate control can be achieved with oral metoprolol or other β blocker, diltiazem, or verapamil.
  - In patients with left ventricular dysfunction or with HFrEF, first-line tx for rate control is a β blocker after fluid status is stabilized; digoxin[BC] with a β blocker or amiodarone[BC] (**Table 29**) can be used as alternatives for rate control. Digoxin has been associated with increased mortality in observational studies of patients with AF. Avoid dronedarone.

- In patients with pre-excitation and AF, digoxin, nondihydropyridine calcium antagonists, and amiodarone are contraindicated.
- For symptomatic patients in whom ventricular rate does not respond to tx, AV node ablation with pacemaker placement can control rate. Continue anticoagulation for ≥2 mo post-ablation; base long-term postablation anticoagulation decisions on stroke risk, bleeding risk, and patient preference (see below).

- Individualize antithrombotic tx to balance reduced stroke risk vs increased bleeding risk. Except in patients with advanced frailty or with severe bleeding risks, the benefits of anticoagulation outweigh the risks.
  - Two risk scoring instruments are used to assess stroke risk ($CHADS_2$, CHA_2DS_2–VASc) and bleeding risk can be assessed using the HAS-BLED score (**Table 28**). CHA_2DS_2–VASc is preferred by cardiologists over $CHADS_2$. CHA_2DS_2–VASc classifies many more older adults (including everyone aged ≥75) as warranting anticoagulant tx than $CHADS_2$.
  - DOACs (apixaban, dabigatran, edoxaban, rivaroxaban) and warfarin can be used in AF. Compared to warfarin, DOAC use lowers rates of all-cause mortality, hemorrhagic stroke, ischemic stroke, and major bleeding; consequently DOACs are preferred over warfarin as first-line agents in nonvalvular AF. Apixaban is associated with lower rates of major bleeding and stroke or embolism when compared to rivaroxaban. Dabigatran and rivaroxaban have higher rates of non–major GI bleeding compared to warfarin.
  - Warfarin is recommended over DOAC use in AF patients with moderate to severe mitral stenosis or a mechanical heart valve (ie, valvular AF).
  - If anticoagulation is contraindicated or not tolerated in patients with $CHADS_2$ or CHA_2DS_2–VASc scores ≥1, use ASA 81–325 mg/d po. Adding clopidogrel 75 mg/d po to ASA lowers stroke risk but also increases risk of major hemorrhage. Both ASA and clopidogrel are less effective for stroke prevention in patients aged ≥75. Another option is percutaneous left atrial appendage occlusion (eg, Watchman device placement), which reduces the risk of hemorrhagic stroke compared to warfarin tx.

Table 28. Risk Instruments to Guide Antithrombotic Treatment in AF

Instrument	What Is Assessed	Score Calculation	Antithrombotic Tx by Score: 0	1	≥2
CHA_2DS_2–VASc	Stroke risk	1 point each for HF, HTN, DM, vascular disease, age ≥65 y, female sex; 2 points each for age ≥75 y, hx of stroke	ASA or no tx	ASA or Anticoagulant[1] or no tx	Anticoagulant[1]
HAS-BLED	Bleeding risk of anticoagulant tx	1 point each for HTN, abnormal renal function, abnormal liver function, prior stroke, prior major bleeding, labile INRs, age ≥65, alcohol use, drug use	If $CHADS_2$ or CHA_2DS_2–VASc score is 1, the risk of bleeding with anticoagulant tx may outweigh the risk of stroke if the HAS-BLED score is >2. If $CHADS_2$ or CHA_2DS_2–VASc score is ≥2, the risk of bleeding from anticoagulant tx may outweigh the risk of stroke if the HAS-BLED score exceeds the $CHADS_2$ or CHA_2DS_2–VASc score.		

[1] Apixaban, dabigatran, edoxaban, rivaroxaban, or warfarin; see **Table 17** and p 44 for dosing, p 39 for selection of anticoagulant.

Rhythm Control

- Consider in patients diagnosed with AF within the previous year regardless of symptoms.
- For patients with unpleasant symptoms or decreased exercise tolerance on rate control tx, rhythm control via direct-current or pharmacologic cardioversion is the preferred tx strategy.
  - For direct-current cardioversion, 3 methods may be used:
    - Early cardioversion (<48 h from onset): proceed with cardioversion; use adjunctive anticoagulation based on risk of thromboembolism (eg, CHA_2DS_2–VASc score).
    - Delayed cardioversion (≥48 h from onset or unknown duration) with transesophageal echocardiography (TEE): perform TEE to exclude intracardiac thrombus; if no thrombus, begin anticoagulation and cardiovert. If thrombus is present, anticoagulation tx should be given for 3 mo before repeat TEE.
    - Delayed cardioversion (≥48 h from onset or unknown duration) without TEE: anticoagulate for at least 3 wk with INR ≥2 before cardioversion; continue anticoagulation for ≥4 wk after cardioversion.
  - Stroke risk should be assessed (**Table 28**), and if indicated, antithrombotic tx should be continued indefinitely after cardioversion due to the high risk for recurrent AF.
- For cardioversion and rhythm maintenance (recommended especially if AF produces symptoms significantly impairing quality of life), catheter AF ablation or rhythm-control drugs (**Table 29**) may be tried.
  - In a nonblinded trial of ablation vs antiarrhythmic drug tx, patients that underwent ablation reported improved quality of life.
  - A meta-analysis of 6 RCTs showed lower recurrence of atrial arrhythmias, less hospitalization, and no difference in serious AEs in AF patients treated with catheter ablation compared to anti-arrhythmic drug tx.
- For patients with infrequent episodes of paroxysmal symptomatic AF, a pill-in-the-pocket strategy can be tried to convert to SR. The patient takes a β blocker or diltiazem followed 30-min later by patient-administered propafenone (450–600 mg po) or flecainide (200–300 mg po).

Table 29. Selected Medications for Rhythm Control in AF

Medication	Maintenance Dosage	Comments (Metabolism)
Amiodarone[BC]	100–200 mg/d po	Most effective antifibrillatory agent; avoid as first-line tx for AF unless patient has HF or LVH; numerous AEs, including pulmonary and hepatic toxic effects, neurologic and dermatologic AEs, hypothyroidism, hyperthyroidism, corneal deposits, warfarin interaction (L)
Flecainide	50–100 mg po q12h	Associated with increased risk of ventricular arrhythmias, dizziness most common side effect (K)
Propafenone IR	150–300 mg po q8h	Contraindicated in patients with ischemic and structural heart disease; AEs include VT and HF (L)
SR	225–425 po q12h	
Sotalol	40–160 mg po q12h	Prolongs QT interval; AEs include torsades de pointes, HF, exacerbation of COPD/bronchospasm (K)

Note: Pretx (30 min before antiarrhythmic administration) with β blocker, diltiazem, or verapamil is recommended.

AORTIC STENOSIS (AS)

Evaluation and Assessment

- Presence of symptoms—angina, syncope, HF (frequently HFpEF)—indicates severe disease and a life expectancy without surgery of <2 y.
- Echocardiography is essential to measure mean aortic valve gradient (AVG) and aortic valve area (AVA).
  - Moderate AS is indicated by an AVG of 20–39 mm Hg and by an AVA of 1–1.5 cm^2.
  - Severe AS is indicated by an AVG ≥40 mm Hg and by an AVA ≤1 cm^2.
- Don't perform echocardiography as routine follow-up for mild, asymptomatic native valve disease in adult patients with no change in signs or symptoms.[CW] Repeat echocardiography 1×/y for asymptomatic moderate AS and q6–12 mo for asymptomatic severe AS.
- ECG and CXR should be obtained initially to look for conduction defects, LVH, and pulmonary congestion.

Management

- Aortic valve replacement (AVR)
  - Indicated for severe AS or symptomatic AS.
  - AVR alleviates symptoms and improves ventricular functioning.
  - In most cases, perform AVR promptly *after* symptoms have appeared.
  - Surgical AVR (SAVR) vs transcatheter aortic valve implantation (TAVI; a percutaneous procedure in the catheterization lab in which an artificial valve is implanted via a catheter):
    - TAVI preferred over SAVR in patients with advanced age; severe lung, liver, or kidney disease; morbid obesity; frailty.
    - SAVR preferred over TAVI in younger patients and those with bicuspid aortic valve or subaortic calcification.
- Pharmacotherapy
  - Based on limited data, unless the patient has a separate indication for anticoagulation, monotx with ASA 75–100 mg/d po has fewer bleeding complications than dual platelet tx with ASA 75–100 mg/d po and clopidogrel 75 mg/d po.
  - Also based on limited data, prescribing an ACEI or ARB after TAVR may be associated with lower mortality and HF admission risk.
  - Avoid vasodilators if possible, unless used with invasive hemodynamic monitoring in patients with acute decompensated severe AS and NYHA class IV HF.

ABDOMINAL AORTIC ANEURYSM (AAA)

- Ultrasound should be performed if aortic diameter is felt to be >3 cm on physical exam.
- Ultrasonographic screening for AAA is recommended once for men aged 65–75 if former or current smoker.
- Management is based on diameter of AAA:
  - <4.5 cm: ultrasound q12mo
  - 4.5–5.4 cm: ultrasound q3–6mo
  - >5.4 cm: surgical referral
- Compared to open repair, endovascular repair is associated with significantly less perioperative morbidity and mortality up to 3 y postoperatively.

PERIPHERAL ARTERIAL DISEASE (PAD)

Evaluation

Hx should include inquiry regarding the following:

- Lower extremity exertional fatigue or pain, or pain at rest
- Poorly healing or nonhealing wounds
- Cardiac risk factors

Physical exam should include the following:

- Palpation of pulses (brachial, radial, ulnar, femoral, popliteal, posterior tibial, and dorsalis pedis)
- Auscultation for abdominal, flank, and femoral bruits
- Inspection of feet
- Skin inspection for distal hair loss, trophic skin changes, and/or hypertrophic nails

Diagnosis established by ABI <0.9 or other test (**Table 30**).

Table 30. Management of PAD

Signs and Symptoms	Useful Tests	Treatment (see below)
Asymptomatic; diminished or absent peripheral pulses	ABI[1]	Risk factor reduction[2]
Atypical leg pain	ABI[1], SABI	Risk factor reduction, antiplatelet tx[2]
Claudication: exertional fatigue, discomfort, pain relieved by rest	ABI[1], SABI, Doppler ultrasound, pulse volume recording, segmental pressure measurement	Risk factor reduction, antiplatelet tx, claudication tx; consider endovascular or surgical revascularization if symptoms persist[2]
Signs and Symptoms	**Useful Tests**	**Treatment (see below)**
Rest pain, nonhealing wound (see also p 330), gangrene	ABI[1], Doppler ultrasound, angiography (MRI, CT, or contrast)	Risk factor reduction, antiplatelet tx, claudication tx, endovascular or surgical revascularization[2]

SABI, stress test (exercise treadmill test or reactive hyperemia for those who cannot walk on a treadmill) with ABI measurement.

[1] Abnormal is <0.9; <0.4 is critical. An ABI >1.40 is also considered abnormal, possibly due to calcified arteries, and may require further testing to rule out arterial stenosis.

[2] Refrain from percutaneous or surgical revascularization of peripheral artery stenosis in patients without claudication or critical limb ischemia.[CW]

Management

Risk Factor Reduction

- Smoking cessation
- Lipid-lowering tx (Dyslipidemia Management, p 51)
- HTN tx (p 54)
- DM tx (Endocrine chapter, p 112)

Antiplatelet Therapy

- ASA 75–325 mg/d po
- Clopidogrel 75 mg/d po if no response or intolerant of ASA

Claudication Therapy

- Walking program (goal: 30–50 min of intermittent walking 3–5 ×/wk)
- Cilostazol 100 mg po q12h, 1 h before or 2 h pc (contraindicated in patients with Class III or IV HFrEF[BC]); second-line alternative tx is pentoxifylline 400 mg po q8h.
- If ACEI not contraindicated, routine use is recommended to prevent cardiovascular AEs in patients with claudication.

SYNCOPE

Table 31. Classification of Syncope

Cause	Frequency, %	Features	Increased Risk of Death
Vasovagal	21	Preceded by lightheadedness, nausea, diaphoresis; recovery gradual, frequently with fatigue	No
Cardiac	10	Little or no warning before blackout, rapid and complete recovery	Yes
Orthostatic	9	Lightheaded prodrome after standing, recovery gradual	No
Medication-induced	7	Lightheaded prodrome, recovery gradual	No
Seizure	5	No warning, may have neurologic deficits, slow recovery	Yes
Stroke, TIA	4	Little or no warning, neurologic deficits	Yes
Other causes	8	Preceded by cough, micturition, or specific situation	No
Unknown	37	Any of the above	Yes

Source: Adapted from Soteriades ES et al. *N Engl J Med* 2002;347:878–885.

Evaluation

- Focus hx on events before, during, and after loss of consciousness; hx of cardiac disease (significantly worsens prognosis of syncope of all causes); careful medication review.
- Focus on cardiovascular and neurologic systems in physical exam.
- ECG and orthostatic BP or pulse check for all patients.
- Characteristics associated with serious outcomes and likely to require urgent or emergent further testing and hospital admission with monitoring include:
  - advanced age, especially >90
  - male sex
  - abnormal ECG
  - exertional syncope
  - hx of palpitations
  - syncope without prodrome
  - hx of HF
  - hx of arrhythmia (VT, symptomatic supraventricular tachycardia, third-degree or Mobitz II AV block, sinus pause >3 sec, symptomatic bradycardia)
  - structural heart disease
  - dyspnea
  - abnormal troponin I
  - persistent abnormal vital signs (eg, SBP <90 mm Hg or >160 mm Hg)
  - significant comorbidity (eg, electrolyte imbalance, severe anemia)

- Additional testing as suggested by initial evaluation:
  - Ambulatory ECG monitoring for further evaluation of arrhythmia
  - Stress testing to investigate ischemic heart disease
  - Echocardiography to investigate structural heart disease
  - Electrophysiologic studies in patients with prior MI or structural heart disease
  - Tilt-table testing for suspected vasovagal cause
  - Head imaging, EEG for suspected neurologic cause
  - Don't perform imaging of the carotid arteries or brain imaging studies (CT or MRI) for simple syncope without other neurologic symptoms.[CW]
  - If suspected orthostatic cause, evaluation for Parkinson disease, autonomic neuropathy, DM, hypovolemia

Management

- Patients with cardiac syncope require immediate hospitalization on telemetry; exclude MI and PE.
- Strongly consider hospital admission for patients with syncope due to neurologic or unknown causes, particularly if concurrent heart disease.
- Patients with syncope due to vasovagal, orthostatic, medication-induced, or other causes can usually be managed as outpatients, particularly if no hx of heart disease.
- Tx is correction of underlying cause.

ORTHOSTATIC (POSTURAL) HYPOTENSION

See also **Table 61**.

Evaluation and Assessment

- Associated with the following symptoms usually after standing: lightheadedness, dizziness, syncope, blurred vision, diaphoresis, head or neck pain, decreased hearing
- Diagnosis: ≥20 mm Hg drop in SBP or ≥10 mm Hg in DBP within 3 min of rising from lying to standing
- Causes
  - Medications, including antihypertensives, antipsychotics, TCAs, MAOIs, acetylcholinesterase inhibitors, SGLT2 inhibitors, anti-Parkinsonian drugs, PDE5 inhibitors (for erectile dysfunction)
  - Autonomic dysregulation (suggested by lack of compensatory rise in HR with postural hypotension): age-related decreased baroreceptor sensitivity, Parkinson disease and related disorders, peripheral neuropathy, prolonged bed rest
  - Hypovolemia
  - Anemia

Management

- Correct underlying disorder, particularly by discontinuing medications that could exacerbate hypotension
- Alter movement behavior: educate patients to rise slowly, flex calf and forearm muscles when standing, stand with one foot in front of other, avoid straining, and elevate head of bed
- Dietary changes: avoid alcohol, maintain adequate fluid intake, increase salt and caffeine intake
- Above-the-knee compression stockings (at least medium compression strength, eg, Jobst)

- Pharmacotherapy:
  - First-line: fludrocortisone: 0.1–0.2 mg po q8–24h; use with caution in patients with HF, cardiac disease, HTN, renal disease, esophagitis, peptic ulcer disease, or ulcerative colitis; watch for fluid overload and hypokalemia.
  - Midodrine: 2.5–10 mg po q8–24h; use with caution in patients with HTN, DM, urinary retention, renal disease, hepatic disease, glaucoma, BPH.
  - Pyridostigmine: 60 mg po q24h; can be used in combination with midodrine 2.5–5 mg/d po.
  - Caffeine: 1 cup of caffeinated coffee q8–12h; alternatively, caffeine tabs 100–200 mg po q8–12h; useful for postprandial hypotension when taken with meals. Avoid in patients with insomnia.[BC]
  - Droxidopa *(Northera)*: 100–600 mg po q8h; use with caution in patients with HTN, cardiac disease, HF, MCI, dementia, Parkinson disease on carbidopa tx.
  - Erythropoietin can be useful for hypotension secondary to anemia if Hb <10 mg/dL.

IMPLANTABLE CARDIAC DEFIBRILLATOR (ICD) PLACEMENT

Indications

- Carefully consider age, life expectancy, and comorbid status for deciding ICD placement. Data are limited in patients aged >65 and suggest no all-cause mortality benefit in patients aged >75.
- Established indications:
  - Cardiac arrest due to VF or VT
  - Spontaneous sustained VT with structural heart disease
  - Spontaneous sustained VT without structural heart disease not alleviated by other tx
  - Unexplained syncope with hemodynamically significant VF or VT inducible by electrophysiologic study when drug tx is ineffective, not tolerated, or not preferred
  - Nonsustained VT, CAD, and inducible VF by electrophysiologic study that is not suppressed by Class I antiarrhythmic
  - LVEF ≤35%, NYHA Class II or III HF, and CAD >40 d after MI
  - ICD + biventricular pacing for advanced HF (NYHA Class III or IV), LVEF ≤35%, and QRS interval ≥120 millisec or mild HF (NYHA Class I or II), LVEF <30%, and QRS interval ≥130 millisec

Contraindications

- Terminal illness with life expectancy <6 mo
- Unexplained syncope without inducible VT or VF and without structural heart disease
- VT or VF due to transient or easily reversible disorder
- End-stage HF (ACC/AHA Stage D) not awaiting cardiac transplant

Complications

- Surgical: infection (1–2%), hematoma, pneumothorax
- Device-related: lead dislodgement or malfunction, connection problems, inadequate defibrillation threshold
- Tx-related: frequent shocks (appropriate or inappropriate), acceleration of VT, anxiety and other psychological stress
- End-of-life planning: discuss and document the circumstances in which the patient would desire the ICD to be turned off. ICDs can be turned off by the cardiologist or the device manufacturer's representative. Don't leave an ICD activated when it is inconsistent with the patient/family goals of care.[CW]

DELIRIUM

DIAGNOSIS

Diagnostic Criteria—Adapted from *DSM-5*

- Core symptom: disturbed consciousness (ie, decreased attention, environmental awareness)
- Cognitive change (eg, memory deficit, disorientation, language disturbance) or perceptual disturbance (eg, visual illusions, hallucinations)
- Three subtypes: hyperactive, hypoactive, and apparently normal alertness but cannot attend
- Rapid onset (hours to days) and fluctuating daily course
- Evidence of a causal physical condition

Predisposing Factors

- Major or Mild Neurocognitive Disorder (Dementia or MCI)
- Advanced age, hearing and visual impairment
- Hospitalization and/or surgery (Postoperative Delirium, p 290)

Prediction of Delirium Risk in Hospitalized Older Patients

- Physical restraints; >3 new medications; Foley catheter; malnutrition; any iatrogenic event
- 1 point each for any, likelihood of delirium based on total: 0 points: 4%; 1–2 points: 20%; ≥3 points: 35%

Evaluation

- Assume reversibility unless proven otherwise.
- Thoroughly review prescription and OTC medications, and alcohol usage.
- Exclude infection and other medical causes.
- Ultra-Brief 2-item (UB-2) bedside test is a screening instrument for rapid initial assessment of delirium but is not diagnostic. The 2 items that tested best were:
  - "What day of the week is it?."
  - "List the months of the year backward starting with December."
- Confusion Assessment Method (CAM): Requires both acute onset and fluctuating course, inattention and either disorganized thinking or altered level of consciousness (90% sensitivity, 60% specificity).
  - CAM–S allows for scoring of delirium severity.
  - For nonverbal patients, use CAM-ICU to assess attention and level of consciousness.
  - The 3D-CAM is a brief verbal or observational assessment tool that can be completed in an average of 3-min and performs very well compared to expert evaluation (>95% sensitivity, 94% specificity).
- Lab studies may include CBC, electrolytes, LFTs, ammonia, UA and urine culture if indicated, thyroid function tests, renal function tests, serum albumin, B_{12}, serum calcium, serum glucose, oxygen saturation, ABG levels, CXR, and ECG.
- Brain imaging and EEG typically not helpful unless evidence of cerebral trauma, possible stroke, focal neurologic signs, or seizure activity.

Mnemonic for Delirium Etiology

D	Drugs
E	Electrolyte disturbances
L	Lack of drugs (withdrawal of sedatives, alcohol, opioids)
I	Infection
R	Reduced sensory input
I	Intracranial disorders
U	Urinary and fecal disorders
M	Myocardial and pulmonary disorders

CAUSES

Table 32. Causes of Delirium (Most Common in Older Adults)

Cause	Examples
Medications (**Table 34**)	*Anticholinergics*[BC] (**Table 35**) Anti-inflammatory agents, including prednisone Benzodiazepines[BC] or alcohol: either acute toxicity or withdrawal Cardiovascular (eg, digoxin, antihypertensives, diuretics) Lithium Opioid analgesics, especially meperidine (Avoid[BC])
Infections	*Respiratory, skin, urinary tract,* others
Metabolic Disorders	Acute blood loss, *dehydration, electrolyte imbalance,* end-organ failure (hepatic, renal), hyperglycemia, *hypoglycemia, hypoxia*
Cardiovascular	Arrhythmia, *HF, MI,* shock
Neurologic	CNS infections, head trauma, seizures, stroke, subdural hematoma, TIAs, tumors
Miscellaneous	Fecal impaction, *postoperative state,* sleep deprivation, urinary retention, pain, immobility

Note: Italicized type indicates the most common causes in older adults.

Table 33. Delirium vs Dementia

	Delirium	Dementia
Onset	Acute	Gradual
Course	Fluctuating	Stepwise deterioration
Attention	Inability to concentrate	May be able to concentrate
Duration	Hours, days, months	Years
Perception	Often impaired	Less frequently impaired
EEG	Diffuse slowing	Normal or slow wave activity common (most prominent in LBD). Focal changes in advanced vascular dementia
Sleep	Disrupted	Less disrupted
Prognosis	Usually improves	Poor

Table 34. Potentially Differentiating Features of Medication-induced Delirium

Factor	Anticholinergic	Serotonin Syndrome	Neuroleptic Malignant Syndrome
Causative medications	Anticholinergic agents	Serotonergic agents	Dopamine antagonists
Physical exam findings	Visual impairment, dry mouth, constipation, urinary retention, increased HR, mydriasis, decreased bowel sounds	Tremor, diarrhea, hyperreflexia, clonus, myoclonic jerks, increased bowel sounds, diaphoresis	Increased EPS, marked rigidity, bradyreflexia, hyperthermia
Lab findings	More commonly no lab findings	More commonly no lab findings	Increased Cr, kinase, leukocytosis, low serum iron

Table 35. Some Drugs with Strong Anticholinergic Properties[BC]

Antidepressants		
Amitriptyline Amoxapine Clomipramine Desipramine	Doxepin (>6 mg) Imipramine Nortriptyline Paroxetine	Protriptyline Trimipramine
Antihistamines		
Brompheniramine Carbinoxamine Chlorpheniramine Clemastine Cyproheptadine Dexbrompheniramine	Dexchlorpheniramine Dimenhydrinate Diphenhydramine Doxylamine Hydroxyzine Meclizine	Pyrilamine Triprolidine
Antimuscarinics (urinary incontinence)		
Darifenacin Fesoterodine Flavoxate	Oxybutynin Solifenacin Tolterodine	Trospium
Antiparkinson agents		
Benztropine	Trihexyphenidyl	
Antipsychotics		
Chlorpromazine Clozapine Loxapine	Olanzapine Perphenazine Promethazine	Thioridazine Trifluoperazine
Antispasmodics		
Atropine products (excludes ophthalmics) Belladonna alkaloids Chlordiazepoxide-clidinium	Dicyclomine Homatropine (excludes ophthalmics) Hyoscyamine products	Methscopolamine Propantheline Scopolamine (excludes ophthalmics)
Skeletal Muscle Relaxants		
Cyclobenzaprine	Orphenadrine	

Note: AGS updated Beers Criteria® for potentially inappropriate medication use in older adults.[BC] American Geriatrics Society 2019 Beers Criteria® Update Expert Panel. *J Am Geriatr Soc* 2019:67(4):674–694.

PREVENTIVE MEASURES

Delirium can be prevented in 30% of cases. (https://www.nice.org.uk/about/nice-communities/social-care/quick-guides/recognising-and-preventing-delirium).

Good nutrition and hydration, early mobility, and meaningful cognitive engagement ("Eat Walk Engage") can significantly reduce the incidence of delirium.

Table 36. Preventive Measures for Delirium[1]

Target for Prevention	Intervention
Cognitive impairment	Orientation protocol: board with names, daily schedule, and reorienting communication
	Therapeutic activities: stimulating activities 3×/d
Sleep deprivation	Nonpharmacologic: warm milk/herbal tea, music, massage
	Noise reduction: schedule adjustments and unit-wide noise reduction; if possible, ensure daylight to maintain circadian rhythm
	Ramelteon 8 mg/d or suvorexant 15 mg/d may prevent delirium in acute care
Immobility	Early mobilization: ambulation or range of motion 3×/d, minimal immobilizing equipment
Visual impairment	Visual aids and adaptive equipment
Hearing impairment	Amplification, cerumen disimpaction, special communication techniques
Dehydration	Early recognition and volume repletion
Infection, HF, hypoxia, pain	Identify and treat medical conditions

[1] May also be valuable for management

See *AGS Clinical Practice Guideline for Postoperative Delirium in Older Adults,* www.geriatricscareonline.org.

MANAGEMENT

Nonpharmacologic Interventions

- Identify and correct underlying cause or contributing factors.
- Relieve distress and maintain safety and vital functions.
- Use families or sitters as first line.
- Physical restraints can lead to serious injury or death and may worsen agitation and delirium.[CW] Use soft physical restraints or mitts only as last resort to maintain patient safety (eg, to prevent patient from pulling out tubes or catheters).

Pharmacotherapy

Avoid antipsychotics for behavioral problems unless nonpharmacological options (eg, behavioral interventions) have failed or are not possible, and the older adult is threatening substantial harm to self or others.[BC]

For acute agitation or aggression that impairs care or safety (other than delirium due to alcohol or benzodiazepine withdrawal), choose from one of the following:

Quetiapine[BC]

- The drug of choice for patients with LBD, Parkinson disease, AIDS-related dementia, or EPS
- Initial dosage 12.5–25 mg po daily or q12h, increase q2d prn to a max of 100 mg/d (50 mg/d in frail older adults). Once symptoms are controlled, administer half the dose needed to control symptoms for 2–3 d; then taper as described above.

Olanzapine

- Although injectable olanzapine is sometimes used, it has higher anticholinergic effects.

Dexmedetomidine

- IV dexmedetomidine is gaining use in ICU patients as a component of sedation tx for delirium or prophylaxis, although trial results are mixed; is sympatholytic and can cause significant hypotension, bradycardia, or both. (See Preoperative and Perioperative Care.)

Cholinesterase inhibitors

- Contraindicated for adjunctive tx of delirium in intensive care (may increase mortality).

Alcohol/Benzodiazepine withdrawal

- Benzodiazepine (eg, lorazepam in dosages of 0.5–2 mg IV q30–60min or po q1–2h and titrated to effect)
- Validated scales are used to guide dosing of benzodiazepines in alcohol withdrawal (Substance-related and Addictive Disorders, p 352).
- Because these agents themselves may cause delirium, gradual withdrawal and discontinuation are desirable.
- If delirium is secondary to alcohol, also use thiamine at 100 mg/d (po, IM, or IV).

PROGNOSIS

- Weeks or months to resolve
- Waxing and waning mental status continues as patient improves, but there will be a general trend toward improvement.
- Persistent symptoms at discharge: 45%; at 1 mo: 33%; at 3 mo: 26%; at 6 mo: 21%.
- Accelerated cognitive decline: Patients with AD may experience a faster rate of cognitive decline after an episode of delirium.
- Prolonged delirium is associated with higher risk of death (2.5× more likely within 1 y compared to those whose delirium has resolved).

DEMENTIA AND COGNITIVE IMPAIRMENT

DEMENTIA SYNDROME (*DSM-5:* MAJOR NEUROCOGNITIVE DISORDER)

Definition

Chronic acquired decline in one or more cognitive domains (learning and memory, complex attention, language, visual-spatial, executive) sufficient to affect daily life.

Estimated Frequencies of Causes of Dementia

- AD: 60–70%
- Other progressive disorders: 15–30% (eg, vascular, Lewy body [LBD], frontotemporal [FTD] including primary progressive aphasia [PPA])
- Completely reversible dementia (eg, severe [psychotic] depression, drug toxicity, metabolic changes, thyroid disease, subdural hematoma, normal-pressure hydrocephalus): 2–5%

Screening

- Dementia is largely unrecognized and underdiagnosed. Clinicians should have a low threshold for triggering an investigation for possible cognitive impairment.
- The value of dementia screening in older adults is controversial. Some professional organizations strongly endorse screening while others do not recommend it, citing lack of evidence of benefit. USPSTF 2020 concluded that evidence was insufficient to recommend either for or against dementia screening.
- Screening for cognitive impairment is a required element of the initial and subsequent Medicare Annual Wellness Visit.
- Suitable screening tests in primary care include the Montreal Cognitive Assessment (MoCA), Mini-Cog (p 2), the Memory Impairment Screen (MIS), General Practitioner Assessment of Cognition (GPCOG), the Informant Questionnaire on Cognitive Decline in the Elderly (IQCODE), the Self-Administered Gerocognitive Examination (SAGE), and the AD8 Dementia Screening Interview. The AGS Cognitive Screening Toolkit includes links to open-access cognitive screening tests (geriatricscareonline.org).
- Brief cognitive tests accurately distinguish AD from normal cognition but are less accurate in distinguishing MCI from AD.

EVALUATION

Identifying and treating secondary physical conditions may improve function.

- Hx: Obtain from family or other caregiver
- Physical and neurologic exam
- Assess functional status: ADLs, IADLs, or using a home-based caregiver scale such as the Dementia Severity Rating Scale (DSRS)
- Assess for depression (PHQ-9, GDS)
- Evaluate mental status for attention, immediate and delayed recall, remote memory, language, visual-spatial cognition, and executive function. Although instruments can be helpful, the diagnosis of dementia requires a clinical assessment.
  - When possible, select and use a single instrument where all who administer have training on its proper use and can receive periodic refresher training.
  - Select an instrument(s) for the populations served:
    - MoCA (mocatest.org) requests that users of the paper version register and complete certification; training is free for students, faculty, and academic researchers, and available to others for a fee.
      - Translated into 35 languages and dialects
      - MoCA Duo test is an app available for a monthly fee; helps standardization, calculates score.

- MoCA-B for patients with low literacy
- MoCA-BLIND eliminates visual components (https://www.mocatest.org/pdf_files/test/MoCA-Test-BLIND.pdf).
- Rowland Universal Dementia Assessment Scale (RUDAS) minimizes effects of cultural learning and language diversity on cognitive performance; provides instructions for interpreters. (dementia.org.au/resources/rowland-universal-dementia-assessment-scale-rudas)
- Repeatable Battery for the Assessment of Neuropsychological Status (RBANS), a 30-min neuropsychological test, best administered by or under the supervision of a psychologist. Useful in detecting and differentiating MCI and early dementia. Materials must be purchased (pearsonassessments.com/search.html); available in Spanish.
- SLUMS (St Louis University Mental Status; slu.edu/medicine/internal-medicine/geriatric-medicine/aging-successfully/pdfs/slums_form.pdf), free online training video recommended before first use and annually for review.
  - Available in 23 languages and dialects.

- See **Table 39** for staging
- Comprehensive evaluation can be billed using cognition and functional assessment code 99483 (p 370)

Clinical Features Distinguishing AD and Other Types of Dementia

- AD: Memory, language, visual-spatial disturbances, indifference, delusions, agitation
  - Frontal variant AD: Prominent executive dysfunction, language impairment and behavioral problems
- FTD
  - Behavioral variant: behavioral disinhibition, apathy, stereotyped compulsive or ritualistic behavior, hyperorality, executive dysfunction with relative sparing of memory
  - Language variant: semantic PPA-progressive loss of word meaning, difficulty naming pictures and objects and nonfluent or agrammatic PPA, gradual impairment of language and difficulty speaking
  - LBD: visual hallucinations, delusions, EPS, fluctuating mental status, increased ADRs to antipsychotic medications. LBD is one of the subcortical dementias, as are Parkinson disease, progressive supranuclear palsy, corticobasal degeneration, and multiple system atrophy. Neurologic features that differentiate these disorders are given in **Table 94**.
- Vascular dementia: abrupt onset, stepwise deterioration, prominent aphasia, motor signs
- LATE 43 (limbic-predominant age-related TDP-43 encephalopathy): newly recognized; may occur in >20% (up to 50%) of adults aged >80; appears clinically similar to late-onset AD; at this writing, no disease biomarker identified through autopsy

Lab Testing

- Routine testing: CBC, TSH, B_{12}, homocysteine, MMA, serum calcium, liver and kidney function tests, electrolytes; HIV, and serologic test for syphilis (selectively)
- Used for research but not clinical practice: genetic testing, commercial "Alzheimer blood tests," and CSF levels (tau and β-amyloid).

Neuroimaging

The likelihood of detecting structural lesions is increased with:

- Onset age <60
- Focal (unexplained) neurologic signs or symptoms
- Abrupt onset or rapid decline (weeks to months)
- Predisposing conditions (eg, metastatic cancer or anticoagulants)

Neuroimaging may detect the 5% of cases with clinically significant structural lesions that would otherwise be missed.

American Academy of Neurology (AAN) recommends at least one structural scan (Non-contrast CT or non-contrast MRI) in the routine evaluation of dementia.

FDG-PET scans are approved by Medicare for atypical presentation or course of AD in which FTD is suspected. See https://www.cms.gov/medicare-coverage-database/view/ncacal-decision-memo.aspx?proposed=N&NCAId=104.

Florbetapir F18 *(Amyvid)* has been approved by the FDA for the detection of amyloid plaques. A positive scan does not establish diagnosis. Medicare does not cover.

Flortaucipir F18 injection *(Tauvid)* has been recently approved by the FDA to estimate the density and distribution of tau neurofibrillary tangles in patients being evaluated for AD. Medicare does not cover.

Amyloid PET, FDG-PET, and CSF test combinations may add accuracy to clinical evaluation.

FUNCTIONAL ASSESSMENT STAGING TOOL (FAST) SCALE

This 16-item scale is designed to parallel the progressive activity limitations associated with AD. Stage 7 identifies the threshold of activity limitation that would support a prognosis of ≤6 mo remaining life expectancy.

(cont.)

FAST Scale Item	Activity Limitation Associated with AD
Stage 1	No difficulty, either subjectively or objectively
Stage 2	Complains of forgetting location of objects; subjective work difficulties
Stage 3	Decreased job functioning evident to coworkers; difficulty in traveling to new locations
Stage 4	Decreased ability to perform complex tasks (eg, planning dinner for guests, handling finances)
Stage 5	Requires assistance in choosing proper clothing
Stage 6	Decreased ability to dress, bathe, and toilet independently
Substage 6a	Difficulty putting clothing on properly
Substage 6b	Unable to bathe properly, may develop fear of bathing
Substage 6c	Inability to handle mechanics of toileting (ie, forgets to flush, does not wipe properly)
Substage 6d	Urinary incontinence
Substage 6e	Fecal incontinence
Stage 7	Loss of speech, locomotion, and consciousness
Substage 7a	Ability to speak limited (1–5 words a day)
Substage 7b	All intelligible vocabulary lost
Substage 7c	Nonambulatory
Substage 7d	Unable to sit up
Substage 7e	Unable to smile
Substage 7f	Unable to hold head up

Source: Sclan S et al. *Int Psychogeriatr* 1992;4(Suppl 1):55–69.

Prognosis

- Variable course from diagnosis, mortality 4–8 y (range 2–20 y). Among nursing-home residents with advanced dementia, 71% die within 6 mo of admission.
- Complications of advanced dementia include pressure ulcers, constipation, pain, and shortness of breath.
- Refer to palliative care if FAST Stage 7.

***DSM-5* CRITERIA FOR MILD NEUROCOGNITIVE DISORDER** (aka Mild Cognitive Impairment [MCI])

- Evidence of modest cognitive decline from a previous level of performance in one or more cognitive domains (**Tables 37 and 38**)
  - concern of the individual, a knowledgeable informant, or the clinician that there has been a mild decline in cognitive function, and
  - a modest impairment in cognitive performance, preferably documented by standardized neuropsychological testing or, in its absence, another quantified clinical assessment

Table 37. Cognitive Domains

Domain	Example of associated skill
Complex attention	Selective and sustained attention
Executive function	Decision making; flexibility; planning; working memory
Language	Object naming; word retrieval; use of speech
Learning and memory	Episodic and semantic memory; short-term and long-term recall
Perceptual/motor	Visual discrimination; spatial ability; hand-eye and body-eye coordination
Social cognition	Nonverbal communication; emotional recognition and regulation

Table 38. Major and Mild Neurocognitive Disorder

	Normal	Mild (MCI)	Major (Dementia)
Memory complaints	+	+	+
Decline in objective cognition	–	+	+
Functional impairment	–	–	+

- The cognitive deficits do not interfere with one's capacity for independence in everyday activities (ie, complex IADLs such as paying bills or managing medications are preserved), but greater effort, compensatory strategies, or accommodation may be required.
- The cognitive deficits do not occur exclusively in the context of a delirium.
- The cognitive deficits are not better explained by another mental disorder (eg, major depressive disorder, schizophrenia).
- In addition to the above, criteria from the National Institute on Aging-Alzheimer's Association for diagnosis of Mild Neurocognitive Disorder (aka MCI) requires at least 2 abnormal neuropsychological test scores (–1.0 to –2.0 SD) based on published norms, corrected for age, education, and premorbid IQ.
- MCI diagnoses may be further classified as amnestic MCI if at least one episodic memory test score is abnormal. If no memory test scores are abnormal, the MCI diagnosis is classified as nonamnestic MCI.
- Demarcations between normal cognition and MCI can be difficult, requiring clinical judgment.

- 12–15% annual conversion of MCI to dementia syndrome; some cases may not progress.
- Depression frequently coexists with MCI, remains underdiagnosed and undertreated, and may contribute to dementia progression.

Table 39. Progression of Alzheimer Disease

Functional Impairment	Cognitive Changes	Behavioral Issues	Complications	Score			
				MMSE	**CDR**	**DSRS**	**FAST**
Mild Cognitive Impairment (preclinical)				26–30	0.5	5–10	3
None	Report by patient or caregiver of memory loss Objective signs of memory impairment Mild construction, language, or executive dysfunction	—	—				
Early, Mild Impairment (y 1–3 from onset of symptoms)				21–25	1	11–24	4
Managing finances Driving Managing medications	Decreased insight Short-term memory deficits Poor judgment	Social withdrawal Mood changes: apathy, depression	Poor financial decisions AEs due to medication errors				
Middle, Moderate Impairment (y 2–8)				11–20	2	25–35	5–6
IADL Difficulty with some ADLs Gait and balance	Disoriented to date and place Worse memory Getting lost in familiar areas Repeating questions	Delusions, agitation, aggression Apathy, depression Restlessness, anxiety, wandering	Inability to remain at home Falls				
Late, Severe Impairment (y 6–12)				0–10	3	36–54	7
ADLs including continence Mobility Swallowing	Little or unintelligible verbal output Loss of remote memory Inability to recognize family/ friends	Motor or verbal agitation, aggression Apathy, depression Sundowning	Pressure sores Contractures Aspiration Pneumonia				

CDR, Clinical Dementia Rating Scale; DSRS, Dementia Severity Rating Scale; FAST, Functional Assessment Staging Tool (p 84); MMSE, Mini-Mental State Examination.

NONCOGNITIVE SYMPTOMS

Psychotic Symptoms (seen in about 20% of patients with AD)

- Delusions may be paranoid (eg, people stealing things, spouse unfaithful)
- Hallucinations (~11% of patients) are more commonly visual

Depressive Symptoms (seen in up to 40% of patients with AD)
- May precede onset of AD
- May cause acceleration of decline if untreated
- Suspect if patient stops eating or withdraws

Apathy (seen in about 50% of patients with AD)
- High prevalence and persistence throughout course of AD
- Causes more impairment in ADL than expected for cognitive status
- High overlap with depressive symptoms but lacks depressive mood, guilt, and hopelessness

Agitation or Aggression (seen in up to 80% of patients with AD)
- A leading cause of nursing-home admission
- Consider superimposed delirium
- Consider pain as a cause in moderate or severe dementia and possible trial of analgesics (Pain chapter, p 252)

Sleep Disorders (seen in 39% of patients with AD)

RISK AND PROTECTIVE FACTORS FOR DEMENTIA

Definite Risks	Possible Risks	Possible Protections
Age	DM	Adequate control of HTN
APOE-E4 (Whites)	Delirium	Mediterranean diet, DASH diet
AF	Heavy smoking	Physical activity
Depression	Hypercholesterolemia	
Down syndrome	HTN	
Family hx	Lower educational level	
Head trauma	Other genes	
	Postmenopausal HT	
	Sleep apnea	
	Stress	

PREVENTION
- Promote brain health by exercise, balanced diet, stress reduction.
- A large 2-y RCT of a multidomain intervention of diet, exercise, cognitive training, vascular risk —suggests that cognitive functioning in at-risk older people can be improved or maintained. Although dementia not prevented rate of cognitive decline was diminished.
- Intensive SBP control (<120 mm Hg) reduced risk of MCI (hazard ratio 0.81) and the combined outcome MCI or dementia (hazard ratio 0.85).
- Antihypertensives that stimulate—as opposed to inhibit—type 2 and 4 angiotensin II receptors had lower rates of incident cognitive impairment. ARBs, thiazide diuretics, and DiCCBs upregulate angiotensin II production and are stimulating. ACEIs, BBs, and non-DiCCBs downregulate angiotensin II production.
- The Lancet Commission on Dementia Prevention estimates that addressing modifiable risk factors over the life course could delay or prevent 40% of dementia cases.

MANAGEMENT

Primary goals of tx are to improve quality of life and maximize functional performance by enhancing cognition, mood, and behavior.

General Treatment Principles

- Identify and treat comorbid physical illnesses (eg, HTN, DM).
- Supervised exercise, whether individual or group, slows disability and prevent falls.
- Vitamin E at 1000 IU 2×/d found to delay functional decline in mild to moderate AD. *Note:* The USPSTF recommends against the use of vitamin E for the prevention of CVD or cancer.
- Avoid anticholinergic medications (**Table 35**).
- Limit prn psychotropic medication use.
- Maximize and maintain functioning (eg, graded assistance: as little help as possible to perform ADLs, practice, and positive reinforcement to increase independence, but with realistic goals).
- Scheduled and prompted toileting (p 174) for UI
- Identify, quantify, and examine the context of any problematic behaviors (is it harmful to patient or others) and environmental triggers (eg, overstimulation, unfamiliar surroundings, frustrating interactions); exclude underlying physical discomfort (eg, illnesses or medication); consider nonpharmacologic strategies.
- Consider referral to hospice (FAST = 7; diminished speech, movement, and consciousness; see Palliative Care and Hospice chapter, **Table 104**).
- The Dementia Management Quality Measurement Set developed by the AAN and the American Psychiatric Association serves as a useful guideline (https://n.neurology.org/content/94/5/210).

Caregiver Issues

- More than 50% develop depression.
- Physical illness, isolation, anxiety, and burnout are common.
- Discuss with patient and family concerns (eg, driving).
- Intervene to decrease hazards of wandering.
- Advise family about sources of care and support, financial and legal issues.
- Intensive education, training, and support of caregivers may delay institutionalization.
- Adult day care for patients and respite services may help.
- Alzheimer's Association offers support, education services (alz.org).
- Family Caregiver Alliance (www.caregiver.org) offers support, education, and information.
- Information about clinical studies can be found at alz.org/research.

Pharmacotherapy of Cognitive Dysfunction

- Patients with a diagnosis of mild or moderate AD should receive a trial of a cholinesterase inhibitor; donepezil also approved for severe AD (**Table 40**).
  - Cholinesterase inhibitors should be prescribed with periodic assessment for cognitive benefits and GI AEs.[CW] Patients should be monitored for weight loss.
  - Only 10–25% of patients taking cholinesterase inhibitors show modest global improvement, but many more have less rapid cognitive decline.
  - Initial studies show benefits of cholinesterase inhibitors for patients with dementia associated with LBD, Parkinson disease, and mixed dementia (AD and vascular). May worsen behavioral variant FTD.
  - Cholinesterase inhibitors may attenuate noncognitive symptoms and delay nursing-home placement.

- AEs increase with higher dosing. Possible AEs include nausea, vomiting, diarrhea, dyspepsia, anorexia, weight loss, leg cramps, bradycardia, syncope, insomnia, and agitation.
- Aducanumab reduces amyloid β plaques in the brain, but evidence is currently equivocal on whether it can slow cognitive decline, Medicare coverage is only available for those enrolled in clinical trials. See AGS guidance geriatricscareonline.org/ProductAbstract/Aducanumab-What-Clinicians-Should-Know/PC0013.
- Lecanemab (*Leqembi*;10 mg/kg q2wk) for patients with MCI or mild AD. CMS coverage pending at press time.

- Patients with moderate to severe AD may benefit from a trial of memantine *(Namenda)*.
  - Side effects minimal (confusion, dizziness, constipation, headache)
  - Several RCTs failed to demonstrate significant advantage to the combination of memantine and donepezil compared with donepezil alone in patients with severe dementia.
  - To evaluate response:
    - Elicit caregiver observations of patient's behavior (alertness, initiative) and follow functional status (ADLs).
    - Follow cognitive status (eg, improved or stabilized) by caregiver's report or serial ratings of cognition (eg, Mini-Cog [p 2]; MMSE).
- D/C medications for cognitive dysfunction when FAST = 7 or lower (p 84).
- Ginkgo biloba is not generally recommended (p 26).
- *Axona* (medium-chain TG) has insufficient evidence to support its value in preventing or treating AD, and long-term effects are uncertain.

Table 40. Medications to Treat Cognitive Dysfunction

Medication	Dosing (Metabolism)
Cholinesterase inhibitors	*Class effects:* Avoid if hx of syncope.[BC]
Donepezil[1,2] (*Adlarity* transdermal pch)	Start at 5 mg/d po or 5 mg/d pch applied 1×/wk, increase to 10 mg/d po or 10 mg/d pch 1×/wk after 1 mo (CYP2D6, -3A4); must be on 10 mg/d po ≥3 mo to consider increasing to 23 mg/d po in moderate to severe AD Those with moderate to severe AD who have been on a stable dose of 10 mg/d for ≥3 mo may be given a trial at 23 mg/d if they are tolerating the 10-mg/d dose. It can be administered concomitantly with memantine; for patients taking memantine, donepezil can be added and then uptitrated to 23 mg, or memantine can be added to donepezil 10 mg before uptitrating the dose to 23 mg. Caution is advocated when using donepezil 23 mg in patients with a low body weight (<55 kg), a hx of GI bleeding, and AV block. (L)
Galantamine[1,3]	Start at 4 mg po q12h, increase to 8 mg po q12h after 4 wk; minimally effective dosage 8 or 12 mg po q12h (CYP2D6, -3A4) (L)
(Razadyne ER)	Start at 1 C/d, preferably with food; titrate as above. Rare complication: Stevens-Johnson syndrome
Rivastigmine *(Exelon)*[1]	Start at 1.5 mg po q12h and gradually titrate up to minimally effective dosage of 3 mg q12h; continue up to 6 mg q12h as tolerated; for pch, start at 4.6 mg/d, may be increased after ≥4 wk to 9.5 mg/d (recommended effective dosage; value of increase to 13.3 mg/d is not established): retitrate if drug is stopped; pch may be helpful if GI AEs on oral meds (K)

(cont.)

Table 38. Medications to Treat Cognitive Dysfunction (cont.)	
Medication	**Dosing (Metabolism)**
NMDA antagonist[2]	
Memantine[4]	Start at 5 mg/d po, increase by 5 mg at weekly intervals to max of 10 mg q12h; if CrCl <30 mL/min, max of 5 mg q12h (K)
XR	Start at 7 mg/d po, increase by 7 mg at weekly intervals to max of 28 mg; if severe renal impairment, max of 14 mg daily (L)
Combination Agent	
Memantine and donepezil *(Namzaric)*	Fixed-dose combination of donepezil and memantine for patients previously stabilized on combination tx of both individual drugs (much more expensive)

[1] Cholinesterase inhibitors. Continue if improvement or stabilization occurs.

[2] Approved by FDA for moderate to severe AD.

[3] Increased mortality found in controlled studies of MCI.

[4] Patients can switch directly from memantine IR 20 mg (10 mg po 2×/d) to memantine XR 28 mg po 1×/d on the day after the last dose of a 10-mg IR tab. Patients with severe renal impairment on memantine IR 5 mg po 2×/d can be switched to memantine XR 14 mg po 1×/d.

Nonpharmacologic Approaches for Problem Behaviors

- Music during meals, bathing
- Walking or light exercise
- Simulate family presence with video or audio tapes
- Pet tx
- Speak at patient's comprehension level
- Bright light, white noise (ie, low-level, background noise)

Approaches for assessment and management of behavioral symptoms of dementia can be found on the UCLA Alzheimer's and Dementia Care Program website (uclahealth.org/dementia).

The evidence base for specific nonpharmacologic approaches using a person-centered approach to care is growing. A nonpharmacologic toolkit for reducing antipsychotic use in nursing homes can be found at nursinghometoolkit.com.

Management of Agitation

- Consider nonpharmacologic approaches first before pharmacotherapy (**Table 41**).
- Steps to reduce nonverbalized pain (p 252).
- Treating cognitive dysfunction (**Table 40**) may slow deterioration, and agitation may worsen if discontinued.
- Low doses of antipsychotic medications have limited role but may be necessary.[BC,CW] Note that this use is off-label and increases risk of death compared with placebo in patients with AD (**Table 110** and **Table 111**). Use rating scale such as the Neuropsychiatric Inventory to assess and quantify symptoms.
- In a placebo-controlled randomized trial, citalopram was found to significantly reduce agitation and caregiver distress. Cognitive and cardiac (QT interval prolongation) AEs at the study dose of 30 mg/d po limits practical application. Appropriate trials for escitalopram have not yet been conducted.
- Limited evidence supports use of dextromethorphan-quinidine (*Nuedexta*)[BC] 20 mg/10 mg po 1×/d.
- Behavioral variant FTD: consider memantine or SSRI.

- Pimavanserin (*Nuplazid*) attenuates psychosis in patients with AD but has same black box warning regarding increased mortality risk. Its use in patients with dementia is considerably less; not FDA approved for AD. Prolongs QT interval, can cause nausea, ataxia, hallucinations, confusion, and peripheral edema.
  - A small clinical trial of persons with dementia who received pimavanserin for psychotic symptoms were less likely to relapse if the drug was maintained compared to discontinuation; may cause QT prolongation and increased risk of hospitalization and death in nursing-home residents.
  - A retrospective cohort study of nursing-home residents with Parkinson disease found pimavanserin use associated with an increased risk of hospitalization after 1 mo and death out to 1 y.

Treatment of Apathy

- Assess and treat underlying depression.
- Cholinesterase inhibitors help.
- Methylphenidate (10 mg bid po) has been found to be safe and efficacious.

Table 41. Pharmacotherapy for Agitation

Symptom	Medication	Dosage
Agitation in context of psychosis	Aripiprazole[BC,1,2]	2.5–12.5 mg/d po
	Olanzapine[BC,1,2]	2.5–10 mg/d po
	Quetiapine[BC,1,2]	12.5–100 mg/d po
	Risperidone[BC,1,2]	0.25–3 mg/d po
Agitation in context of depression	SSRI[BC] (eg, citalopram, escitalopram, sertraline)	10–20 mg/d po (citalopram) 5–10 mg/d po (escitalopram) 25–100 mg/d po (sertraline)
Anxiety, mild to moderate irritability	Buspirone[3] Trazodone[4]	15–60 mg/d po 50–100 mg/d po
Refractory agitation or aggression	Carbamazepine[BC,5]	300–600 mg/d po
	Divalproex sodium[BC,6]	500–1500 mg/d po
	Olanzapine[BC,2,7]	2.5–5 mg IM
Sexual aggression, impulse-control symptoms in men	SSRIs[BC], second-generation antipsychotics,[BC] or divalproex[BC]	See dosages above
	If no response, estrogen	0.625–1.25 mg/d po
	Medroxyprogesterone	100 mg IM/wk

[1] Avoid.[BC]

[2] Increased risk of mortality and cerebrovascular events compared with placebo; use with particular caution in patients with cerebrovascular disease or hypovolemia.

[3] Can be given q12h; allow 2–4 wk for adequate trial.

[4] Small divided daytime dosage and larger bedtime dosage; watch for sedation and orthostasis.

[5] Monitor serum levels; periodic CBCs, platelet counts secondary to agranulocytosis risk. Beware of drug-drug interactions.

[6] Can monitor serum levels; usually well tolerated; check CBC, platelets for agranulocytosis, thrombocytopenia risk in older adults.

[7] For acute use only; initial dose 2.5–5 mg, second dose (2.5–5 mg) can be given after 2 h, max of 3 injections in 24 h (max daily dose 20 mg); should not be administered for >3 consecutive d.

DEPRESSION

EVALUATION AND ASSESSMENT

Major depression occurs in approximately 2% of people aged ≥55 and increases with age; 15% may have clinically significant depressive symptoms without major depression.

Recognizing and diagnosing late-life depression can be difficult. Older adults may complain of lack of energy or other somatic symptoms, attribute symptoms to old age or other physical conditions, or neglect to mention them to a healthcare professional.

Consider screening with Patient Health Questionnaire 2 (PHQ-2):

- Over the past 2 wk, have you often had little interest or pleasure in doing things?
- Over the past 2 wk, have you often been bothered by feeling down, depressed, or hopeless?

Score each item: 0 = not at all, 1 = several days, 2 = more than half the days, 3 = nearly every day; a score ≥3 indicates high probability of depressive disorder.

Follow-up and/or assess tx with PHQ-9, clinician-rated Cornell Scale for Depression in Dementia or self-rated scale such as the GDS (collateral source version available).

Medical Evaluation

TSH, B_{12}, calcium, liver and kidney function tests, electrolytes, UA, CBC

DSM-5 Criteria for Major Depressive Disorder (Abbreviated)

Five or more of the following criteria have been present during the same 2-wk period and represent a change from previous functioning; at least one of the symptoms is either depressed mood ***or*** loss of interest or pleasure. Do not include symptoms that are clearly due to a medical condition. The following mnemonic (SIGECAMPS) captures the main symptoms:

S **S**leep disturbance
I Loss of **I**nterest or pleasure in usual activities
G Excessive feelings of **G**uilt or worthlessness
E Decreased **E**nergy and increased fatigue
C Diminished ability to think or **C**oncentrate
A **A**ppetite change with weight loss/gain
M **M**ood is low most days
P **P**sychomotor agitation or retardation
S **S**uicidal ideation

The *DSM-5* criteria are not specific for older adults; cognitive symptoms may be more prominent, and concurrent medical disorders are common.

Subsyndromal Depression

Subsyndromal depression does not meet full criteria for major depressive disorder and may include adjustment disorders and milder depression with anxiety symptoms but can be serious and associated with functional impairment. In older adults, subsyndromal depression may actually reflect major depression not diagnosed by current diagnostic criteria and may require pharmacotherapy and nonpharmacologic intervention.

Prolonged Grief Disorder

Persistent and pervasive grief response 12 mo after bereavement, characterized by persistent longing, yearning, or preoccupation with the deceased accompanied by ≥3 of

8 other symptoms: disbelief, intense emotional pain, feeling of identity confusion, avoidance of reminders of the loss, feelings of numbness, intense loneliness, meaninglessness, or difficulty engaging in ongoing life. May affect 10% of bereaved. Grief-focused CBT has been found to help.

MANAGEMENT

Tx should be individualized on the basis of hx, past response, and severity of illness as well as concurrent illnesses.

Nonpharmacologic Interventions

For mild to moderate depression (PHQ-9 scores 4–9) or in combination with pharmacotherapy: CBT, mindfulness-based CBT, interpersonal tx, problem-solving tx, repetitive transcranial magnetic stimulation (rTMS), intermittent theta burst stimulation (iTBS), transcranial direct current stimulation (tDCS).Bright light tx in morning may be helpful for seasonal depression.

CBT can be effectively delivered in group, telephone, guided self-help (internet based), or individual formats. Unguided self-help CBT has been shown to be significantly less effective.

Recently, mindfulness-based CBT performed via Internet or by phone has been found to reduce the risk of relapse in patients with major depressive disorder. For patients with major depression with mild to moderate dementia, problem adaptive therapy (PATH) may be helpful. PATH is a home-based tx that integrates problem-solving approaches with alternate strategies, environmental adaptations, and caregiver participation to improve the regulation of emotion. Supportive tx for cognitively impaired patients focuses on expression of affect, understanding, and empathy.

Physical activity and a Mediterranean diet have been found to help manage depression.

For severe pharmacological-resistant or psychotic depression, consider ECT (p 96).

Pharmacotherapy

For mild, moderate, or severe depression: the duration of tx should be 12 mo after remission for patients experiencing their first depressive episode. Most older adults with major depression require maintenance antidepressant tx. Ensure an adequate initial trial of 4–6 wk after titrating up to therapeutic dosage; if inadequate response, consider switching to a different first-line agent of a different class or second-line or combination of medications from different classes (see below).

SSRIs may increase hemorrhagic stroke risk; low initial dosages and monitoring are recommended, especially in patients at risk of stroke. Check serum sodium before starting SSRI and after a few weeks of tx; high index of suspicion for hyponatremia. SSRIs are also associated with increased risk of GI and postsurgical bleeding as well as accelerating osteoporosis and increasing fracture risk (NNH is 85 after 1 y, 46 after 2 y). Conversely, lithium appears to lower the risk of osteoporosis caused by bipolar disorder itself. Do not prescribe CYP2D6 inhibiting SSRIs (fluoxetine, paroxetine) with oxycodone because they increase overdose risk.

Choosing an Antidepressant (Table 42)

First-line Therapy: SSRI[BC] (consider sertraline, escitalopram), bupropion, or SNRI[BC] (desvenlafaxine, duloxetine, venlafaxine)

Second-line Therapy: Consider mirtazapine or vilazodone. Mirtazapine may be useful in patients with insomnia or marked weight loss. Combination tx using a reuptake inhibitor (ie, SSRI, SNRI) with an antagonist of presynaptic α2-autoreceptors (mirtazapine or trazodone) is more effective than monotx for first-line tx of acute severe depression and for patients for whom monotx fails.

Do not combine 2 serotonergic drugs.

Third-line Therapy: Consider augmentation of first- or second-line antidepressants with second-generation atypical antipsychotics[BC] (aripiprazole, brexpiprazole, quetiapine), buspirone, bupropion, lithium[BC], or vortioxetine (**Table 43**).

Esketamine *(Spravato)* nasal spray: FDA approved for tx-resistant depression. Geriatric substudy did not indicate statistically significant efficacy. Side effects include dissociation, autoscopy, suicidal ideation, dizziness, nausea, sedation, vertigo, hypoesthesia, anxiety, panic attacks, paranoia, lethargy, increased BP, vomiting, and feeling drunk.

Maintenance Treatment

After symptoms have remitted, pharmacotherapy should be maintained for 1 y after a single episode of depression, 2 y after 2 episodes, and at least 3 y for 3 or more episodes or consider indefinite maintenance.

- When stopping antidepressants, a gradual reduction in dose over at least 1 mo is recommended.
- Patients should be monitored carefully for discontinuation symptoms (flu-like syndrome, hyperarousal) or depression relapse.
- Discontinuation symptoms may be severe if medication is stopped abruptly or has a short half-life.

Table 42. Antidepressants Used for Older Adults

Class, Medication	Initial Dosage	Geriatric Dosage	Comments (Metabolism, Excretion)
SSRIs	*Class AEs*: EPS, hyponatremia, increased risk of upper GI bleeding, suicide (early in tx), lower BMD and fragility fractures, risk of toxicity if methylene blue or linezolid co-administered. Avoid if hx of falls or fracture; caution if hx of SIADH.[BC] (L, K [10%])		
Citalopram	10–20 mg po qam	20 mg/d po	20 mg/d is max dosage in adults aged >60; risk of QTc prolongation
✓Escitalopram	10 mg/d po	10 mg/d po	10 mg/d is max dosage in adults aged >60; risk of QTc prolongation
Fluoxetine	5 mg po qam	5–60 mg/d po	Long half-lives of parent and active metabolite may allow for less frequent dosing; may cause more insomnia than other SSRIs; CYP2D6, -2C9, -3A4 inhibitor (L)
Fluvoxamine	25 mg po qhs	100–300 mg/d po	Not approved as an antidepressant in US; greater likelihood of GI AEs; CYP1A2, -3A4 inhibitor (L)
Paroxetine	5 mg po	10–40 mg/d po	Increased risk of withdrawal symptoms (dizziness); anticholinergic AEs; CYP2D6 inhibitor (L)
Paroxetine hydrochloride	12.5 mg/d po	12.5–37.5 mg/d po	Increase by 12.5 mg/d no faster than 1×/wk (L)
✓Sertraline	25 mg po qam	50–200 mg/d po	Greater likelihood of GI AEs (L)

(cont.)

Table 42. Antidepressants Used for Older Adults (cont.)			
Class, Medication	**Initial Dosage**	**Geriatric Dosage**	**Comments (Metabolism, Excretion)**
SNRIs			Avoid if hx of falls or fracture; caution if hx of SIADH.[BC]
✓◆Duloxetine	20 mg/d po, then 20 mg po q12h	40–60 mg po q24h or 30 mg po q12h	Most common AEs: nausea, dry mouth, constipation, diarrhea, urinary hesitancy; contraindicated if CrCl <30
✓Venlafaxine	25–50 mg po q12h	75–225 mg/d po in divided doses	Low anticholinergic activity; minimal sedation and hypotension; may increase BP and QTc; may be useful when somatic pain present; EPS, withdrawal symptoms, hyponatremia (L)
XR	75 mg po qam	75–225 mg/d po	Same as above
✓Desvenlafaxine	50 mg/d po	50 mg po; max 400 mg po	Active metabolite of venlafaxine; adjust dosage when CrCl <30 (L, K [45%])
Additional Medications			
✓Bupropion	37.5–50 mg po q12h	75–150 mg po q12h	Consider for SSRI, TCA nonresponders; safe in HF; may be stimulating; can lower seizure threshold. Avoid.[BC] (L)
Bupropion hydrochloride SR	100 mg po q12h or q24h	100–150 mg po q12h	
Bupropion hydrochloride ER	150 mg/d po	300 mg/d po	
Levomilnacipran *(Fetzima)*	20 mg po q24h × 2 d	40 mg po q24h max; 120 mg/d po	SNRI (L, K [58%])
Lithium	150 mg/d po	300–900 mg/d po Levels 0.4–0.8 mEq/L	Risk of CNS toxicity; cognitive impairment; hypothyroidism; interactions with diuretics[BC], ACEIs, CCBs, NSAIDs
Methylphenidate	2.5–5 mg po at 7 AM and noon	5–10 mg po at 7 AM and noon	Short-term tx of depression or apathy in physically ill older adults; used as an adjunct. Avoid if insomnia. (L)
Mirtazapine	7.5 mg po qhs	15–45 mg/d po	May be quite sedating but this may diminish as dosage is increased; increased appetite; ODT (SolTab) available (L)
Vilazodone *(Viibryd)*	10 mg/d po for 7 d, then 20 mg/d	40 mg/d po	Metabolized by CYP3A4; limited geriatric data; AEs: diarrhea and nausea
Vortioxetine *(Trintellix)*		5–10 mg po q24h max; 20 mg/d po	SSRI with 5-HT1A agonist and 5-HT3 antagonist activity (L)
TCAs			Avoid.[BC]
Desipramine	10–25 mg po qhs	50–150 mg/d po	Therapeutic serum level >115 ng/mL (L)
Nortriptyline	10–25 mg po qhs	75–150 mg/d po	Therapeutic window (50–150 ng/mL) (L)

✓ = preferred for treating older adults. ◆ = Also has primary indication for neuropathic pain.
CrCl unit = mL/min.

Antidepressants to Avoid in Older Adults to Avoid Excessive AEs or Drug Interactions[BC]

- Amitriptyline
- Amoxapine
- Doxepin
- Imipramine
- Ketamine
- Maprotiline
- Protriptyline
- St John's wort
- Trimipramine

Electroconvulsive Therapy (ECT)

Generally safe and very effective. Potential complications include temporary confusion, anterograde and retrograde amnesia, arrhythmias, aspiration, falls, pneumonia.

Major AEs and death after ECT are infrequent and may occur in about 10 of 10,000 patients and after 0.4 per 10,000 ECT treatments, respectively.

Indications: Severe depression when a rapid onset of response is necessary; when depression is resistant to drug tx; for patients who are unable to tolerate antidepressants, have previous response to ECT, have psychotic depression, severe catatonia, or depression with Parkinson disease. Evaluation: Before ECT, perform CXR, ECG, serum electrolytes, and cardiac exam. Additional tests (eg, stress test, neuroimaging, EEG) are used selectively.

Contraindications:

- Increased intracranial pressure
- Intracranial tumor
- MI within 3 mo (relative)
- Stroke within 1 mo (relative)

Consider Maintenance ECT:

- Hx of ECT-responsive illness
- Resistance or intolerance to medications alone
- Serious medical comorbidity
- More effective than pharmacotherapy after successful ECT

Repetitive Transcranial Magnetic Stimulation (rTMS) and Theta Burst Stimulation (TBS)

- Repetitive magnetic pulses are directed to the brain at low frequency (1 Hz) for rTMS or high frequency (10 Hz) and patterned pulses for TBS. Tx sessions last between 19 min and 48 min for rTMS and between 3–4 min for TBS. A full course of tx is typically 30 sessions.
- Placebo-controlled studies have demonstrated moderate effect sizes for tx-resistant depression in younger adults and appear safe with minimal adverse effects.
- Emerging data shows clinically meaningful effectiveness of bilateral rTMS and bilateral TBS in tx-resistant late-life depression.

Depression and Parkinson Disease

Patients with Parkinson disease and depression may benefit more from nortriptyline than SSRIs. Pramipexole may also reduce depressive symptoms independent of effect on motor symptoms (also p 241).

Psychotic Depression

- Psychosis accompanying major depression; increased disability and mortality
- ECT is the tx of choice
- Olanzapine 15–20 mg/d po added to sertraline 150–200 mg/d po significantly improves remission rate vs placebo.

BIPOLAR DISORDER

See **Table 43**.

- 5–19% of mood disorders in older adults.
- Usually begins in early adulthood, family hx.
- 10% may develop after age 50.
- Distinct period of abnormally and persistently elevated, expansive, or irritable mood for longer than 1 wk.
- Symptoms may include racing thoughts, pressured speech, decreased need for sleep, distractibility, grandiose delusions.
- A single manic episode is sufficient for a diagnosis if secondary causes are excluded.
- Late-onset mania may be secondary to head trauma, stroke, delirium, other neurologic disorders, alcohol abuse, or medications (eg, corticosteroids, L-DOPA, thyroxine).
- Use aripiprazole, lurasidone, olanzapine, quetiapine, risperidone, or ziprasidone for acute mania (**Table 110**) and D/C antidepressants if taking.
- If depression emerges in bipolar disorder, lamotrigine or lurasidone may be helpful.
- Initiate long-term tx (**Table 44**) as soon as patient is able to comply with oral tx.

Table 43. Medications for Management of Bipolar Disorders

	Mania		Depression	
Medication	***Acute***	***Maintenance***	***Acute***	***Maintenance***
Atypical antipsychotics	All +	Aripiprazole + Olanzapine +/–	Quetiapine + Olanzapine +/– Lamotrigine + Lurasidone +	Quetiapine + Olanzapine + Lamotrigine + Lurasidone +
Mood stabilizers				
Lithium	+	+	+	+
Valproate	+	+/–	–	+/–
Carbamazepine	+	+/–	?	+/–
Antidepressants				
SSRIs	Avoid	Avoid	+	+
TCAs	Avoid	Avoid	–	–

+ = evidence to support use; +/– = some evidence to support use; – = evidence does not support use; ? = has not been studied.

Table 44. Long-term Treatment of Bipolar Disorders[1]

Medication	Initial Dosage	Geriatric Dosage	Comments
Lithium	150 mg/d po	300–900 mg/d po Levels 0.4–0.8 mEq/L	Risk of CNS toxicity; cognitive impairment; hypothyroidism; interactions with diuretics, ACEIs, CCBs, NSAIDs[BC]
Carbamazepine	100 mg po q12h	800–1200 mg/d po Levels 4–12 mcg/L	Many drug interactions; may cause SIADH[BC]; risk of leukopenia, neutropenia, agranulocytosis, thrombocytopenia; monitor CBC; drowsiness, dizziness

(cont.)

Table 44. Long-term Treatment of Bipolar Disorders[1] (cont.)			
Medication	**Initial Dosage**	**Geriatric Dosage**	**Comments**
Valproic acid	125 mg po q12h	750 mg/d po in divided doses Levels 50–125 mcg/L	Can cause weight gain, tremor, several drug interactions; risk of hepatotoxicity, hyponatremia, neutropenia, pancreatitis, thrombocytopenia; monitor LFTs, electrolytes, and platelets. Avoid concurrent use of ≥3 CNS agents.[BC]
Lamotrigine	25 mg/d po	100–200 mg/d po	D/C if rash; interaction with valproate (when used together, begin at 25 mg po q48h, titrate to 25–100 mg po q12h); prolongs PR interval; in patients with clinically important structural or functional heart disorders can increase risk of serious arrhythmias; somnolence, headache common
Lurasidone	20 mg with food	20–80 mg/d	Has not been well studied in older adults. Max dose 120 mg/d; if CrCl = 50: 80 mg/d (L, F, K)

[1] Limited evidence base in older adults. See healthquality.va.gov (also **Table 96**). CrCl unit = mL/min.

DERMATOLOGIC CONDITIONS

DERMATOLOGIC CONDITIONS COMMON IN OLDER ADULTS

For dermatologic images, visit medicine.uiowa.edu/dermatology/education/clinical-skin-disease-images.

Skin Cancers and Precancerous Conditions

As with any cancer, the course of tx should be balanced with the patient's wishes, current quality of life, and life expectancy (eg, Mohs surgery in the last year of life).

Actinic Keratosis

Erythematous, flat, rough, scaly papules 2–6 mm; may be easier felt than seen; precancerous (can develop into SCC); cutaneous horn may develop; affects sun-exposed areas, including lips (actinic cheilitis)

Risk Factors: UV light exposure (amount and intensity), increased age, fair coloring, immunosuppression

Prevention: Limit UV light exposure, use sunscreen with UVA and UVB coverage, wear protective clothing

Treatment Choices: Cryotherapy (for tx of 1–3 lesions) or topical

- Topical 5-FU *(Carac* crm 0.5% or *Tolak* crm 4% daily × 4 wk, *Efudex* crm 5% q12h × 2–4 wk, *Fluoroplex* crm 1% to face, 5% elsewhere, q12h × 2–4 wk) to entire area affected
- Aminolevulinic acid *(Levulan Kerastick* 20%) applied to lesions with PDT after 14–18 h, repeat in 8 wk. Curettage with or without electrosurgery
- Imiquimod 2.5% and 3.75% pk *(Zyclara)*. Apply 1 or 2 pk to face or scalp (not both) qhs × 14 d, wash off with soap and water after 8 h. Rest 14 d, then repeat another 14 d. Max 56 pk/2 cycles
- Imiquimod 5% pk *(Aldara)*. Apply 1 or 2 pk to face or scalp (not both) qhs × 16 d, wash off with soap and water after 8 h. Rest 14 d, then repeat another 14 d. Max 56 pk/2 cycles
- Second-line tx: Ingenol mebutate 0.015% gel *(Picato)*, diclofenac 3% gel *(Solaraze)*, tirbanibulin 1% oint *(Klisyri)*
- Other tx options: Chemical peels (trichloroacetic acid), dermabrasion, laser tx

Basal Cell Carcinoma

Can affect any body surface exposed to the sun, most often head and neck

Types

- Nodular (most common): pearly papule or nodule over telangiectases with a rolled border; may contain melanin
- Superficial: scaly erythematous patch or plaque, may contain melanin
- Morpheaform: indurated, whitish, scar-like plaque with indistinct margins

Risk Factors

- Exposure to UV radiation (sun, tanning beds), especially intense intermittent exposure during childhood or adolescence
- Physical factors: fair skin, light eye color, red or blonde hair
- Exposure to ionizing radiation, arsenic, psoralen, UVA radiation, smoking
- Immunosuppression (eg, after solid-organ transplant)

Prevention: Avoid sun exposure, use sunscreen with UVA and UVB coverage, wear protective clothing

Treatment: (for localized control)

- Surgical: Mohs micrographic surgery (first-line for facial lesions), cryosurgery, excision, curettage and electrodessication
- Nonsurgical: radiation tx, imiquimod 5% crm applied to superficial lesions 5 d/wk × 6 wk (not for use on face, hands, or feet); PDT; 5-FU crm or sol q12h × 3–6 wk or longer; vismodegib 150 mg po q24h until disease progresses or unacceptable toxicity (L, F 92%). Imiquimod, 5-FU useful for older patients who may not tolerate surgical interventions.

Melanoma

Less common than nonmelanoma lesions; usually asymptomatic

Clinical Features

Asymmetry: a line down the center of the lesions does not create a mirror image

Border: irregular, ragged, fuzzy, or scalloped

Color: nonuniform throughout the lesion; red, blue, black, gray, or white

Diameter: >6 mm (considered relatively insensitive as an independent factor)

Evolution: change in size, shape, or color

Patients with changing pigmented lesions that meet ABCDE criteria should be referred to dermatology.

Types

- Lentigo maligna: most often located on atrophic, sun-damaged skin; irregular-shaped tan or brown macule; slow growing
- Superficial spreading: occur anywhere; irregular-shaped macule, papule, or plaque; coloration varies
- Nodular: a rapidly growing, often black or gray papule or nodule
- Acral lentiginous: located on the palms, soles, or nail beds; dark brown or black patch; more common in Hispanic, Black, and Asian individuals

Risk Factors

- Very fair skin type
- Family hx
- Dysplastic or numerous nevi
- Sun exposure; blistering sunburns as a child

Prevention: Avoid sun exposure, use sunscreen with UVA and UVB coverage, wear protective clothing

Treatment

- Surgical excision; advanced: ipilimumab, vemurafenib, dabrafenib plus trametinib, pembrolizumab, nivolumab
- If BRAF V600 mutant variants: combination immunotherapy (eg, nivolumab + ipilimumab)

Squamous Cell Carcinoma (SCC)

- Erythematous papule, plaque, or nodule with keratotic scale; maybe tender
- Scaling or crusting may be present.
- May develop in nonhealing wounds or scars (Marjolin ulcers)

Risk Factors: Cumulative sun exposure, age, immunosuppression, exposure to ionizing radiation or arsenic

Treatment

- Surgical excision, cryotherapy, electrosurgery
- Ionizing radiation is an alternative.
- 5-FU crm or sol q12h × 4–8 wk or longer (off-label) tx for SCC in situ (Bowen disease); not for invasive cutaneous SCC.
- Imiquimod 5% for Bowen disease: apply q24h × 5 d/wk, before normal sleeping hours × 6 wk; leave on skin for ~8 h, then remove with mild soap and water. Maximum to be prescribed: 36 pk during the 6-wk tx period. Alternative (if surgery refused): 5-FU crm q12h × 2–8 wk.

Infectious Conditions

Bed Bugs

Bugs reside in mattresses, bedding, furniture, clothing, and luggage. Typical bite reaction appears as a 2- to 5-mm erythematous papule or wheal with a central hemorrhagic punctum; may appear in multiple red papules in a linear pruritic eruption. Older adults may be less prone to reactions.

Treatment (cdc.gov/parasites/bedbugs)

- Symptomatic tx of bites: topical steroids (eg, triamcinolone acetonide 0.1%); topical or oral anti-itch medication (eg, oral antihistamines)
- Infestation eradication: vacuuming, heat-treating, or wrapping mattresses. Professional extermination is advised.

Cellulitis

Ill-defined erythema, pain, blisters, and exudates; most often affects lower dermis and subcutaneous tissue, commonly the legs; group A streptococci and *Staphylococcus aureus* most frequent pathogens

Treatment (Oral)

- Incise and drain abscesses (first antibiotic dose 60 min before if high risk for endocarditis)
- Empiric tx if MRSA is suspected:
  - TMP-SMX[BC] doxycycline, minocycline, or clindamycin
- Empiric tx if MRSA plus other gram-positive or gram-negative organisms, or anaerobes suspected:
  - TMP-SMX[BC] + amoxicillin-clavulanate
  - Doxycycline/minocycline + amoxicillin-clavulanate
  - Doxycycline /minocycline + levofloxacin + metronidazole
  - Clindamycin + amoxicillin-clavulanate
  - Clindamycin + ciprofloxacin
  - Tailor tx to culture and sensitivity results when available
  - Drain abscess
- Compression tx: if applied often, cellulitis has resolved for recurrent cases.

Folliculitis

Multiple small, erythematous papules and pustules surrounding a hair; most often affects areas with coarse, short hair (ie, neck, beard, buttocks, thighs)

Treatment

- Mild localized cases—topical antibiotic: cleanser (eg, benzoyl peroxide), mupirocin 2%, or clindamycin

- Extensive or severe cases—oral dicloxacillin, cephalexin, doxycycline, TMP-SMZ,[BC] or clindamycin

Impetigo

Very contagious; nonbullous and bullous variants; honey-colored crusts on face around nose and mouth

Treatment

- Small, localized lesions: topical mupirocin 2% q8h × 7–10 d, topical retapamulin 1% oint *(Altabax)* q12h × 5 d
- Widespread: oral dicloxacillin, cephalexin, erythromycin, clarithromycin, TMP-SMX,[BC] or clindamycin × 7 d

Rosacea

Vascular and follicular dilatation; mild to moderate; can accompany seborrhea; can affect face (nose, chin, cheeks, forehead) or eyes (dryness, blepharitis, conjunctivitis)

Prevention: Avoid triggers (stress, prolonged sun exposure and exercise, hot and humid environment, alcohol, hot drinks, spicy foods); may be worsened by vasodilators, niacin, or topical corticosteroids. Wear sunscreen with UVA and UVB coverage (SPF ≥15) or sunblock with titanium and zinc oxide. See rosacea.org.

Treatment

Topical (for mild cases and maintenance)

- When pustules and papules are present

Preferred tx

- Azelaic acid 15% gel *(Finacea)* q12–24 h or 20% crm *(Azelex, Finevin)* q12h
- Ivermectin 1% crm *(Soolantra)* q24h
- Metronidazole 0.75% crm q12h or 1% crm or gel *(Noritate, Metrogel)* q24h

Alternative tx

- Benzoyl peroxide 2.5%, 5%, 10% crm, gel, wash, soap q12–24h
- Clindamycin 1% lot q12h
- Sodium sulfacetamide 10% + sulfa 5% (*Rosula* aqueous gel, *Clenia* crm, foaming wash) q12–24h, avoid if sulfa allergy or kidney disease (K)
- Erythromycin 2% sol q12h
- Minocycline 1.5% q24h

When flushing and redness (facial erythema) are present

- Brimonidine 0.5% gel *(Mirvaso)* q24h
- Oxymetazoline 1% crm *(Rhofade)* q24h for persistent facial erythema
- Tretinoin 0.025% crm or liquid, 0.01% gel qhs

Oral (for moderate to severe papulopustular rosacea)

Tx duration 6–12 wk.

- Tetracycline
- Doxycycline
- Minocycline
- Clarithromycin[BC]
- Metronidazole × 4–6 wk
- Erythromycin[BC]
- Azithromycin

Scabies

Burrows, erythematous papules or rash, dry or scaly skin, pruritus (worse at night); spread by close, skin-to-skin or sexual contact; can affect interdigital webs, flexor aspects of wrists, axillae, umbilicus, nipples, genitalia. Diagnostic confirmation by microscopic exam of skin scrapings in mineral oil for feces, eggs, or mites. Symptoms may be delayed 6 wk postexposure.

Treatment

- Infestation can result in epidemics; treat all contacts including family members and treat environment, including laundering clothing and bedding in hot water, dry cleaning, or sealing in an airtight plastic bag × 3 d.
- Oatmeal baths, topical corticosteroids, or emollient creams for symptom relief
- Apply topical products from head to toe:

Preferred tx

- Permethrin 5% crm, apply qhs, wash off after 8–14 h, repeat in 7–10 d if symptomatic or if live mites were found
- Ivermectin *(Stromectol)* 200 mcg/kg po, may repeat 1× in 1 or 2 wk

Alternative tx

- Crotamiton 10% crm, lot *(Eurax)*, less effective, apply to the entire body below the neck, repeat in 24 h and leave on for 48 h after second application.
- Ivermectin 1% lot applied from the neck down, wash off after 8–14 h; repeat in 1 wk if symptomatic.
- Spinosad 0.9% topical sus applied from the neck down, including bald areas of the scalp; wash off after ≥6 h.

Crusted (Norwegian) Scabies

Persons with dementia and immunocompromised persons may be at greater risk; long-term care facilities may experience outbreaks.

Treatment: Topical permethrin 5% or benzoyl benzoate 5% q24h × 7 d, then 2×/wk until cured ***plus*** oral ivermectin 200 mg/kg po dose on days 1, 2, 8, 9, and 15 (plus days 22 and 29 if severe infestation).

Inflammatory Conditions

Atopic dermatitis (Eczema)

Chronic and pruritic with dry skin, erythema, oozing, crusting, and lichenification.

Treatment

- Avoid environmental triggers (eg, heat and low humidity), harsh soaps, detergents, and contact allergens.
- Maintain skin hydration with barrier creams or ointments (eg, petrolatum based) that have little or no water content. Apply after bathing.
- Topical corticosteroids applied 1 or 2×/d
- Mild eczema: lowest to low potency corticosteroid cream or ointment (**Table 47**)
- Reserve moderate and high potency corticosteroids for moderate disease and flare-ups.
- Avoid applying moderate- and higher-potency corticosteroids to the face and skin folds; if needed, no more than 5–7 d. Skin atrophy can result.

- Topical tacrolimus 0.1% or 0.03% ointment 2×/d or pimecrolimus 1% crm 2×/d for patients who do not respond or cannot tolerate topical corticosteroids. Can be applied to the face or intertriginous areas.
- Topical crisaborole *(Eucrisa)* 2% oint 2×/d for mild to moderate atopic dermatitis
- Treat skin infections (eg, *Staph aureus* and herpes simplex)
- Treat pruritus with oral antihistamines.
- Phototherapy (eg, UV light), oral cyclosporine, dupilumab, methotrexate, azathioprine are reserved for severe cases.

Bullous Pemphigoid

An autoimmune, subepidermal blistering disease; incidence increases with age. Typical presentation is an extremely pruritic eruption with symmetrical and widespread, tense and clear fluid–filled blisters. Commonly affected areas include flexural areas, the lower trunk, and mucous membranes. Medications including diuretics, analgesics, antibiotics, and ACEIs are causes. Refer when ocular, esophageal, pharyngeal, or laryngeal mucosal involvement.

Treatment

- Often self-limited, but can last of months to years.
- Localized lesions: Topical super-potency corticosteroids (eg, clobetasol propionate 0.05% crm)
- Extensive lesions: Systemic glucocorticoids (eg, prednisone 0.5–0.75 mg/kg/d po) for >2 wk after cessation of new blisters and pruritus, and 80% of blisters have healed.
- Azathioprine 0.5–2.5 mg/kg/d has been used for patients for whom systemic glucocorticoids are best avoided.
- Doxycycline 100 mg po 2×/d; tetracycline 500 mg po 4×/d, or minocycline 100 mg po 2×/d) with nicotinamide 500 mg po 4×/d is another alternative tx. Duration until clear, usually 4–8 wk.

Neurodermatitis

Generalized or localized itching, redness, scaling; can affect any skin surface

Treatment: Mid- to higher-potency topical corticosteroids (**Table 47**); exclude other causes (eg, allergies, irritants, xerosis)

Pemphigus vulgaris

An autoimmune, intraepidermal blister disease; most often affecting middle-aged adults. Higher mortality than bullous pemphigoid. Bullae are flaccid, easily rupture, and leave erosions that are slow to resolve. Mucous membranes and skin are commonly affected areas. Blistering can be induced by applying pressure to the edge of blister or normal skin (Nikolsky sign).

Diagnosis: Rule out idiopathic or drug-induced pemphigoid. Biopsy lesion for hematoxylin and eosin staining, biopsy perilesional area for direct immunofluorescence, and draw serum for ELISA and indirect immunofluorescence.

Treatment

- First line: Systemic glucocorticoids (eg, prednisone or prednisolone po 1–1.5 mg/kg/d [up to 2.5 mg/kg]). Expect cessation of blistering in 2–3 wk. Begin dose taper 7 d after blistering ceases.
- Alternate first line (for refractory cases or when glucocorticoid is contraindicated):
  - Rituximab 1000 mg IV × 2 doses 2 wk apart +/- glucocorticoid or +/- immunoglobulin. Rituximab maintenance dose (if needed): 50 mg IV at 12 mo, then q6mo.

- Nonsteroid adjuvants with glucocorticoid (when glucocorticoid-sparing is desired):
  - Azathioprine 2.5 mg/kg/d po × 2 mo, then 50 mg/d
  - Mycophenolate mofetil 1 g q12h po; 720 mg SR q12h

Psoriasis

Well-defined, erythematous plaques covered with silver scales; severity varies; can affect all skin areas, nails (pitting)

Treatment

- Topical corticosteroids, UV light, PUVA, methotrexate, cyclosporine, etretinate, sulfasalazine, tazarotene gel 0.05%, 0.1%, anthralin preparations, and tar + 1–4% salicylic acid, tapinarof *(Vtama)* 1% crm q24h.
- Topical tacrolimus, pimecrolimus *(Elidel)* are nonsteroidal alternatives for facial and intertriginous lesions.
- Calcipotriene for nonfacial areas
- Cyclosporine, methotrexate, and biological agents for extensive and recalcitrant disease (See Rheumatoid Arthritis, p 227)
- Older adults with psoriasis treated with cyclosporine have been shown to be at increased risk for deteriorating kidney function.

Seborrheic Dermatitis

Greasy, yellow scales with or without erythematous base; common in Parkinson disease and in debilitated patients; can affect nasal labial folds, eyebrows, hairline, sideburns, posterior auriculare, and midchest

Treatment

- Hydrocortisone 1% or 2% crm q12h or triamcinolone 0.1% oint q12h × 2 wk
- Scalp: shampoo containing selenium sulfide, zinc, or tar
- Ketoconazole 2% crm 1–2×/d, or other topical azole antifungal, or ciclopirox if *Malassezia* colonization on the face or scalp
- Oral azole antifungals have shown limited benefit when multiple patches are present.
- Topical cyclosporine or tacrolimus for refractory cases

Pruritus

- Common symptom of many systemic, dermatologic, neuropathic, and psychiatric disorders
- Common causes in old age: dry skin, atopic dermatitis, eczema, contact dermatitis, drug reactions, infection
- Systemic causes include renal and liver disease, thyrotoxicosis, DM, and malignancies (eg, Hodgkin and non–Hodgkin lymphoma, polycythemia vera, mycosis fungoides)

Evaluation

- Pruritis with primary skin lesion
  - skin biopsy, KOH test for fungal infection, etc
- Pruritis without skin lesions
  - hx of thyroid, liver, or renal disease, HIV infection, or malignancy, medication, travel, psychiatric and substance use disorder; presence in other household members

Treatment

- Nonpharmacologic: skin moisturizers, cool environment, reduce contact with skin irritants, reduce stress, and apply physical barriers and trim nails to prevent damage from scratching
- Pharmacotherapy, topical
  - Calamine or 4% menthol lotion as cooling counterirritant
  - Capsaicin 0.075% crm q6h when pruritus due to neuropathic or renal etiologies
  - Crisaborole 2% oint *(Eucrisa)* q12h
  - Tacrolimus 0.03% or 0.1% oint q12h; 6-wk trial
  - Pimecrolimus 1% crm q12h; 6-wk trial
  - Pramoxine 1% crm q6-8h
  - Compounded product of ketamine (5% or 10%), amitriptyline (2% or 5%), and lidocaine (2% or 5%) has been reported to provide relief for various types of pruritus, despite a small and weak evidence base.
  - Topical and oral antihistamines have not shown consistent benefit.

Urticaria

Hives

- Uniform, red edematous plaques surrounded by white halos, can affect any skin surface
- Treatment
  - Identify cause
  - Oral H_1 antihistamines (**Table 117**) or oral H_2 antihistamines
  - Oral glucocorticoids[BC] (eg, prednisone 40 mg po q24h)
  - Doxepin (po[BC] or topical 5%) for refractory cases

Angioedema

- Larger, deeper than hives; can affect lips, eyelids, tongue, larynx, GI tract
- Treatment
  - Oral H_1 antihistamines (**Table 117**)
  - Oral glucocorticoids[BC]
  - For severe reactions, epinephrine 0.3 mL of a 1:1000 dilution *(EpiPen)* SC

Cholinergic

- Round, red papular wheals; can affect any skin surface
- Treatment
  - Hot shower may relieve itching
  - Oral H_1 antihistamines (**Table 117**) 1 h before exercise

Fungal Conditions

Candidiasis

Erythema, pustules, or cheesy, whitish matter in body folds; satellite lesions

Treatment: See intertrigo; topical antifungals (**Table 46**)

Intertrigo

Moist, erythematous lesions with local superficial skin loss; satellite lesions caused by *candida*; can affect any place 2 skin surfaces rest against one another (eg, under breasts, between toes)

Treatment

- Keep area dry.
- Topical antifungals (**Table 46**), absorbent pwd, 1–2% hydrocortisone or 0.1% triamcinolone crm q12h × 1–2 d if inflamed

Onychomycosis

Thickening and discoloration; affects nails *(Tinea unguium); Tinea rubrum* most common in people with DM; candida, mold, and bacteria are other causes

Treatment: Obtain nail specimens for lab culture to confirm diagnosis before prescribing itraconazole or terbinafine. Treat affected family members to decrease risk of reinfection.

Table 45. Onychomycosis Medications

Drug	Site	Cure Rate	Comment (Metabolism)
Itraconazole C: 100 S: 100 mg/mL	Toenails Fingernails	Complete cure rate[1] 23%; Mycologic cure rate[2] with pulse tx 63%	Contraindicated in HF (L)
Fluconazole T: 50, 100, 150, 200 S: 10, 40 mg/mL	Toenails Fingernails	Mycologic cure rate 48%	(L)
Efinaconazole *(Jublia)* sol: 10%	Toenails	Complete cure rate 17.8%; mycologic cure rate 55.2%	
Terbinafine[OTC] T: 250	Toenails Fingernails	Complete cure rate 48%; mycologic cure rate 76%	Avoid if CrCl <50, acute or chronic liver disease; choice for people with DM
Ciclopirox S: 8%	Toenails and fingernails	Complete cure rate 8%	
Tavaborole *(Kerydin)* S: 5%	Toenails		Effective against *T rubrum* and *T mentagrophytes sp.*

[1] Complete cure = negative mycologic analysis and normal nail

[2] Mycologic cure = negative fungal culture and negative KOH exam of the target toenail

KOH, potassium hydroxide; CrCl unit = mL/min.

- OTC lacquers (eg, *Fungi-Nail*) treat the fungus around the nail but do not penetrate the nail
- Laser tx: improves appearance; not covered by insurance

Other Conditions

Hair Loss (Alopecia)

Types of Hair Loss

- Cicatricial alopecia: results in permanent hair loss; primarily secondary to inflammatory conditions of the scalp

- Nonscarring alopecia: hair loss is not permanent, because follicles are not destroyed; includes androgenic alopecia (male and female pattern hair loss) and telogen effluvium (acute or chronic hair loss secondary to major physical and psychological stresses, diet, medication, thyroid disorders, and iron deficiency anemia)
- Structural hair loss: brittle or fragile hair that breaks easily or appears not to grow due to exposure to chemicals, heat, or excessive brushing or teasing

Assessment and Evaluation

- Patient hx: hair loss, medical, and family
- Visual exam of scalp, hair, and other body sites
- Referral to dermatology: hair pull test, trichoscopy, etc

Female Pattern Hair Loss *(androgenic alopecia)*

- Presentation: primarily involves the frontal scalp and vertex of the scalp; scarring, inflammation, and scale are absent.
- Treatment
  - First line: topical minoxidil 2% or 5% sol q12h, or 5% foam ½ cap q24h; time to effect 4 mo; adequate trial 12 mo
  - Second line: lack of response to minoxidil or hyperandrogenism
    - Spironolactone 50–200 mg po q24h; adequate trial 6 mo
    - Finasteride 2.5–5 mg po q24h; adequate trial 6 mo
    - Flutamide 62.5–250 mg q24h; adequate trial 6 mo

Note: Topical finasteride 0.25% with topical minoxidil 3% has proven superior to minoxidil 3% alone in 30 postmenopausal women.

Male Pattern Hair Loss *(androgenic alopecia)*

- Presentation: usually begins in the temporal scalp, midfrontal scalp, or vertex area of the scalp; rate of loss varies from periods of high to low hair loss
- Treatment (in order of relative efficacy)
  1. Dutasteride 0.5 mg po q24h
  2. Finasteride 5 mg po q24h or topical 1% q24h
  3. Minoxidil 5 mg po q24h
  4. Finasteride 1 mg po q24h
  5. Topical minoxidil 5% sol q12h or 5% foam q12h
  6. Topical minoxidil 2% sol q12h
  7. Minoxidil 0.25 mg po q24h

Skin Maceration

Erythema; abraded, excoriated skin; blisters; white and silver patches; can affect any area constantly in contact with moisture, covered by occlusive dressing or bandage; skin folds, groin, buttocks

Prevention and Treatment

- Eliminate cause of moisture.
- Toileting program for incontinence (p 166)
- Condom catheter
- Indwelling catheter (reserve for most intractable conditions)
- FI collector
- Protect skin from moisture.
- Clean gently with mild soap after each incontinent episode.

- Apply moisture barrier (eg, *Vaseline, ProShield Plus, Smooth and Cool, Calmoseptine*).
- Use disposable briefs that wick moisture from the skin; use linen incontinence pads when disposable briefs worsen perineal dermatitis.

Xerosis

Dull, rough, flaky, cracked; nummular; can affect all skin surfaces

Treatment

- Increase humidity
- Avoid excess bathing, sponges, brushes, and use of bath oils, which can lead to falls from slippery feet
- Tepid water in baths or showers
- Oatmeal baths
- Apply emollient oint (eg, *Aquaphor*) or crm (eg, *Eucerin*) immediately after bathing
- Hydrocortisone 1% oint

DERMATOLOGIC MEDICATIONS

Table 46. Topical Antifungal Medications[1]

Medication	Dermatologic Indications
Butenafine[OTC]	*Tinea pedis, T cruris, T corporis, T versicolor*
Ciclopirox	*Tinea pedis, T cruris, T corporis, T versicolor*; candidiasis; scalp seborrhea; onychomycosis
Clotrimazole[OTC]	Candidiasis, dermatophytoses; superficial mycoses
Econazole nitrate	Candidiasis; *Tinea cruris, T corporis, T versicolor*
Ketoconazole	Candidiasis; seborrhea; *Tinea cruris, T corporis, T versicolor*
Luliconazole	*Tinea pedis, T crusis*
Miconazole[OTC]	*Tinea cruris, T corporis, T pedis*
Naftifine	*Tinea cruris, T corporis, T pedis*
Nystatin	Mucocutaneous candidiasis
Oxiconazole *(Oxistat)*	*Tinea corporis, T cruris, T pedis, T versicolor*
Sertaconazole *(Ertaczo)*	*Tinea pedis*
Sulconazole *(Exelderm)*	*Tinea corporis, T cruris, T versicolor*
Terbinafine[OTC]	*Tinea cruris, T corporis, T pedis, T versicolor*
Tolnaftate[OTC]	*Tinea cruris, T corporis, T pedis*
Undecylenic acid *(Fungi-Nail*[OTC]*, MycoNail)*	*Tinea pedis*, ringworm (except nails and scalp)
Topical Antifungal Medication plus Corticosteroid	
Clotrimazole 1% Betamethasone 0.05%	*Tinea corporis, T pedis, T cruris*
Iodoquinol 1%, 2% plus Hydrocortisone 1%	Dermatosis
Nystatin 100,000 U Triamcinolone 0.1%	*Cutaneous candida*

[1] Dosing frequency and tx duration can vary by indication and formulation. Consult prescribing information.

Table 47. Topical Corticosteroids		
Medication	**Strength and Formulations**	**Frequency of Applications**
Lowest Potency		
Hydrocortisone	0.5%[OTC], 1%[OTC], 2.5% crm, oint, lot, sol	q6–8h
Low Potency		
Alclometasone dipropionate[1]	0.05% crm, oint	q8–12h
Desonide	0.05% crm, oint	q6–12h
Fluocinolone acetonide	0.01% crm, sol	q6–12h
Triamcinolone acetonide	0.025%, 0.1% crm, oint, lot	q8–12h
Midpotency		
Betamethasone dipropionate	0.05% lot	q6–12h
Betamethasone valerate	0.1% crm	q6–12h
Clobetasone butyrate	0.05% crm	q8h
Clocortolone pivalate	0.1% crm	q8h
Desoximetasone	0.05% crm	q12h
Fluocinolone acetonide	0.025% crm, oint	q6–12h
Flurandrenolide *(Cordran)*	0.05% crm, oint, lot, tape	q12–24h
Fluticasone propionate	0.05% crm, lot, 0.005% oint	q12h
Hydrocortisone butyrate	0.1% oint, sol	q12–24h
Hydrocortisone valerate	0.2% crm, oint	q6–8h
Prednicarbate	0.1% crm, oint	q12h
Higher Potency		
Amcinonide	0.1%, crm, oint, lot	q8–12h
Betamethasone dipropionate	0.05% augmented crm	q6–12h
Betamethasone dipropionate	0.05%, crm, oint	q6–12h
Betamethasone valerate	0.1% oint	q6–12h
Clobetasol propionate	0.02% crm	q12h
Desoximetasone	0.25% crm, oint; 0.05% gel	q12h
Diflorasone diacetate	0.05%, crm, oint	q6–12h
Fluocinonide	0.05% crm, oint, gel	q6–12h
Fluticasone propionate	0.1% oint	q6–12h
Halcinonide	0.1% crm, oint	q8–24h
Mometasone furoate[1]	0.1% crm, lot, oint	q24h
Triamcinolone acetonide	0.5% crm, spr	q8–12h

(cont.)

Medication	Strength and Formulations	Frequency of Applications
Super Potency		
Betamethasone dipropionate	0.05% oint, lot, gel (augmented)	q6–12h
Clobetasol propionate	0.05% crm, oint, lot, gel, shp, spr	q12h
Diflorasone diacetate	0.05% optimized oint	q8–24h
Fluocinonide	0.1% oint, oily crm	q6–12h
Halobetasol propionate	0.05% crm, oint	q12h

Table 47. Topical Corticosteroids (cont.)

[1] Hydrocortisone (all forms), alclometasone, and mometasone are nonfluorinated.

HYPOTHYROIDISM

Common Causes

- Autoimmune (primary thyroid failure)
- After tx for hyperthyroidism
- Pituitary or hypothalamic disorders (secondary thyroid failure)
- Medications, especially amiodarone (rare after first 18 mo of tx) and lithium

Screening for hypothyroidism in asymptomatic older persons is controversial

Evaluation

TSH (up to 7.5 mU/L is normal in adults aged 80 and older), and if high, repeat TSH and free T_4

Pharmacotherapy

- Tx of subclinical hypothyroidism (TSH 5–10 mIU/L, normal free T_4 concentration, and no overt symptoms) does not improve hypothyroid symptoms, tiredness, cognitive function, depression, or quality of life. Most experts recommend treating if TSH ≥10 mIU/L.
- If patient is receiving tx without a clear indication and TSH is normal or low, can reduce dose by half and recheck in 4–6 wk with further reductions or discontinuation based on results.
- Levothyroxine is given on empty stomach 30 min before breakfast, 1 h before a different meal, or hs (at least 2 h after last meal), which is more potent. Start at 25–50 mcg po and increase by 12- to 25-mcg intervals q6wk with repeat TSH testing until TSH is in normal range. Prescribe product from same manufacturer for individual patients for consistent bioavailability. Recheck TSH in 6 wk if there is a change in formulation, although switching among generics rarely affects TSH. If adherence is a problem, can be given weekly or 2×/wk.
- Combinations of levothyroxine and L-triiodothyronine (T_3) are not recommended.
- Thyroid USP is not recommended. (Avoid.[BC]) To convert thyroid USP to thyroxine: 60 mg USP = 100 mcg thyroxine.
- For myxedema coma: Load T_4 400 mcg IV or 100 mcg q6–8h for 1 d, then 100 mcg/d IV (until patient can take orally) and give stress doses of corticosteroids (p 124); then start usual replacement regimen.
- If patients are npo and must receive IV thyroxine, dose should be half usual po dose.
- If tx has been interrupted for <6 wk and without an intercurrent cardiac event or marked weight loss, previous full replacement dose can be resumed.
- Monitor TSH level at least q12mo (ASCE/ATA) in patients on chronic thyroid replacement tx. Don't measure total or free T_3.[CW]
- Normal TSH ranges are higher in older persons and higher target (eg, 4–10 mIU/L) may be appropriate.

HYPERTHYROIDISM

Common Causes

- Graves disease
- Toxic nodule
- Toxic multinodular goiter
- Medications, especially amiodarone (can occur any time during tx)

Evaluation

Older persons are less likely to have heat intolerance, tremor, nervousness, or goiter but more likely to have weight loss, dyspnea, constipation, AF, and moderate to severe ophthalmopathy.

TSH (biotin supplements can interfere with assay, suggesting hyperthyroidism), free T_4

- If TSH is low (<0.3) and free T_4 is normal, recheck TSH in 4–6 wk; if TSH is still low, check free T_3.
- If TSH is low and free T_4 or free T_3 is high, or free T_3 alone is high, check radioactive iodine uptake and, if thyroid nodularity, thyroid scan.
- If TSH is low, high T_4, and normal free T_3 suggests concurrent nonthyroidal illness, amiodarone tx, or exogenous T_4 administration.
- If cause is not obvious, check thyrotropin-receptor antibodies (TRAb), radioactive iodine uptake, or thyroidal blood flow on ultrasonography. If nodules on exam, also get radioactive iodine uptake.

Table 48. Causes of Hyperthyroidism Based on Thyroid Function Test Patterns

Diagnosis	TSH	Free T_4	T_3
Subclinical hyperthyroidism	↓	Normal	Normal
Overt hyperthyroidism	↓	↑	↑
T_3 toxicosis	↓	Normal	↑
T_4 toxicosis (also seen with amiodarone)	↓	↑	Normal
Critical illness	↓	Normal[1] or ↓	Normal or ↓
TSH-induced hyperthyroidism	↑	↑	↑

[1] May be difficult to distinguish whether due to critical illness or superimposed hypothyroidism.

Management

In older adults, treat both symptomatic hyperthyroidism and subclinical hyperthyroidism (low TSH and normal serum-free T_4 and T_3 concentrations confirmed by repeat testing in 3–6 mo) if TSH <0.1 mIU/L. If TSH 0.1–0.5 mIU/L and underlying CVD or low BMD, treat or closely monitor.

Nonpharmacologic Interventions

Radioactive iodine ablation is the usual tx of choice for older persons but surgery (which works faster but more likely to become hypothyroid) or medical tx are options. Pretreat with methimazole and β blockers before iodine ablation if symptomatic or if free T_4 > 2–3× normal. If active or severe ophthalmopathy, give prophylactic glucocorticoids or choose surgery. Monitor free T_4 and total T_3 within 1–2 mo after tx. Pretreat with methimazole and β blockers before surgery. Give potassium iodide in immediate preoperative period. After surgery, measure calcium or intact PTH, stop antithyroid drugs, and taper β blockers.

Pharmacotherapy (commonly used but less effective)

- β blockers (p 66) if symptomatic hyperthyroidism; may add methimazole if severe symptoms or risk of hyperthyroid complications.
- Methimazole: first-line drug tx; start 5–20 mg po q8h, then adjust. If used as primary tx, continue for 12–18 mo then D/C or taper if TSH is normal. Check CBC, LFTs before starting.
- Propylthiouracil: Use only if allergic to or intolerant of methimazole; can cause serious liver injury; start 100 mg po q8h, then adjust up to 200 mg po q8h prn. Check CBC, LFTs before starting.
- When dose has stabilized, follow TSH per hypothyroid monitoring.

EUTHYROID SICK SYNDROME

Definition

Abnormal thyroid function tests in nonthyroidal illness

Evaluation

- Do not assess thyroid function in acutely ill patients unless thyroid dysfunction is strongly suspected.
- Low T_3, high reverse T_3, low T_4, low or high TSH may be seen.
- If TSH is very low (<0.1 mIU/L in high-sensitivity assays), hyperthyroidism is likely.
- If TSH is very high (>20 mIU/L), hypothyroidism is likely.
- Do not treat low T_3 or T_4 in absence of clinical symptoms.
- If thyroid disease is not strongly suspected, recheck in 3–6 wk.

SOLITARY THYROID NODULE

See digital text.

HYPERCALCEMIA

Common Causes

- Primary hyperparathyroidism
- Malignancy
- Thyrotoxicosis
- Increased calcium intake (rare unless also CKD or milk-alkali syndrome)
- Hypervitaminosis D
- Lithium
- Thiazide diuretics
- Granulomatous diseases

Evaluation

- Confirm hypercalcemia with ionized calcium or calcium corrected for albumin
- Measure intact PTH
  - If high (or normal but ≥20 pg/mL), measure 24-h urinary calcium excretion. If high, primary hyperparathyroidism. If low, familial hypocalciuric hypercalcemia. Also check Cr and 25(OH)D.
  - If low (<20 pg/mL), measure PTHrP, 1,25(OH)2D, and 25(OH)D. If PTHrP is high, workup for malignancy. If normal and 1,25(OH)2D is high, get CXR to look for granulomatous diseases. If normal and 25(OH)D is high, probably due to medications (eg, thiazide diuretics, lithium, teriparatide, abaloparatide), vitamins (vitamin A, calcitriol), supplements. If all are normal, consider other causes (eg, myeloma).

Management

Treat underlying cause, if possible.

Nonpharmacologic Interventions

Asymptomatic primary hyperparathyroidism: surgery if any of the following: serum calcium >1.0 mg/dL above upper limits of normal, eGFR <60 mL/min, BMD T score <-2.5 or prior fragility or vertebral fracture, 24h Ca excretion >400 mg/d, nephrolithiasis, nephrocalcinosis. In a cohort study, parathyroidectomy was associated with lower risk of any fracture and hip fracture in older adults. If no surgery, avoid thiazide diuretics, lithium, excessive vitamin D (maintain 25[OH]D 20–30 ng/mL), dehydration, bedrest, or physical inactivity.

Pharmacotherapy

If symptomatic or Ca >14 mg/dL:

- Isotonic saline 200–300 mL/h and then adjusted to maintain 100–150 mL/h urine output. Effective within 12–48 h. Loop diuretics if CKD or HF.
- Calcitonin 4 (IU/kg IM or SC), short term in addition to saline, if needed. Effective within 12–48 h.
- Zoledronic acid (4 mg IV over 15 min) or pamidronate (50–90 mg IV over 2 h) effective by 48–96 h.
- Other tx are reserved for refractory hypercalcemia (eg, denosumab, cinacalcet) or specific causes (glucocorticoids for some lymphomas and granulomatous disease). Denosumab may be valuable but if CrCl <30 mL/min, may precipitate hypocalcemia.

If surgery criteria are met, but patient is not a candidate for surgery, specific tx that either targets hypercalcemia (cinacalcet) or reduced bone mass (see Osteoporosis chapter) may be considered.

DIABETES MELLITUS

Definition and Classification (ADA)

DM is a group of metabolic diseases characterized by hyperglycemia resulting from defects in insulin secretion, insulin action, or both.

Type 1 (DM1): Caused by an absolute deficiency of insulin secretion. As persons with DM1 age, insulin may be more difficult to use because of cognitive or functional impairment and caregivers may assume increased importance. Continuous glucose monitoring is approved by Medicare and can be beneficial to older adults.

Type 2 (DM2): Caused by a combination of resistance to insulin action and an inadequate compensatory insulin secretory response. DM2 is a progressive disorder requiring higher dosages or additional medications over time.

Screening—Screen asymptomatic adults aged ≥35 (ADA); repeat at 3-y intervals (only if overweight or obese [USPSTF]).

Criteria for Diagnosis—One or more of the following:

- Symptoms of DM (eg, polyuria, polydipsia, unexplained weight loss) plus casual plasma glucose concentration ≥200 mg/dL
- Fasting (no caloric intake for ≥8 h) plasma glucose ≥126 mg/dL
- 2-h plasma glucose ≥200 mg/dL during an oral glucose tolerance test with equivalent of 75 g anhydrous glucose dissolved in water
- Unless hyperglycemia is unequivocal, diagnosis should be confirmed by repeat testing (2 abnormal tests from same sample or 2 separate samples).
- A1c >6.5. *Note:* A1c can be falsely lowered by any condition that shortens erythrocyte survival or decreases mean erythrocyte age (eg, hemolysis, tx for iron, B_{12}, folate deficiency, or erythropoietin tx) and falsely increased when RBC turnover is low (eg, iron, B_{12}, or folate deficiency, anemia), asplenia; CKD can increase or decrease A1c.

Prediabetes (a minority progress to DM2 over 6 y but monitoring at least yearly is recommended)

Any of the following:

- Impaired fasting glucose: defined as fasting plasma glucose ≥100 and <126 mg/dL
- Impaired glucose tolerance: 2-h plasma glucose 140–199 mg/dL
- A1c 5.7–6.4%

Prevention/Delay of DM2 in Patients with Prediabetes

- Lifestyle modification (most effective), including smoking cessation
  - Weight loss (target 7% loss) if overweight
  - Reduction in total and saturated dietary fat
  - High dietary fiber (14 g fiber/1000 kcal) and whole grains
  - Mediterranean diet and extra-virgin olive oil
  - Exercise (at least 150 min/wk of moderate activity, such as walking)
  - Medicare Diabetes Prevention Program for persons without DM or ESRD who have BMI ≥25 (≥23 if East Asian) and have prediabetes. Program includes a minimum of 10 intensive core sessions of a CDC-approved curriculum over 6 mo in a group-based, classroom-style setting followed by less intensive follow-up meetings monthly for 1–2 y to help ensure that the participants maintain healthy behaviors. Monitor A1c at least yearly.
- Pharmacotherapy (typically combined with lifestyle modifications). Drugs may be helpful in preventing DM2, but the impact on future CVD events is unclear; it is unknown whether early tx confers benefit versus withholding tx until DM develops.
  - Metformin (850 mg po q12h) (best long-term evidence but less effective than lifestyle modification)
  - Valsartan[BC] (beginning 80 mg/d po and increased to 160 mg/d po after 2 wk as tolerated) slightly reduces risk of developing DM but does not reduce rate of cardiovascular events.
  - Weight-loss medications if overweight or obese (see Malnutrition chapter)

Management of Diabetes

Hospital

- Target glycemic control:
  - If critically ill, 140–180 mg/dL, which usually requires IV insulin infusion.
  - If noncritically ill, there are no clear evidence-based guidelines, but fasting <140 mg/dL and random <180 mg/dL are suggested (might be relaxed if severe comorbidities [ADA]).
  - If good nutritional intake, scheduled basal and prandial insulin doses with correction doses with rapid-acting analog (aspart, glulisine, or lispro).[BC]
    - If npo or poor oral intake, basal plus correction dose with rapid-acting analog (aspart, glulisine, or lispro) every 4 h only.
  - If insulin-naive, patient can initiate insulin at total daily dose of 0.3 U/kg, half as long-acting (basal) and half as rapid-acting before each meal.
- Correction dose for older persons is 1 unit for every 40–50 mg/dL in excess of 140 mg/dL.
- Point-of-care blood glucose monitoring is used to guide insulin dosing.

Perioperative

- Check preoperative A1c.
- The day before surgery, continue all DM medications, including metformin; reduce long-acting nighttime basal insulin by 25%.
- The day of surgery, give ½ dose of basal and intermediate-acting insulins. Hold short-acting insulin and noninsulin drugs until patient resumes oral intake.
- Intraoperative goal is <180 mg/dL without causing hypoglycemia.
- Postoperative goals are 100–140 mg/d (preprandial), and 100–180 mg/dL (random).

Nursing home: Providers should be called for blood glucose <70 mg/dL (immediately), 70–100 mg/dL, >250 mg/dL, readings are too high for the glucometer, or if patient is sick, with vomiting, symptomatic hyperglycemia, or poor oral intake. Do not use sliding-scale insulin in chronic glycemic management.[BC, CW]

Dying patients: D/C hypoglycemics for patients with DM2. For patients with DM1, small amount of basal insulin may prevent acute hyperglycemic complications.

Outpatient Settings

Evaluate and Treat Comorbid Conditions and Provide Preventive Care *(AGS, ADA):* Depression (p 92), polypharmacy (p 16), cognitive impairment (p 82), UI (p 165), falls (p 136), pain (p 252) (AGS), PAD (claudication hx and assessment of pedal pulses) (p 73), sleep disorders (p 342). Stress test if cardiac symptoms or abnormal ECG (p 62). In men, if symptoms of hypogonadism, consider screening with morning testosterone.

- Assess risk of DM complications including ASCVD, CKD, and hypoglycemia.
- Use shared decision-making to set goals for glucose and BP control and self-management.
- Tx of comorbid conditions should be individualized based on life expectancy, patient preferences, and tx goals.
  - Manage HTN (BP goal <130/80 mm Hg [ACC] and for high risk [ADA] and <140/90 mm Hg [lower risk ADA]; also HTN, p 54) including an ACEI or ARB (first-line if CAD or proteinuria), dihydropyridine CCB, or thiazide diuretic (ACEI or ARB if albuminuria). If patient is Black, CCB or thiazide diuretic is preferred as initial tx (JNC 8). Promote DASH diet.
  - Assess 10-y ASCVD risk and treat lipid disorders (p 51). If on statin with controlled LDL-C but elevated TG (135–499 mg/dL), consider adding icosapent ethyl (ADA).
  - ASA 75–162 mg/d po if hx of heart disease but not for primary prevention[BC]; if allergic, clopidogrel 75 mg/d po. Consider dual antiplatelet tx after ACS or percutaneous coronary intervention, high ischemic risk and low bleeding risk. [ADA]
- If DM2 and K ≤5 and CKD, consider finerenone 20 mg/d if eGFR ≥60 and 10 mg/d if eGFR ≥25 to <60 to prevent CKD progression, HF hospitalization, and CVD death.
- Vaccinations (see Prevention chapter)
  - Consider hepatitis B vaccination.

Goals of Glycemic Treatment (ADA, AGS) **(Table 49)**

- In older persons and patients with cognitive dysfunction, individualize tx to avoid hypoglycemia and polyuria.
- The effects of tight control in DM2 on microvascular and macrovascular complications are uncertain.
- The benefit of achieving biomarker (eg, A1c, BMI, SBP, LDL-C) targets is less for older persons.
- At end of life, focus should be to avoid symptoms and complications from glycemic management.

Nonpharmacologic Interventions

- Patient and family education for self-management (reimbursed by Medicare)
- Individualize medical nutrition tx to achieve tx goals (diet plus exercise is more effective than diet alone)
  - Macronutrient (carbohydrate, protein, and fat) distribution based on individualized assessment of current eating patterns, preferences, and metabolic goals.
  - The amount of dietary saturated fat, cholesterol, and trans fat is the same as that recommended for the general population.
  - Decrease consumption of sugar and nonnutritive sweetened beverages.
  - Carbohydrate intake from vegetables, fruits, whole grains, legumes, and dairy products—with an emphasis on foods higher in fiber and lower in glycemic load—should be advised over intake from other carbohydrate sources, especially those that contain added sugars.

- Mediterranean diet high in monounsaturated fatty acids may be beneficial in glycemic control and cardiovascular risk reduction.
- Limit alcohol intake to ≤1 drink/d.

• Smoking cessation

• Exercise for ≥150 min/wk, resistance training 3×/wk if not contraindicated, balance and flexibility training

• Weight loss if overweight or obese. For younger and healthier older adults, consider bariatric surgery if DM with BMI ≥40, BMI 35–39 when hyperglycemia is inadequately controlled with lifestyle changes and medical tx, and BMI 30.0–34.9 if hyperglycemia is not controlled with oral or injectable medications. See Malnutrition chapter.

• Psychosocial assessment and care

Table 49. Goals of Treatment for Older Patients with Diabetes Mellitus

Patient Health	A1c goal	FPG or PPG, mg/dL	Bedtime glucose, mg/dL	BP goal, mm Hg	Lipid Tx
Healthy[1,CW]	7.0–7.5%	80–130	80–180	<140/90	Statin
Complex/intermediate[2]	<8.0%	90–150	100–180	<140/90	Statin
Very complex/poor health[3]	Avoid reliance on A1c	100–180	110–200	<150/90	Consider statin
Receiving SNF rehab	Avoid using A1c	Target glucose 100–200 mg/dL		Per above categories of patient health	

FPG, fasting plasma glucose; PPG, postprandial glucose; SNF, skilled nursing facility.

[1] Older adults who are functional, cognitively intact, and have life expectancy >10 y. Avoid using medications to achieve an A1c <7.5% in most older adults.[CW]

[2] Multiple (3+) coexisting chronic illness or 2+ IADL impairments or mild to moderate cognitive impairment

[3] LTC or end-stage chronic illnesses or moderate to severe cognitive impairment or 2+ ADL dependencies

Pharmacotherapy for DM1 (ADA)

• Most should be treated with multiple daily injections of prandial and basal insulin or continuous infusion.

• Most should use rapid-acting insulin analogs to reduce hypoglycemia risk.

• Consider continuous glucose monitoring.

• Patients should receive education to match doses to carbohydrate intake, premeal glucose, and physical activity.

Pharmacotherapy for DM2 (ADA)

• If diet and exercise have not achieved target A1c in 6 mo, begin drug tx. Reinforce lifestyle modifications at every visit.

• *Monotherapy* (A1c <9): Metformin (reduce dose in Stage 3 CKD; avoid in Stage 4 CKD) beginning 500 mg po q12h or q24h; can titrate up q5–7d to max of 2000 mg/d po if no AEs and blood glucose uncontrolled. GLP-1 receptor agonists and SGLT2 inhibitors are appropriate initial tx if coexisting or high risk for ASCVD, HF, or CKD.

• *Dual therapy* (A1c ≥9): If A1c target is not achieved after 3 mo of monotx. Choice is based on circumstances.
  - **If high risk of or established ASCVD,** drug choice: SGLT2i (eg, empagliflozin, canagliflozin, dapagliflozin) or GLP-1 RA (eg, liraglutide, semaglutide, or dulaglutide) are first choice.

◦ **If high risk of or established HF,** drug choice: SGLT2i (eg, empagliflozin, canagliflozin, dapagliflozin) are first choice. If SGLT2i are not tolerated or eGFR is not adequate, liraglutide, semaglutide, or dulaglutide is preferred.
◦ **If high risk of or established CKD,** SGLT2i (eg, empagliflozin, canagliflozin, dapagliflozin) or GLP-1 RA (eg, liraglutide, semaglutide, dulaglutide) are first choice.
◦ If compelling need to minimize hypoglycemia, consider specific drug and patient factors in selecting drug (**Table 50**) in the following classes:
  ▪ SGLT2i: lower mortality compared to DPP-4 inhibitors
  ▪ GLP-1 RA: lower mortality compared to DPP-4 inhibitors and also preferred over insulin as first injectable choice. Also promote weight loss.
  ▪ DPP-4 enzyme inhibitors
  ▪ Thiazolidinediones[BC]
◦ If compelling need to minimize weight gain or promote weight loss, GLP-1 RA or SGTLT2i
◦ If cost is a major issue, sulfonyl urea, thiazolidinedione or some insulins

- *Switch dual therapy drugs or triple therapy:* If fails to achieve target A1c after 3 mo of dual tx
- If A1c remains above target, consider adding basal insulin. Maintain metformin, if tolerated.

Table 50. Noninsulin Agents for Managing Diabetes Mellitus[1]

Medication	Comments (Metabolism)
Biguanide	Decrease hepatic glucose production; lower A1c by 1–2%; do not cause hypoglycemia
Metformin *XR*	Contraindicated if eGFR <30 and use with caution if 30–45. If already taking and eGFR drops to 30–45, monitor KFTs. Hold before contrast radiologic studies and do not administer for 48 h after imaging if eGFR <60. HF, COPD, ↑ LFTs; may cause weight loss, B_{12} deficiency. XR form may be helpful if GI intolerance. (K)
♥SGLT2 Inhibitors (SGLT2i)	Decreases glucose reabsorption from kidney; lowers A1c by 0.5–1.0%; may cause weight loss (0.1–4 kg) and has increased risk of ketoacidosis, AKI, genital mycotic infections, UTIs, gallbladder or biliary disease, increased LDL, and fracture risk
♥Canagliflozin *(Invokana)*	Initial dose 100 mg and no more than 100 mg if eGFR 45–59; (L). If albuminuric CKD, reduces risk of CVD if high cardiovascular risk and risk of progressive kidney disease
♥Dapagliflozin *(Farxiga)*	Should not be used if eGFR <45 (L). If patient has or is at risk of ASCVD, reduces hospitalization for HF and progression of CKD.
♥Empagliflozin *(Jardiance)*	Should not be used if eGFR <45 (L). May reduce HF hospitalizations, cardiovascular and all-cause mortality, and progression of renal disease in patients with established CVD.
Ertugliflozin *(Steglatro)*	Should not be used if eGFR <60. No trials on cardiovascular or renal outcomes (L, K)
GLP–1 Receptor Agonists (GLP–1 RA) Albiglutide *(Tanzeum)*	Cardiovascular benefits if established or risk for ASCVD. Hypoglycemia common if combined with sulfonylurea or insulin. Lowers A1c by 0.7–1%; less likely to cause hypoglycemia than insulin or sulfonylureas; can cause nausea, vomiting, diarrhea, and weight loss. Risks include acute pancreatitis and possibly medullary thyroid cancer.
Dulaglutide *(Trulicity)*	When added to standard regimen, reduces MI, nonfatal stroke, or cardiovascular deaths and reduces new macroalbuminuria, decline in eGFR, or chronic renal replacement tx.

(cont.)

Table 50. Noninsulin Agents for Managing Diabetes Mellitus[1] (cont.)	
Medication	**Comments (Metabolism)**
Exenatide *(Byetta)*	Avoid if CrCl <30 (K)
ER *(Bydureon)*	Avoid if CrCl <30 (K)
Liraglutide *(Victoza)*	Lowers rates of CVD and all-cause mortality and composite outcome (cardiovascular mortality, nonfatal MI, nonfatal stroke) (L); 3-mg dose used for weight loss does not provide additional glucose lowering beyond 1.8-mg dose
Lixisenatide *(Adlyxin)*	Reduce new onset and progressive macroalbuminuria
Semaglutide *(Ozempic, Rybelsus)*	Starting dose is 0.25 mg 1×/wk for 4 wk. Reduces persistent macroalbuminuria and nephropathy but increased retinopathy. SC preparation reduces major cardiovascular AEs (driven by reduction in nonfatal stroke).
Dual GIP/GLP-1 Receptor Agonist	
Tirzepatide *(Mounjaro)*	More effective than semaglutide in reducing A1c but clinical trial CVD outcomes pending.
DPP–4 Enzyme Inhibitors	Protect and enhance endogenous incretin hormones; lower A1c by 0.5–1%; do not cause hypoglycemia, weight neutral; no effect on major adverse cardiovascular outcomes
Alogliptin	(K)
Linagliptin *(Tradjenta)*	(L)
Saxagliptin *(Onglyza)*	(K)
Sitagliptin *(Januvia)*	(K)
α-Glucosidase Inhibitors	Delay glucose absorption; lower A1c by 0.5–1%; can cause hypoglycemia and weight gain
Acarbose	GI AEs common, avoid if Cr >2 mg/dL, monitor LFTs (gut, K)
Miglitol	Same as acarbose but no need to monitor LFTs (L, K)
Thiazolidinediones	Insulin resistance reducers; lower A1c by 0.5–1.5%; ↑ risk of HF; avoid if NYHA Class III or IV cardiac status[BC]; D/C if any decline in cardiac status; weight gain. Avoid if taking insulin, osteoporosis, falls, fractures, or macular edema. Check LFTs at start, q2mo during first year, then periodically; avoid if clinical evidence of liver disease or if serum ALT levels >2.5× upper limit of normal; may increase risk of fractures in women (L, K)
Pioglitazone	(L)
Rosiglitazone *(Avandia)*	(L)
Meglitinides	Increase insulin secretion; lower A1c by 1–2%; can cause hypoglycemia and weight gain
Nateglinide	Give 30 min ac. Should not be administered if patient is skipping a meal.
Repaglinide *(Prandin)*	Give 30 min ac, adjust dosage at weekly intervals, potential for drug interactions, caution in hepatic, renal insufficiency (L). Should not be administered if patient is skipping a meal.

(cont.)

Medication	Comments (Metabolism)
Amylin Analog	
Pramlintide *(Symlin)*	Lowers A1c by 0.5%; nausea common; reduce premeal dose of short-acting insulin by 50% (K)
Second-Generation Sulfonylureas	Increase insulin secretion; lower A1c by 1–2%; can cause hypoglycemia and weight gain; use of clarithromycin, levofloxacin, trimethoprim-sulfamethoxazole, metronidazole, and ciprofloxacin are associated with increased risk of hypoglycemia
Glimepiride[BC]	Numerous drug interactions, long-acting (L, K)
✓ Glipizide	Short-acting (L, K)
XL	Long-acting (L, K)
Other	
Bromocriptine *(Cycloset)*	Start 0.8 and increase 0.8 weekly; lowers A1c by 0.5% (L)
Colesevelam *(Welchol)*	Give with meals; lowers A1c by 0.5%; not absorbed (GI)

Table 50. Noninsulin Agents for Managing Diabetes Mellitus[1] (cont.)

[1] Many combination drugs are available. ✓ = preferred for treating older adults; ♥ = useful in managing HfrEF; CrCl unit = mL/min; eGFR unit = mL/min

- Insulin. D/C sulfonylureas and meglitinides when insulins are started. Insulin analogs are not more effective than regular insulin, are much more expensive and have higher incidence of hypoglycemia.
  - Begin with basal insulin (intermediate at bedtime or long-acting at bedtime or morning) 10 U or 0.1-0.2 U/kg; can increase by 2–4 U q3d depending on fasting blood glucose. 30–50 U is often needed. When fasting blood glucose is at goal, recheck A1c in 2–3 mo. If hypoglycemia or fasting blood glucose <70 mg/dL, reduce dose by 4 U or 10%, whichever is greater. If above target A1c, check before lunch, dinner, and bedtime blood glucose concentrations and add rapid-acting (beginning at 4 IU/d or 10% of basal dose before largest meal); can combine with intermediate-acting insulin (**Table 51**).
  - Simplification of insulin regimens (consider if severe or recurrent hypoglycemia, unable to manage complexity)
    - If patient is on basal insulin, mealtime insulin, or both, can change basal from bedtime to morning.
    - If on premixed insulin, use 70% of total dose as basal only in the morning.
    - If mealtime insulin >10 U/dose, decrease dose by 50% and add noninsulin agent then titrate insulin down.
    - If <10 U/dose, D/C mealtime insulin and add noninsulin agents.
  - Timing for prandial insulin: if blood glucose is in the 100s, give 10 min before eating; if blood glucose is in the 200s, give 20 min before eating; if blood glucose is in the 300s, give 30 min before eating.
  - If using fixed daily insulin doses, carbohydrate intake on a day-to-day basis should be consistent with respect to time and amount.
    - Use 4-mm, 32-gauge needle if BMI <40 kg/m^2 and 8-mm, 32-gauge needle if BMI >40 kg/m^2. Inject at 90° without a pinch.
    - Injection sites for human insulin: fastest onset is abdomen and slowest onset is thigh.

Table 51. Insulin Preparations				
Preparation	**Onset**	**Peak**	**Duration**	**Number of Injections/d**
Rapid-acting				
Insulin glulisine *(Apidra)* 100 U/mL (3 mL)	20 min	0.5–1.5 h	4–5 h	3
Insulin lispro 100 U/mL (3 mL) 200 U/mL (3 mL)	15 min	0.5–1.5 h	3–5 h	3
Insulin aspart 100 U/mL (3 mL, 10 mL)	25 min	1–3 h	3–5 h	3
(Fiasp)	4 min	1 h	3–5 h	3
Inhaled *(Afrezza)*[1] 4 U, 8 U, 12 U	12 min	35–55 min	1.5–3 h	3
Regular[2] 100 U/mL (3 mL, 10 mL) 500 U/mL (3 mL, 20 mL)	0.5–1 h	1–5 h	4–12 h	1–3
Intermediate- or Long-acting (NPH has higher risk of hypoglycemia compared to long-acting analogs in DM2.)				
NPH[2] 100 U/mL (3 mL, 10 mL)	1–2 h	4–8 h	12 –24 h	1–2
Insulin detemir *(Levemir)* 100 U/mL (3 mL, 10 mL)	1–2 h	6–12 h	12–24 h depending on dose	1–2
Insulin glargine[3]		No peak		
100 U/mL (3 mL)	1–4 h		24 h	1
300 U/mL (1.5 mL)	1–6 h		24–36 h	1
Intermediate- or Long-acting (NPH has higher risk of hypoglycemia compared to long-acting analogs in DM2.) (continued)				
Insulin degludec *(Tresiba)* 100 U/mL (3 mL) 200 U/mL (3 mL)	1–9 h	No peak	42 h	1
Combinations				
Insulin isophane and regular insulin inj *(70/30)* 100 U/mL (3 mL, 10 mL)	isophane 1.5 h	2–12 h	24 h	1–2
Insulin aspart protamine and insulin aspart (70/30)		See individual drugs		
Insulin lispro protamine suspension and insulin lispro *(50/50; 75/25)* 100 U/mL (3 mL, 10 mL)		See individual drugs		
Long-acting combined with GLP-1 receptor agonists				
Insulin glargine/lixisenatide *(Soliqua)* 100 U/33 mcg/mL (3 mL)	1–4 h	No peak	See individual drugs	1–2
Insulin degludec/liraglutide *(Xultophy)* 100 U/3.6 mg/mL (3 mL)	1–9 h	No peak	See individual drugs	

[1] Available as 4-unit and 8-unit single-use cartridges administered by inhalation

[2] Also available as mixtures of NPH and regular in 50:50 proportions

[3] To convert from NPH dosing, give same number of units 1×/d. For patients taking NPH q12h, decrease the total daily units by 20%, and titrate on basis of response. Starting dosage in insulin-naive patients is 10 U 1×/d hs.

Glucose Monitoring

- If multiple daily injections or using insulin pump, blood glucose monitoring before meals and snacks, occasionally postprandially, at bedtime, before exercise, when patient suspects low blood glucose, after treating low blood glucose until patient is normoglycemic, and before critical tasks such as driving.
- In patients with DM1, continuous glucose monitoring is associated with modest improvement of A1c and reduced risk of hypoglycemia. May be beneficial in DM2 if multiple daily insulin injections or frequent hypoglycemia.
- Self-monitoring of blood glucose (SMBG) in patients with DM2 who are not receiving insulin does not improve A1c or quality of life; do not recommend.[CW]
- There is no consensus about the frequency of SMBG patients on insulin. Medicare only approves up to 3×/d.

Hypoglycemia

- Risk factors: tx-associated hypoglycemia (most common with insulin, sulfonylurea, α-glucosidase inhibitors, and meglitinides); polypharmacy; impaired kidney or liver function; longer DM duration; frailty, older age, or cognitive impairment; impaired counterregulatory responses
  - Level 1 (<70 mg/dL and ≥54 mg/dL): Treat with fast-acting carbohydrate (eg, glucose tabs, hard candy, paste *[Insta-Glucose]*) or instant fruit that provides 15–20 g of glucose.
  - Level 2 (<54 mg/dL): Treat with glucagon 0.5–1 mg SC or IM or 3 mg nasal powder *(Baqsimi) or dasiglucagon (Zegalogue) 0.6 mg SC*. In medical settings, 25–50 g of D50 IV restores glucose quicker.
  - Level 3: altered mental and/or physical function that requires assistance from another person for recovery with no specific glucose threshold. Treat with glucagon.
- Recheck blood glucose in 15 min. Repeat up to 3× until blood glucose is >100. If blood glucose remains <100, seek medical attention.
- If hypoglycemia unawareness or >1 episodes of severe hypoglycemia, reevaluate regimen.

Monitoring (abridged ADA)

Initial and Annually

- Screen for depression, anxiety, and disordered eating
- Assess for cognitive impairment if aged ≥65
- Height, weight, and BMI (and at every follow-up visit)
- BP (and at every follow-up visit), orthostatic BP measures on initial visit and when indicated
- Foot exam including visual inspection (and at every visit), checking pedal pulses and asking about claudication, and annual monofilament testing plus determination of either temperature or pinprick sensation or vibration.
- Comprehensive dilated eye and visual exams by an ophthalmologist or optometrist who is experienced in the management of diabetic retinopathy
- A1c if results are not available in past 3 mo, or 6 mo if meeting glycemic goals
- If not performed within the past year: lipid profile, LFTs, spot urinary albumin:Cr ratio, serum Cr, and eGFR, vitamin B_{12} if on metformin, serum potassium if on ACEI, ARB, or diuretics
- If second-generation antipsychotics are being used, changes in weight, glycemic control, and cholesterol levels should be carefully monitored.

ADRENAL INSUFFICIENCY

Common Causes

Secondary (more common; mineralocorticoid function is preserved, no hyperkalemia or hyperpigmentation, dehydration is less common)

- Abrupt discontinuation of chronic glucocorticoid administration
- Megestrol acetate
- Brain irradiation
- Traumatic brain injury
- Pituitary tumors

Primary (less common)

- Autoimmune
- Tuberculosis
- Metastatic cancer

Evaluation

- Basal (morning) plasma cortisol >18 mcg/dL excludes adrenal insufficiency, and <3 mcg/dL is diagnostic.
- ACTH stimulation test: tetracosactrin *(Synacthen Depot)* 250 mcg IV; best administered in the morning; peak value at 30–60 min >18 mcg/dL is normal, <15 mcg/dL is diagnostic.
- If adrenal insufficiency is diagnosed with high ACTH (eg, >100 pg/mL), insufficiency is primary.

Pharmacotherapy

For corticosteroid dose equivalencies, see **Table 52**.

Table 52. Corticosteroids

Medication	Approx Equivalent Dose, mg	Relative Anti-inflammatory Potency	Relative Mineralocorticoid Potency	Half-life, h
Betamethasone	0.6–0.75	20–30	0	36–54
Cortisone	25	0.8	2	8–12
Dexamethasone	0.75	20–30	0	36–54
Fludrocortisone[1]	NA	10	4	12–36
Hydrocortisone	20	1	2	8–12
Methylprednisolone	4	5	0	18–36
Prednisolone	5	4	1	18–36
Prednisone	5	4	1	18–36
Triamcinolone	4	5	0	18–36

NA, not available.

[1] Usually given for orthostatic hypotension at 0.1 mg q8–24h (max 1 mg/d) and at 0.05–0.2 mg/d for primary adrenal insufficiency.

- For acute adrenal insufficiency, begin tx with dexamethasone if no previous diagnosis, while completing diagnostic evaluation. If previously diagnosed, IV hydrocortisone 100 mg IV bolus followed by 50 mg IV q6h × 24 h.

- For chronic adrenal insufficiency, hydrocortisone po in 2 or 3 divided doses (total dose of 10–12 mg/m^2/d). Alternatives are dexamethasone or prednisone. If primary adrenal insufficiency, add fludrocortisone to glucocorticoids. Adjust fludrocortisone dose to lower the plasma renin activity to the upper normal range. In women with impaired mood or well-being despite tx, consider DHEA 50 mg/d.
- Stress doses of corticosteroids for patients with severe illness, injury, or undergoing surgery: In emergency situations, do not wait for test results. Give hydrocortisone 100 mg IV bolus (or if patient has not been previously diagnosed, dexamethasone 4 mg IV bolus). Also treat with IV fluids (eg, saline). For less severe stress (eg, minor illness), double or triple usual oral replacement dosage for 3 d.
- For minor surgery (eg, hernia repair), hydrocortisone 25 mg/d on day of surgery and return to usual dosage on the following day.
- For moderate surgical stress (eg, cholecystectomy, joint replacement), total 50–75 mg/d on the day of surgery and the first postoperative day, then usual dosage on the second postoperative day.
- For major surgical procedures (eg, cardiac bypass), total 100–150 mg/d given in divided doses for 2–3 d, then return to usual dosage.

EYE DISORDERS

VISUAL IMPAIRMENT

Definition

Visual acuity 20/40 or worse; severe visual impairment (legal blindness) 20/200 or worse in the better eye.

Visual Acuity	*Examples of Problems with Daily Tasks*
20/50	Reading newspaper print
20/70	Reading large print
20/100	Writing checks
20/400	Reading paper currency

Evaluation

- Acuity testing
  - Near vision: check each eye independently with glasses using handheld Rosenbaum card at 14″ or Lighthouse Near Acuity Test at 16″. *Note:* Distance must be accurate.
  - Far vision: Snellen wall chart at 20′
- Visual fields (by confrontation)
- Ophthalmoscopy
- Emergent referral for acute change in vision
- Medication review for drugs associated with ocular adverse effects (eg, amiodarone, minocycline, sildenafil, tamoxifen, bisphosphonates, hydroxychloroquine, antipsychotics, SSRIs, lithium, topiramate, carbamazepine, TCAs) and agents with anticholinergic properties

Prevention

Biennial full eye exams for people aged >65, at diagnosis and every 1–2 y for people with DM (see Diabetic Retinopathy below).

SPECIFIC CONDITIONS ASSOCIATED WITH VISUAL IMPAIRMENT

Refractive Error

- The most common cause of visual impairment. Incorrect refraction may account for 20% of IADL dysfunction.
- Correction with multifocal lenses increases risk of falls.

Cataracts

Lens opacity on ophthalmoscopic exam. Risk factors: age, sun exposure, smoking, corticosteroids, DM, alcohol, low vitamin intake, quetiapine. Smoking cessation reduces risk for cataract extraction.

Nonpharmacologic Interventions

- Reduce UV light exposure.
- Criteria for cataract extraction:
  - If visual function no longer meets the patient's needs and cataract surgery is likely to improve vision.
  - When cataract coexists with lens-induced disease (eg, glaucoma) or other eye disease requiring unrestricted monitoring (eg, diabetic retinopathy).

- Cataract extraction, other considerations:
  - Benefits include reduced fall risk with the first but possibly not with the second extraction.
  - Dry eye can be exacerbated by cataract surgery. Treat dry eye before and after surgery to reduce complications.
  - The risk of bleeding is small when antithrombotic agents are continued in the perioperative period (p 285).
  - Do not perform preoperative medical tests for eye surgery without specific indications. Reasonable indications include an ECG in patients with heart disease, serum K^+ in patients on diuretics, and serum glucose in patients with DM.[CW] Outpatient eye surgery is ***not*** associated with increased risk of MI.

Age-related Macular Degeneration (AMD)

Atrophy of cells in the central macular region of retinal pigmented epithelium; on ophthalmoscopic exam, white-yellow patches (drusen) or hemorrhage and scars in advanced stages. AMD has "wet" and "dry" forms.

- Risk factors: age, smoking, sun exposure, family hx, White race (14% of White Americans by age 80). In observational studies, high calcium intake (diet and supplements) reduces risk of progression to late-stage AMD.
- Patients with AMD have double the rate of depression and those with depression perceive greater vision-related disability compared to peers with AMD and no depression; evaluate for depression annually and treat.
- Dry AMD: Accounts for 85–90% of cases, is characterized by abnormalities in the retinal pigment with focal drusen, and has a natural hx of slow gradual loss of vision; may convert to the wet form.
- Wet AMD or neovascular type: Often causes rapid visual loss; causes 90% of severe visual loss in AMD. Early intervention when the dry form converts to the wet form saves vision.

Nonpharmacologic Interventions

- Smoking cessation
- Monitor daily for conversion from dry to wet form using Amsler grid.
- Patients with large drusen most at risk of conversion to wet AMD.
- Dietary modification reduces risk of progression to neovascular AMD: high intake of beta-carotene, vitamin C, zinc, n-3 long-chain polyunsaturated fatty acids, and fish.

Pharmacotherapy of Wet AMD

- Vascular endothelial growth factor (VEGF) inhibitors and inhibitor-like drugs reduce neovascularization (eg, bevacizumab, ranibizumab, aflibercept, or brolucizumab); all given intravitreal; maintain vision in the majority and improves it in a significant minority.
- Frequency of injections (often monthly) impedes adherence with tx. Brolucizumab *(Beovu)* is longer acting (q2–3mo).
- Refillable ocular implant *(Susvimo)* for continuous administration of ranibizumab needs refilled q24wk; must have prior response to VEGF inhibitors; higher rate of endophthalmitis than other VEGF injectables.
- Complications of the intraocular injections include uveitis, cataract, increased IOP, retinal detachment or endophthalmitis, and visual loss in 1–2% of patients.
- Most patients can receive intraocular VEGF inhibitors while taking anticoagulants and antiplatelet agents, but tx must be individualized.
- Patients have serious problems with depression despite effective VEGF inhibitor tx.

Pharmacotherapy of Both Wet and Dry AMD

- In intermediate or more advanced stages of dry AMD and all stages of wet AMD, AREDS2 preparation (zinc oxide 80 mg, cupric oxide 2 mg, lutein 10 mg, zeaxanthin 2 mg, vitamin C 500 mg, and vitamin E 400 IU) in divided doses q12h reduces risk of progression with effectiveness ≥ AREDS1 without increase in lung cancer seen with AREDS1.

Table 53. Ophthalmologic Indications for VEGF Inhibitors

Agent	AMD	Neovascular (wet) AMD	Diabetic macular edema	Diabetic retinopathy	Macular edema[1]	Myopic choroidal neovascularization
Aflibercept	x		x	x	x	
Bevacizumab	OL		OL			
Brolucizumab		x				
Pegaptanib		x				
Ranibizumab	x	x	x	x	x	x

x, FDA label indication; OL, off-label; [1] after retinal vein occlusion

Diabetic Retinopathy: Proliferative Retinopathy and Macular Edema

Retinopathy: microaneurysms, dot and blot hemorrhages on ophthalmoscopy with proliferative retinopathy ischemia and vitreous hemorrhage.

Macular edema: intraretinal fluid (edema) and thickening involving the macula; is a vision-threatening complication of DM and can occur at any stage or severity of diabetic retinopathy.

Risk factors: chronic hyperglycemia, smoking. Screen all patients with DM2 at the time of diagnosis, and at least annually if any retinopathy is found; if none at baseline, rescreen every 2 y.

Management

- Annual ophthalmologic evaluation determines the level of retinopathy (ie, mild, moderate, severe), whether retinopathy is proliferative or nonproliferative, and whether macular edema is present.
- The combination of these features determines the follow-up interval of 1–12 mo.
- VEGF inhibitors are first-line tx for diabetic macular edema; treat monthly for 6 mo then as needed; achieves stability for 5 y. VEGF inhibitors for proliferative retinopathy requires q2–4wk injections long-term, which reduces adherence. Panretinal photocoagulation remains an important tx with equivalent visual outcomes.

Diabetic Management to Reduce Risk or Progression of Retinopathy

Tailor glycemic control based on comorbidities and life expectancy (Diabetes, p 115); BP control <140/80 mm Hg; benefits of lipid control have not been established.

Glaucoma

An optic neuropathy that may or may not be associated with elevated IOP. Findings include optic cupping and nerve damage, and loss of peripheral visual fields. Tx targets reducing IOP regardless of baseline pressure.

- Risk factors: Black race, age, family hx, increased ocular pressures. Most common cause of blindness in Black Americans. Most patients need 6-mo follow-up appointments.

- Primary open-angle glaucoma is asymptomatic until severe visual loss occurs. Initial tx may be either pharmacologic or laser surgery; more severe damage prompts earlier surgery.
- Angle-closure glaucoma, while a less common disease, has both acute and chronic variants, and is painful if acute, requiring emergent management.
- Angle-closure glaucoma is a surgical disease, although topicals are used preoperatively to control IOP.

Nonpharmacologic Interventions

- Open angle—selective laser trabeculoplasty (SLT) is first-line nonpharmacologic tx based on patient preference, adherence issues, intolerance to topical agents. Best results if SLT is used before topical agents.
- Surgical procedures (filtration, shunts, etc) have complications such as scarring and visual loss. Newer minimally invasive procedures may reduce complications.
- Angle closure (both acute and chronic)—laser peripheral iridotomy

Pharmacotherapy—reduces aqueous inflow or increases outflow

- Prostaglandin analogs are first line followed by β blockers (**Table 54**).
- Combining drugs from different classes reduces pressure more than monotx.
- Patients receiving oral β blockers do not benefit from adding the topical; the combination increases AEs.
- Administration: Patients must use proper technique both for benefit and to avoid systemic ADRs, ie, instill 1 gtt under lower lid, close eye for at least 1 min to reduce systemic absorption; repeat if a second drop is needed. Systemic absorption is further reduced by teaching the patient to compress the lacrimal sac for 15–30 sec after instilling a drop. Always wait 5 min before instilling a second type of drop. Eyedrop cups assist patients with tremor or other reasons that make instillation difficult.

Table 54. Medications Commonly Used for Treating Glaucoma

Medication	Adverse Effects (metabolism)
Prostaglandin Analogs (bottles with turquoise caps) ✓Bimatoprost, ✓Latanoprost, Latanoprostene, Tafluprost, ✓Travoprost drops	First-line tx *Systemic AEs:* few, if any *Class AEs:* change in eye color and periorbital tissues, hyperemia, itching (L)
β Blockers (bottles with blue or yellow caps) ✓Betaxolol, ✓Carteolol, ✓Levobunolol, ✓Metipranolol, ✓Timolol drops	*Systemic AEs:* hypotension, bradycardia, HF, bronchospasm, anxiety, depression, confusion, hallucination, diarrhea, nausea, cramps, lethargy, weakness, masking of hypoglycemia, sexual dysfunction. Use with caution in asthma, bradycardia, COPD, HF, or when taking oral β-blockers. Betaxolol may cause fewer systemic effects than the nonselective alternatives, but is less effective at lowering IOP. (L) *Ocular AEs:* rarely cause stinging, itching, redness, and blurred vision

(cont.)

Table 54. Medications Commonly Used for Treating Glaucoma (cont.)	
Medication	**Adverse Effects (Metabolism)**
Carbonic Anhydrase Inhibitors	
Topical (bottles with orange caps) ✓Brinzolamide, ✓Dorzolamide drops	*Systemic AEs:* bitter taste *Ocular AEs:* eye irritation, redness, avoid after corneal transplant (K)
Oral Acetazolamide, Methazolamide po	*Systemic AEs:* fatigue, weight loss, bitter taste, paresthesias, depression, COPD exacerbation, cramps, nausea, diarrhea, kidney failure, blood dyscrasias, hypokalemia, myopia, renal calculi acidosis; not recommended in kidney failure. Acetazolamide (K), Methazolamide (L, K)
Combinations (May improve adherence when both agents required)	
Dorzolamide/timolol, Brimonidine/timolol, Brinzolamide/brimonidine drops	See individual agents
Rho Kinase Inhibitor	
Netarsudil *(Rhopressa)* drops	*Systemic AEs:* not reported *Ocular AEs:* hyperemia, corneal verticillata, conjunctival hemorrhage (eye)

✓ = preferred for treating older patients.

Note: Patients may not know names of drugs but instead refer to them by the color of the bottle cap. The usual colors are listed above.

ADDITIONAL CONSIDERATIONS IN MANAGEMENT OF EYE DISORDERS

Topical Steroid Treatment

Are prescribed for serious ocular inflammatory disorders and long-term use requires monitoring by an ophthalmologist. Serious and potentially vision-threatening adverse effects can occur from chronic topical corticosteroid use.

Low-vision Services

- Address the full range of functional visual impairment from blindness to partial sight. Refer patients with uncompensated visual loss that reduces function. Participation may reduce depression.
- Recommend and provide training on technology to reduce impairment (afb.org/blindness-and-low-vision/using-technology)
  - General technology (eg, computers, smart phones, GPS devices)
  - Assistive technology are those designed specifically for persons with vision impairment
    - Screen readers, screen magnifiers, and video magnifiers
    - Spectacle-mounted telescopes for distance vision, including driving
    - Closed-circuit television to enlarge text
    - Tablet and smartphone apps are an inexpensive substitute for text-to-speech conversion, lighted magnifiers, big clocks, etc.
    - *Spotlight Text* is an eBook reader app for readers with vision loss and has a book share with >250,000 books.
- Environmental modifications that improve function include color contrast, floor lamps to reduce glare, motion sensors to turn on lights, talking clocks, spoken medication reminders.
- Many states have "Services for the Visually Impaired" through the health department.

Dual Sensory Impairment (DSI)

- 9–21% of adults aged >70 have loss of both vision and hearing; tx of both may improve quality of life.
- Compared with single-sensory impairment, DSI is more often associated with depression, poor self-rated health, reduced social participation, IADL and cognitive impairment, and higher mortality (OR=1.6–2.2 at 10 y).
- Nursing home residents with DSI have higher risk of behavioral problems and faster cognitive decline (unless they remain socially engaged).
- Persons with dementia and DSI have greater functional impairment than persons with dementia and either no sensory impairment or DSI.
- Management currently limited to vibrating devices such as alarm clocks, doorbells, smoke alarms, etc.
- Rehab should be designed by a team of providers from audiology and visual rehab.

RED EYE

The "red eye" is an eye with vascular congestion: some conditions that cause this pose a threat to vision and warrant prompt ophthalmologic referral (**Table 55**).

Initial evaluation: check visual acuity, pupil reactivity; note if painful, corneal ulcer, or exudate in the anterior chamber (**Table 55**).

- Acute conjunctivitis, allergic conjunctivitis, and foreign bodies are common causes of red eye. Diagnosis and tx of acute and allergic conjunctivitis are discussed below.

Table 55. Signs and Symptoms of Serious Conditions in Patients with Red Eye

Red Flag Signs and Symptom	Potentially Dangerous Condition(s)
Lid or lacrimal sac swelling or proptosis	Orbital cellulitis, orbital tumor
Subnormal visual acuity, foreign-body sensation, severe pain, photophobia, or circumcorneal hyperemia (ciliary flush)	Keratitis, anterior uveitis; acute angle-closure glaucoma; endophthalmitis, episcleritis, and scleritis
Proptosis, chemosis, visual loss, and ophthalmoplegia	Cavernous sinus arteriovenous fistula

Acute Conjunctivitis

Symptoms: Red eye, foreign-body sensation, discharge, photophobia

Signs: Conjunctival hyperemia and discharge

Etiology: Viral, bacterial, chlamydial

Viral Versus Bacterial:

Viral—profuse tearing, minimal exudate, preauricular adenopathy common, monocytes in stained scrapings and exudates; may be part of URI. Extremely contagious; wash hands frequently and use separate towels to avoid spread.

Bacterial—moderate tearing, profuse exudation, preauricular adenopathy uncommon, bacteria and polymorphonuclear cells in stained scrapings and exudates

Both—minimal itching, generalized hyperemia, occasional sore throat, and fever

Management: Most are viral; do not treat viral infections with antibiotics; if diagnosis is uncertain, patients may be followed closely for worsening that would warrant antibiotics.[CW]

- Treat viral infections with artificial tears and cool compresses.

- If purulent discharge, suspect bacterial. Many cases resolve without antibiotics and without adverse effect on visual function. Antibiotics reduce duration of symptoms. Some recommend use of erythromycin or polymyxin/trimethoprim. Avoid quinolones, which are expensive and select resistant organisms (**Table 56**). If severe, obtain culture and Gram stain, then start tx.
- If signs and symptoms do not improve in 24–48 h on tx for bacterial conjunctivitis, refer to ophthalmologist.
- If severe purulence or if patient wears contact lenses, refer to ophthalmologist immediately.

Table 56. Treatment for Acute Bacterial Conjunctivitis[1]

Medication/Formulations[2]	Comments
First Line (inexpensive, narrow spectrum)	
Erythromycin 5 mg/g oint	Good if staphylococcal blepharitis is present
Trimethoprim and polymyxin 1 mg/mL, 10,000 IU/mL sol	Well tolerated but some gaps in coverage
Second Line (more expensive, broad spectrum); preferred in contact lens wearers	
Besifloxacin *(Besivance)* 0.6% sol	Very broad spectrum, a first choice in severe cases, well tolerated, expensive
Ciprofloxacin 0.3% sol, 0.3% oint	See besifloxacin
Gatifloxacin 0.3% sol	See besifloxacin
Moxifloxacin 0.5% sol	See besifloxacin
Ofloxacin 0.3% sol, 0.3% oint	See besifloxacin
Tobramycin 3 mg/g oint, 3 mg/mL sol	Well tolerated but more corneal toxicity

[1] Do not use steroid or steroid-antibiotic preparations in initial tx.

[2] In mild cases, solution is applied q6h and gel or oint q12h for 5–7 d. In more severe cases, solution is applied q2–3h and oint q6h; as the eye improves, solution is applied q6h and oint q12h.

Allergic Conjunctivitis

Symptoms: Prominent itching, watery discharge accompanied by nasal stuffiness often seen with allergic rhinitis (p 310).

Signs: Bilateral eyelid edema, conjunctival bogginess, and hyperemia.

Etiology: IgE–mediated hypersensitivity to airborne allergen

Management:

Mild to Moderate Symptoms

- Dilute and clear allergen with liberal use of refrigerated artificial tears.
- Topical H_1 antihistamine with mast cell stabilizing properties are the most effective agents, compared to mast cell stabilizers or topical NSAIDs (**Table 57**); 2 wk of tx required for full effectiveness. If symptoms are seasonal, begin tx 2–3 wk before pollen season.
- A daily-wear drug-eluting monovision contact lens *(Acuvue Theravision with Ketotifen)* is an option for people with both a need for contact lens and tx for allergic conjunctivitis (ie, no need to remove lens to instill gtt).
- Nasal steroids reduce ocular symptoms to some degree (**Table 117**).
- Oral antihistamines may aggravate symptoms if there is a concomitant dry eye.

Severe or Persistent Symptoms

- If symptoms persist after 3 wk of topical antihistamine/mast cell stabilizer, refer to an ophthalmologist to confirm diagnosis.
- Topical steroids (eg, loteprednol) may be necessary but should be prescribed only by an ophthalmologist.
- The OTC vasoconstrictor/antihistamines are for short-term use only (**Table 57**).
- Recurrent or severe symptoms may benefit from desensitization; refer to allergist.

Table 57. Topical Therapy for Allergic Conjunctivitis

Category/Medication	Adverse Events[1]/Comments
H_1 Antihistamine/Mast Cell Stabilizers (effective within a few minutes)	
Alcaftadine [OTC]	*Class effects*: Itching, erythema, headache, rhinitis, dysgeusia, cold syndrome, headache, keratitis
Azelastine	
Bepotastine *(Bepreve)*	
Cetirizine	
Epinastine	
Ketotifen[OTC, 2]	
Olopatadine	May be more effective than ketotifen
NSAID (less effective than H1 antihistamines)	
Ketorolac	Ocular irritation, burning[2]
Mast Cell Stabilizers (slower onset of action better for prevention than symptom management)	
Lodoxamide *(Alomide)*	Ocular irritation, burning
Cromolyn sodium	Ocular irritation, burning
Nedocromil	Headache, ocular irritation, burning
Vasoconstrictor/Antihistamine combinations (for short-term <2 wk use only)	
Pemirolast *(Alamast)*	Headache, rhinitis, flu-like symptoms, ocular irritation, burning
Naphazoline[OTC] (0.1%, 0.12%, 0.2%)	*Class effects:* Caution in heart disease, HTN, BPH, narrow angle glaucoma; chronic use can cause follicular reactions or contact dermatitis
Pheniramine maleate (0.3–0.315%)/naphazoline hydrochloride (0.025–0.027%)[OTC]	
Tetrahydrozoline (0.05%)[OTC]	

[1] Most contain benzalkonium chloride and may cause stinging, which can be reduced by refrigerating drops.

2 Preservative (benzalkonium chloride) -free preparations available

BLEPHARITIS

Inflammation of the eyelid margin that causes eye irritation; may affect inner portion of the eyelid (posterior blepharitis) or the base of the eyelashes (anterior blepharitis).

Inflammation causes instability of tear film and abnormal secretions that have a toxic effect on the ocular surface, promoting bacterial growth. Long-term inflammation leads to gland dysfunction, fibrosis, and damage to the eyelid and ocular surface.

Symptoms: generally chronic recurrent symptoms, which vary over time, involving both eyes. These include:

- Red, swollen, or itchy eyelids
- Crusting of eyelashes in the morning
- Gritty or burning sensation
- Excessive tearing
- Flaking/scaling of the eyelid skin

Diagnosis is clinical, based on findings of bilateral red and irritated eyelid margins with crusting or flakes on the lashes or lid margins. If the diagnosis is unclear, refer to ophthalmology.

Management: Good lid hygiene is the mainstay of tx.

- **Mild to moderate symptoms**: Tx is symptomatic with warm compresses (5–10 min, 2–4×/d), lid massage (gentle circular motion against the eye), lid washing (with very dilute baby shampoo, rinse thoroughly, or use commercial preparation), and artificial tears (for dryness).
- **Severe or refractory symptoms**: Patients who do not respond to the above measures or those with severe symptoms need topical or oral antibiotic tx and need referral to ophthalmology.

PTOSIS

Ptosis occurs due to dysfunction of the muscles that raise the eyelid or their nerve supply.

- Acquired ptosis is most commonly caused by aponeurotic ptosis as a result of senescence, dehiscence, or disinsertion of the levator aponeurosis.
  - Risk factors: age, chronic inflammation, intraocular surgery, prolonged use of contact lenses
  - Tx is most often surgical and indicated when ptosis is severe enough to interfere with vision.
  - Nonsurgical tx includes mechanical support of the affected lid(s) with a ptosis crutch, which is a bar placed along the inside of an eyewear frame that supports the drooping eyelid. The crutch creates a fold above the eye, tucking the lid in, and raising it above the pupil.
- Other causes of ptosis to consider in older people include myasthenia gravis, drug induced (pregabalin, high-dose opioids), oculomotor nerve palsy (often in people with DM2), and Horner syndrome.

DRY EYE DISEASE (DED)

Symptoms: itchy or sandy eyes (foreign-body sensation), visual impairment, excess tearing.

Signs: symmetrical conjunctival injection, blepharitis, entropion, ectropion, reduced blink

Etiology: altered tear film composition, reduced tear production, poor lid function, environment, drug-induced causes (eg, anticholinergics, estrogens, SSRIs, diuretics), or diseases such as Sjögren syndrome; refer to ophthalmology for diagnostic assistance.

Management:

- Application of warm compresses softens secretions in obstructed meibomian excretory ducts.

- Artificial tear formulations are administered q1–6h prn.
  - There are limited data on whether different OTC artificial tears provide similar relief of signs and symptoms when compared with each other or placebo.
  - However it appears that 0.2% polyacrylic acid-based artificial tears (*Viscotears* gel) are more effective at managing dry-eye symptoms than 1.4% polyvinyl alcohol-based artificial tears (eg, *Opti-Lube*) in 2 trials that assessed this comparison.
  - Preservatives may cause eye irritation. Preservative-free preparations should be recommended if frequency of use is more often than q6h. Ointment preparations can be used at night or also during the day in severe cases.
- Hydroxypropyl cellulose ophthalmic insert gradually released over 24 h (eg, *Lacrisert*) by prescription or OTC is FDA approved for moderate to severe DED.
- Environmental strategies: room humidifiers, frequent blinking, and swim goggles or moisture chambers fit to eyeglasses are all helpful.
- Scleral contact lenses reduce dry eye. Must be fit by an experienced contact lens provider.
- Pharmacotherapy (when unresponsive to the above measures):
  - Cyclosporine ophthalmic emulsion 0.05% and 0.09% (Cequa) 1 gtt OU q12h. Indicated when tear production is suppressed by inflammation. May take 4–6 wk to achieve results. Must have a complete eye exam before prescribing.
  - Lifitegrast 5% *(Xiidra)*, an integrin antagonist, improves symptoms in mild to severe cases. Dose: 1 gtt q12h, ADRs: eye irritation, bad taste in 25%. Patients should be monitored by an ophthalmologist.
  - Varenicline nasal spray *(Tyrvaya)*, a cholinergic agonist, 1 spr intranasal 2×/d, increases tear production. ADRs are sneezing, cough, throat, and nasal irritation.
- Surgery:
  - Temporary or permanent punctal occlusion; do not place punctal occlusion for mild dry eye before trying other medical tx.[CW]
  - Eyelid abnormalities should be surgically corrected to recreate normal lid architecture. Surgery is also used on normal eyelids to reduce ocular surface area and reduce tear evaporation.

FALLS

DEFINITION

An event that results in a person coming to rest inadvertently on the ground, floor, or other lower level without known loss of consciousness (WHO, 2018; AGS/BGS Clinical Practice Guideline: Prevention of Falls in Older Persons, 2010). Excludes falls from major intrinsic event (eg, seizure, stroke, syncope), which should be evaluated and managed.

ETIOLOGY

Typically multifactorial. Composed of intrinsic (eg, poor balance, weakness, chronic illness, visual or cognitive impairment), extrinsic (eg, polypharmacy), and environmental (eg, poor lighting, no safety equipment, loose carpets) factors. Commonly a nonspecific sign for one of many acute illnesses in older adults.

SCREENING

Fall risk screening is an important first step in fall prevention, but must be followed by a thorough assessment and the development of a plan that tailors person-centered interventions to address identified risk factors. Fall risk screening or assessment is a quality measure included in the CMS MACRA and Medicare Annual Wellness Visit.

Screen for fall risk as part of routine primary healthcare visit (at least annually). Risk of falling significantly increases as the number of risk factors increases. Falls occur frequently in ambulatory residents in long-term care and in acute care settings.

- Ask 3 questions to determine risk (yes to any question suggests increased fall risk)
  - Feel unsteady when standing or walking?
  - Worries about falling?
  - Has fallen in past year? (If yes, ask "How many times?" and "Were you injured?")
- Use a fall risk screening tool to identify risk factors (see below)
- Complete *Stay Independent* brochure: a 12-question tool to identify risk

Table 58. Toolkits and Tools Available to Guide Falls Screening, Assessment, and Tailored Intervention

Setting	Title (url)
Community	Stopping Elderly Accidents, Deaths and Injuries [STEADI] (cdc.gov/Steadi; cdc.gov/steadi/training.html) Stay Independent brochure (cdc.gov/steadi/pdf/STEADI-Brochure-StayIndependent-508.pdf)
Nursing facilities	AHRQ Safety Program for Nursing Homes: On-Time Falls Prevention (ahrq.gov/patient-safety/settings/long-term-care/resource/ontime/fallspx/intro.html) The Morse Fall Scale
Hospitals	AHRQ (ahrq.gov/professionals/systems/hospital/fallpxtoolkit/index.html) The Morse Fall Scale

ASSESSMENT

- Assess for modifiable risk factors and fall hx.
- Assess for risk factors (**Table 59**) using a multidisciplinary team, such as PT and OT, if problems with gait, balance, or lower extremity strength are identified.
- See **Figure 6** for recommended assessment strategies. USPSTF does not recommend multifactorial assessment, although small benefit (6% reduction in fall risk; 11% when risk factors managed).

- USPSTF recommends assessing for the following risk factors for falls in older adults: age, hx of falls, and impairments in mobility, gait, and balance
- Reassess yearly or any time patient presents with an acute fall

Table 59. Risk Factors and Medications Associated with Falls (in those with at least one fall during follow-up)

Risk Factor Category and OR	Specific Risk Factor	Evaluation
Falls ≥1.5	Hx of falls; fear of falling	Assess fear of falling using 7-item *Falls Efficacy Scale-International* (FES-I). Measures levels of concern about falling during physical and social activities on a 1- to 4-point Likert scale (sites.manchester.ac.uk/fes-i/)
Pain ≥1.5	Number of chronic musculoskeletal pain sites; pain (yes/no)	Pain intensity scale; *Brief Pain Inventory*—Pain Interference Scale; pain distribution; assess for antalgic gait; note higher pain severity
Pain <1.5	Moderate to severe foot pain[1]	Assess feet or footwear issues
Medical conditions ≥1.5	Parkinson disease; rheumatic disease, orthostatic BP	See **Table 61** for symptoms
Medical conditions <1.5	UI[1]; arthritis; depression/anxiety; comorbidity[1]	PHQ2/9; GAD7
Activity/Balance ≥1.5	Balance limits activity; homebound; walking aid use; gait deficit; many problems moving around; ADL difficulty-physical	Functional gait: observe chair sit to stand, walking (stride length, speed, symmetry), turning, TUG test; volitional and reactive step test Mobility: observe use and fit of assistive device (eg, cane, walker) or personal assistance, extent of ambulation Balance: semi-tandem, and full-tandem stance; presence of forward head posture; Functional Reach test; Berg Balance Scale (especially retrieve object from floor); Short Physical Performance Battery (SPPB) Neither Functional Reach Test, Single Leg Stance Test, or Tinetti Performance-Oriented Mobility Assessment are able to consistently predict falls. Do not substitute for comprehensive falls risk assessment, but use to identify and track balance impairment
Activity/Balance <1.5	IADL difficulty-physical	
Sensory ≥1.5	Vertigo	See Dizziness, p 234
Sensory <1.5	Visual deficit, particularly unilateral visual loss[1]; hearing impairment[1]; glaucoma	See Eye Disorders and Hearing Impairment; Snellen Chart; Brief Hearing Loss Screener; whisper test
Cognitive/Psychiatric ≥1.5	Poor self-rated health; depression	PHQ-2

(cont.)

Table 59. **Risk Factors and Medications Associated with Falls (in those with at least one fall during follow-up) (cont.)**

Risk Factor Category and OR	Specific Risk Factor	Evaluation
Cognitive/Psychiatric <1.5	Cognitive impairment[1]	Cognition: assess frontal-lobe cognitive function (MiniCog) to identify impaired executive function and judgment that can impact fall risk
Medications ≥1.5	≥2 CNS-active agents (Avoid >3 CNS-active agents[BC]); NSAIDs; non-TCA/non-SSRI (SNRI[BC]); polypharmacy; other sedatives (Avoid[BC]), hypnotics; anticonvulsants (Avoid[BC]); antiarrhythmics (Class 1A)	Identify medications that increase fall risk[BC] (**Table 61**)
Medications <1.5	TCA[1] (Avoid[BC])/SSRI; benzodiazepines[BC]; opioids; antipsychotics[1]; antihypertensives; loop diuretics	Risk-benefit analysis for opioids as both pain and opioids increase fall risk
Other medications associated with ND	Skeletal muscle relaxants (Avoid[BC]); systemic glucocorticoids	Identify medications that increase fall risk[BC] (**Table 61**)

OR, odds ratio; ND, no data on OR unable to calculate.

[1] increased OR to 1.5 or greater for recurrent fallers[BC]

EVALUATION OF FALL

Diagnose and treat underlying cause. Exclude acute illness or underlying systemic or metabolic process (eg, infection, electrolyte imbalance) as indicated by hx, exam, and lab studies. Determine if fall is syncopal or nonsyncopal (Syncope, p 74). Evaluate impact of cognition.

History

- Circumstances of fall (eg, activity at time of fall, location, time, footwear at time of fall, lighting)
- Associated symptoms (eg, lightheadedness, vertigo, syncope, weakness, confusion, palpitations, joint pain, joint stability, feelings of pitching [common in Parkinson disease], foot pain, ankle instability); functional status
- Relevant comorbid conditions (eg, prior stroke, parkinsonism, cardiac disease, DM, seizure disorder, depression, anxiety, hyperplastic anemia, sensory deficit, OA, osteoporosis, hyperthyroidism, glucocorticoid excess, GI or chronic renal disease, myeloma)
- Medication review, including OTC medications and alcohol use; note recent changes (p 17)

Physical Exam

- Vital signs: postural pulse and BP lying and 3 min after standing, temperature
- Head and neck: visual impairment (especially poor acuity; reduced contrast sensitivity; decreased visual fields; cataracts): if dizziness, check for motion-induced vertigo and nystagmus (Dix-Hallpike test); bruit
- Musculoskeletal: arthritic changes, motion or joint limitations (especially lower extremity joint function), postural instability, skeletal deformities, podiatric problems, muscle strength

- Neurologic: slower reflexes, altered proprioception, altered mental status (focus on frontal-lobe impairment and impact on making poor choices), focal deficits, peripheral neuropathy, gait or balance disorders, hip flexor weakness, instability, tremor, rigidity
- Cardiovascular: heart arrhythmias, cardiac valve dysfunction (peripheral vascular changes, pedal pulses)

Figure 6. Assessment and Prevention of Falls

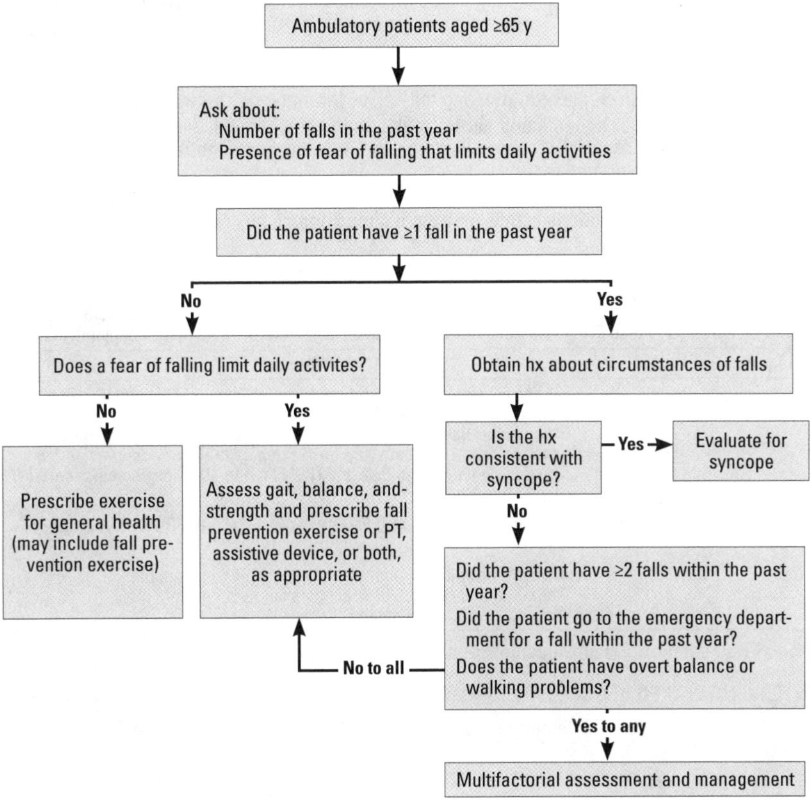

Source: Ganz et al. *N Eng J Med.* 2020;382(8):734–743. Reprinted with permission.

Diagnostic Tests

- Lab tests for people at risk include CBC, serum electrolytes, BUN, Cr, glucose, B_{12}, thyroid function
- Bone densitometry in all women aged >65 except those on osteoporosis tx or those who have osteopenic fragility fractures. Although BMD is not a risk factor for falls, it does affect serious fall-related outcomes (see Osteoporosis, p 246).
- Cardiac workup if symptoms of syncope or presyncope (Syncope Evaluation, p 74)

- Imaging: neuroimaging if head injury or new, focal neurologic findings on examination or if a CNS process is suspected; spinal imaging to exclude cervical spondylosis or lumbar stenosis in patients with abnormal gait, neurologic exam, or lower extremity spasticity or hyperreflexia

PREVENTION OF FALLS

See **Figure 6** for recommended prevention strategies.

Recommendations below are primarily based on studies of community-dwelling older adults with limited evidence from RCTs regarding single or multifactorial interventions in the long-term care setting or in cognitively impaired patients.

- Educate on fall prevention.
- Use multifactorial strategies for lowering fall risk by targeting risk factors (**Table 61**).
  - Consider balance of benefits and harms of identified interventions, based on circumstances of prior falls, comorbid medical conditions, and patient values, in providing comprehensive intervention.
  - Multiple component interventions are most effective across care settings (↓ risk 21% [USPSTF 2018]). Reductions in falls may not be accompanied by reductions in fall-related injuries.
  - No evidence for benefit of hip protectors or medication review in long-term care facilities.
- Refer to community exercise or fall prevention program.

Table 60. Evidence-based Programs Advocated by the CDC and/or Administration for Community Living

Program	Details
Exercise	• *Tai chi: Moving for Better Balance* (or similar tai chi classes), *Otago Exercise Program, Stay Safe, Stay Active* • Otago home-based exercise available at med.unc.edu/aging/cgec/exercise-program/videos and for *Strategies to Reduce Injuries and Develop Confidence in Elders* (STRIDE) stride-study.org/home-excercise/
Multifactorial education programs	*Stepping On*, Prevention Of Falls in the Elderly Trial (PROFET), *A Matter of Balance*
Other	cdc.gov/homeandrecreationalsafety/Falls/compendium.html • Visually impaired (eg, VIP Trial home safety program) • Walking on ice and snow (eg, *Yaktrax Walkers*)

- See Prevention (p 291) or Musculoskeletal Disorders (p 213) for details on exercise.

INTERVENTIONS TO REDUCE FALL RISK FACTORS

- Develop tailored tx plan including recommended interventions as appropriate to reduce fall risk.

FALL MANAGEMENT

- Use strategies to prevent future falls by addressing risk factors (**Table 61**).
- Treat osteoporosis (see Osteoporosis chapter).
- Maintain anticoagulation. Assess risk of anticoagulation (see HAS-BLED in Cardiovascular chapter, **Table 28**). In most cases, benefits of anticoagulation tx outweigh risks (see Antithrombotic Therapy and Thromboembolic Disease [p 39]).

Table 61. Strategies for Lowering Fall Risk	
Factors	**Suggested Interventions (Outcome Reduction[1])**
General Risk	Offer: exercise program to include exercises that address balance and stability, plus resistance (strength), flexibility, and endurance. Exercise combination most effective in reducing # of fallers: anticipatory control, dynamic stability, functional stability limits, reactive control, and flexibility. • medical assessment before starting • tailor to individual capabilities; consider strengths, weaknesses, and injury risk • initiate with caution in those with limited mobility not accustomed to physical activity • progress slowly, appropriate to ability and competence • maintain regular, comfortable, yet challenging plan • provide environment that builds self-efficacy • prescribed by qualified healthcare provider • regular review and progression ↓ risk 11% [USPSTF 2018] ↓ risk 15%; ↓ rate 23% [Cochrane 2019] Tai Chi: ↓ risk 29%, ↓ rate 22% [Cochrane] Aerobic + strength + balance 2–3×/wk (↓ risk 12%) Provide exercise program resources (eg, NIA Exercise Booklet, Otago resources) or refer to local senior exercise program (↓ risk of fall 17%; ↓ risk of injurious falls 49%) Group exercise in community [requires ability to travel, stand independently, and engage in ≥30 min of activity] Home-based exercise program [requires adequate training and progression for safe/effective exercise dose]. Home-based e-health balance exercise programs (eg, *Standing Tall*). Education and information, CBT intervention to decrease fear of falling and activity avoidance (limited evidence [Cochrane]) Telehealth combined with exercise and smart home systems are effective in reducing falls Manage pain and anxiety to reduce fear of falling
Medication-related Factors (Consider deprescribing [see Appropriate Prescribing, p 16 and digital text for further guidance])	
Use of benzodiazepines, sedative-hypnotics, antidepressants, or antipsychotics; opioids	Consider agents with less risk of falls Avoid if hx of falls or fracture[BC] Taper and D/C medications, as possible (see Appropriate Prescribing chapter) Address sleep problems with nonpharmacologic interventions (p 330) Educate regarding appropriate use of medications and monitoring for AEs
Recent change in dosage or number of prescription medications or use of ≥4 prescription medications or use of other medications associated with fall risk	Review medication profile and reduce number and dosage of all medications, as possible (Withdrawal of antipsychotics: no ↓ risk; ↓ rate 66% [Cochrane]) Monitor response to medications and to dosage changes

(cont.)

Table 61. Strategies for Lowering Fall Risk (cont.)	
Factors	**Suggested Interventions (Outcome Reduction[1])**
Mobility-related Factors (cont.)	
Environmental hazards (eg, improper bed height, cluttered walking surfaces, lack of railings, poor lighting)	Refer to OT for home safety evaluation, modifications, and adaptive equipment Improve lighting, especially at night Remove floor barriers (eg, loose carpeting) Replace existing furniture with safer furniture (eg, correct height of beds/chairs, more stable) Install support structures, especially in bathroom (eg, railings, grab bars, elevated toilet seats) Use nonslip bathmats (↓ risk 12%; ↓ rate 19%; more effective delivered by OT [Cochrane])
Impaired gait, balance, or transfer skills	Provide exercise guidance (See above under General Risk). Refer to PT for comprehensive evaluation and rehabilitation. Refer to PT or OT for gait training, transfer skills, use of assistive devices, balancing, strengthening and resistance training, and evaluation for appropriate footwear. Home-based PT must meet definition of "homebound" by CMS to be reimbursed by Medicare.
Impaired gait, balance, or transfer skills (cont.)	Cane fitting: top of the cane should be at the top of the greater trochanter or at the break of the wrist when patient stands with arms at side; when the patient holds the cane, there is approximately a 15° bend at the elbow. Canes are most often used to improve balance but can also be used to reduce weight-bearing on the opposite leg. Walker fitting: walkers are prescribed when a cane does not offer sufficient stability. Front-wheeled walkers allow a more natural gait and are easier for cognitively impaired patients to use. Four-wheeled rolling walkers (ie, rollators) have the advantage for a smoother faster gait, but require more coordination because of the brakes; however, they are good for outside walking because the larger wheels move more easily over sidewalks. Refer to podiatrist for evaluation and management of foot or ankle issues that affect mobility and balance.
Impaired leg or arm strength or range of motion, or proprioception	Refer to PT or OT
Medical Factors	
Parkinson disease, OA, depressive symptoms, impaired cognition, carotid sinus hypersensitivity, other conditions associated with increased falls	Optimize medical tx Monitor for disease progression and impact on mobility and impairments Address issues related to anxiety and impulsiveness, which may increase fall risk Determine need for assistive devices Use bedside commode if frequent nighttime urination cannot be managed by other methods Cardiac pacing in patients with carotid sinus hypersensitivity who experience falls due to syncope (See Syncope, p 74) (↓ rate 27%, but not risk [Cochrane])

(cont.)

Table 61. Strategies for Lowering Fall Risk (cont.)	
Factors	**Suggested Interventions (Outcome Reduction[1])**
Postural hypotension: drop in SBP ≥20 mm Hg (or ≥20%) with or without symptoms, within 3 min of rising from lying to standing	See orthostatic postural hypotension, p 75
Visual (Eye Disorders, p 126)	Refer to ophthalmologist for evaluation and management of vision-related issues Cataract extraction (first eye cataract removal, rate ↓ 34%, but not second eye) Avoid wearing multifocal lenses while walking, particularly up stairs

[1] risk of falls = # people falling; rate of falling = # falls per person

DYSPHAGIA

See also p 281.

Types, Presentation, and Patient Complaints

Table 62. Dysphagia Complaints

Classification	Presentation and Signs	Common Causes
Oral	Inability to move food or medication from mouth to pharynx. Food deposits in cheeks	Dementia
Pharyngeal	Impaired involuntary food transport pharynx to esophagus with airway protection. Coughing, choking, or nasal regurgitation	Stroke, Parkinson disease, CNS tumor, ALS, local strictures, Zenker diverticulum, dementia
Esophageal	Sensation that food is stuck in the throat	Impaired esophageal motility, obstruction, medication

Evaluation

Physical exam and history

- Oral cavity, head, neck, and supraclavicular region
- All cranial nerves with emphasis on nerves V, VII, IX, X, XI, XII
- Review medications for those that can decrease saliva production (eg, anticholinergics)
- Referral to speech-language pathologists

Diagnostic tests (as indicated)

- Modified barium swallow or videofluoroscopy to assess swallowing mechanism; may document aspiration; usual initial test before upper endoscopy (oral-pharyngeal)
- Fiberoptic endoscopic evaluations of swallowing (FEES) provides detailed evaluation of lesions in oropharynx, hypopharynx, larynx, and proximal esophagus; also visualizes pooled secretions or food
- Upper endoscopy in patients with esophageal dysphagia (esophageal)
- Esophageal manometry in combination with barium radiography; more useful for assessment of esophageal dysphagia and usually when a motility disorder is suspected or upper endoscopy is inconclusive (esophageal)

Management

- Identify and treat underlying cause (eg, endoscopic dilation, cricopharyngeal myotomy, botulinum toxin injection in cricopharyngeal muscle)

Oral-Pharyngeal

- Dietary modifications based on recommendation of speech pathologist or dietitian that are consistent with the patients and families wishes and quality of life. Thickening liquids may increase risk of dehydration, and compliance with altered food consistencies may be poor.
- Swallowing rehabilitation, eg, multiple swallows, tilt head back and place bolus on strong side, or chin tuck
- Avoid rushed or forced feeding
- Sit upright at 90°

- Elevate head of the bed at least 30°
- Review medications and administration for unsafe practices, eg, crushing enteric-coated or ER formulations (see Appropriate Prescribing, p 16)

Esophageal

- Symptomatic presbyesophagus responds to esophageal dilatation
- Botulinum toxin for severe esophageal spasms
- Neuromuscular electrical stimulation (NMES)

Fluid and Food Consistencies and Thickening Agents

Table 63. Food Consistencies[1,2]

Category	Consistency	Descriptor
0	Thin	Water; flows like water
1	Slightly thick	Thicker than water, flows through a straw, nipple, or syringe (eg, infant formula; primarily used in pediatrics)
2	Mildly thick	Nectar-like: thin enough to be sipped through a straw, off a spoon, or from a cup, but still spillable (eg, eggnog, buttermilk); 2–3 tsp (10–15 mL) of thickening powder to ½ cup (120 mL) of liquid
3	Moderately thick	Honey-like: thick enough to be drunk from a cup, eaten with a spoon, too thick for a straw without effort, not able to independently hold its shape (eg, yogurt, tomato sauce); no chewing required; 3–5 tsp (15–25 mL) of thickening powder to ½ cup (120 mL) of liquid
4	Extremely thick	Pureed, spoon-thick: pudding-like, must be eaten with a spoon (eg, thickened applesauce); 5–6 tsp (25–30 mL) of thickening powder to ½ cup (120 mL) of liquid
5	Minced & moist	Can be eaten with a spoon, fork, or chopsticks (with dexterity); minimal chewing required
6	Soft & bite-sized	Can be eaten with a spoon, fork, or chopsticks; can be mashed with spoon or fork, no knife required
7	Regular	Normal, everyday foods

[1] Based on the International Dysphagia Diet Standardization Initiative (IDDSI; iddsi.org)

[2] Thickening agents are starch- or gum-based. Liquids thickened with modified starch continue to thicken or over-thicken over time. The thicker the product, the less consumed and the greater risk for dehydration, UTI, and fever.

Note: In patients with dementia, the evidence is conflicting whether nectar- or honey-like thickened liquids reduce the risk for aspiration pneumonia compared to chin-down posture alone.

GASTROESOPHAGEAL REFLUX DISEASE (GERD)

Evaluation and Assessment

Empiric tx is appropriate when hx is typical for uncomplicated GERD.

- Upper GI endoscopy (if symptoms are chronic or persist despite 6–8 wk management with PPI or H2RA, atypical presentation, dysphagia, iron-deficiency anemia, bleeding)
- Ambulatory pH testing: confirm diagnostic when symptoms persist despite normal endoscopy and to monitor adequacy of pH suppressive tx
- Esophageal manometry when normal upper GI endoscopy and esophageal dysphagia

Risk Factors

- Obesity
- Hiatal hernia
- Use of estrogen, nitroglycerin, tobacco
- Genetic predisposition

Symptoms Suggesting Complicated GERD and Need for Evaluation

- Dysphagia
- Bleeding
- Weight loss
- Anemia
- Choking, cough, shortness of breath, hoarseness
- Chest pain
- Pain with swallowing
- Vomiting

Management

Universal Lifestyle and Dietary Interventions Supported by Evidence

- Avoid lying down for 3 h after eating
- Change diet (selective elimination of triggers: spicy, fatty, or acidic foods; carbonated beverages; coffee; tea)
- Elevate head of the bed using 6–8 in blocks
- Lose weight (if overweight)

Recommendations for Treatment-Naive Patients with Mild, Intermittent Symptoms

- Universal lifestyle and dietary interventions
- As needed H2RA
- As needed antacids

Other Interventions

- Consider antireflux surgery (concerns about long-term PPI exposure, hiatal hernia, or intractable symptoms, regurgitation symptoms without motility disorders; not recommended for PPI nonresponders)

Pharmacotherapy of GERD

Treatment with PPIs: reserve for severe or frequent symptoms or erosive esophagitis

- Initial tx: 8 wk with 1×/d PPI with morning meal; use lowest effective dose to achieve symptom control.
- Maintenance tx if symptoms remain after stopping or if complicated by erosive esophagitis or Barrett esophagus
- Long-term use is associated with bone loss and fractures, CAP, hypomagnesemia, and vitamin B_{12} deficiency.
- To discontinue, lowering dose, frequency, or both (eg, 2×/d to 1×/d or every other day) weekly may help prevent symptom rebound.
- PPIs more effective than H_2 antagonists for tx and maintenance
- See deprescribing.org for an algorithm for deprescribing PPIs (deprescribingnetwork.ca)

Treatment-resistant GERD

- PPI q12h × 6–8 wk; consider rabeprazole or esomeprazole if CYP2C19 polymorphism suspected (ie, lack of response to other PPIs).
- Additional diagnostic evaluation (ambulatory pH testing, manometry)
- Transoral incisionless fundoplication when regurgitation symptoms are dominant; may not eliminate the need for long-term PPI tx.
- Laparoscopic Nissen fundoplication works best for typical GERD when at least a 50% response to PPIs.

Table 64. Pharmacotherapy of GERD[CW]	
Medication (Metabolism, Excretion)	**Comments**
PPIs [BC]	
Dexlansoprazole (L) ✓Esomeprazole magnesium[OTC] (L) Esomeprazole strontium (L) ✓Lansoprazole[OTC] (L) ✓Omeprazole[OTC] (L) ✓Pantoprazole (L) ✓Rabeprazole (L)	PPIs more effective than H_2 antagonists for tx and maintenance. Associated with osteopenia/osteoporosis Prolonged exposure may increase risk of fractures, community-acquired pneumonia, *C difficile* diarrhea, hypomagnesemia; reduce vitamins C and B_{12} concentrations, kidney disease, and gastric atrophy. Monitor magnesium if taken long-term or with digoxin. Omeprazole and esomeprazole strongest inhibitors of CYP2C19, pantoprazole is the weakest.
H_2 Antagonists (for less severe GERD)(Avoid[BC] in patients with delirium)	
Cimetidine[OTC] (K, L)	Cimetidine inhibits CYP1A2, -2D6, -3A4
✓Famotidine[OTC] (K)	
Nizatidine (K)	
Prokinetic Agents (No role in absence of gastroparesis)	
✓Domperidone (L)	Domperidone is available in the United States only through an Investigational New Drug application for compassionate use in patients refractory to other tx (fda.gov).
Metoclopramide[BC] (K, F)	Risk of EPS; avoid unless for gastroparesis

✓ = preferred for treating older adults CrCl unit = mL/min

[CW]Use lowest dose needed to achieve symptom control.

PEPTIC ULCER DISEASE

Causes

Helicobacter pylori is the major cause. NSAIDs are the second most common cause.

Diagnosis of *H pylori*

- Endoscopy with biopsy (definitive)

Noninvasive testing

- Urea breath test
- Fecal antigen test
- Serology: poor specificity and sensitivity; cannot differentiate between past and current infection
- PPIs, antibiotics, and bismuth-containing products interfere with testing (except serology). Hold PPIs and bismuth for ≥1–2 wk and antibiotics ≥4 wk before testing.

Who Should be Tested and Treated if Tested Positive

- Active peptic ulcer disease or hx of peptic ulcer disease without *H pylori* eradication
- Low-grade gastric mucosa-associated lymphoid tissue (MALT) lymphoma or hx of endoscopic resection of early gastric cancer
- Long-term, low dose ASA (consider)
- Before initiating long-term NSAID
- Unexplained iron-deficiency anemia
- Idiopathic thrombocytopenia purpura

- After tx for *H pylori* infection to confirm eradication, testing should be performed ≥30 d after completing tx and while the patient is not taking a PPI.
- Review patient's chronic medications for drug interactions before selecting regimen; many potential drug interactions and ADRs.

Table 65. Pharmacotherapeutic Management of *H pylori* Infection

Regimen	Duration	Comments
Bismuth Quadruple Therapy		Consider if penicillin allergy or previous macrolide exposure
PPI[1] po q12h *plus* Bismuth subsalicylate 525 mg po q6h *plus* Metronidazole 250–500 mg po q6h *plus* Tetracycline 500 mg po q6h *(Helidac)*	10–14 d	Preferred first-line regimen Components prescribed separately Bismuth subsalicylate T: 262; C: 262, 527 mg/15 mL
Concomitant Quadruple Therapy		
PPI[1] po q12h *plus* Clarithromycin[BC,2] 500 mg po q12h Amoxicillin 1000 mg po q12h Metronidazole 500 mg po q12h	10–14 d	Preferred first-line regimen
Clarithromycin Triple Therapy		Preferred if no previous macrolide exposure
PPI[1] po q12h *plus* Clarithromycin[BC,2] 500 mg po q12h *plus* Amoxicillin 1000 mg po q12h ***or*** Metronidazole 500 mg po q12h if penicillin allergy	14 d	Example: *PrevPac* (includes lansoprazole 30 mg); Omeclamox-Pak (includes omeprazole) Preferred when clarithromycin resistance is <15% and patients with no previous macrolide exposure
Other		
Vonoprazan 20 mg po q12h Amoxicillin 1000 mg po q12h Clarithromycin[BC,2] 500 mg q12h	14 d	Available as *Voquezna Triple Pak* or *Dual Pak* (vonoprazan and amoxicillin)

[1] Esomeprazole is dosed 40 mg q24h.

[2] Clarithromycin may increase the risk of cardiac AEs and death in patients with CAD. Clarithromycin is a strong inhibitor of CYP3A4 and P-glycoprotein. Small increased risk of major hemorrhage if used in combination with a DOAC.

Source: Adapted from Chey WD et al. *Am J Gastroenterol.* 2017;112:212–238.

Medications

Bismuth subsalicylate (for complete information, see **Table 68**)

Antibiotics: For complete information, see **Table 80**.

PPIs: See **Table 64**.

Duration of use for complicated duodenal ulcers 4–12 wk depending on location and cause

Duration of use may need to be extended when:

- Peptic ulcer size is >2 cm and age >50 or multiple comorbidities
- *H pylori*–negative, NSAID-negative ulcers
- >2 recurrent peptic ulcers per year
- Continued NSAID use

STRESS-ULCER PREVENTION IN HOSPITALIZED OLDER ADULTS

Risk Factors (Prophylaxis if >1 present)

- Hx of GI ulceration or bleed in past year
- Mechanical ventilation for >48 h (major risk factor)
- Coagulopathy (platelets <50,000/μL, INR >1.5, or PTT >2 × control) (major risk factor)
- Chronic liver disease
- Major trauma, shock, head or spinal injury, or burns over >35% BSA
- Prophylaxis indicated; also if ≥2 of the following are present:
  - Sepsis
  - ICU stay >1 wk
  - Occult GI bleeding × >6 d
  - Glucocorticosteroid >250 mg hydrocortisone or equivalent

Prophylaxis

- PPIs preferred (**Table 64**)
- H_2 antagonists (**Table 64**)
- Sucralfate 1 g po q6h
- Antacids 30–60 mL po q1–2h
- Enteral feedings

Key Points

- Prophylaxis has not been shown to reduce mortality.
- No one regimen has shown superior efficacy.
- Choice of regimen depends on access to and function of GI tract and presence of nasogastric suction.
- D/C H_2 antagonists, PPIs, and other tx for stress-ulcer prevention when risk factors are eliminated, ICU discharge, or before transfer to SNF or discharge from hospital.

IRRITABLE BOWEL SYNDROME (IBS)

Signs and Symptoms

Symptoms should be present ≥12 wk.

Consistent with IBS:

- Abdominal pain
- Bloating
- Constipation
- Diarrhea

Not Consistent with IBS:

- Weight loss
- First onset after age 50
- Nocturnal diarrhea
- Family hx of cancer or inflammatory bowel disease
- Rectal bleeding or obstruction
- Lab abnormalities
- Presence of fecal parasites
- Unexplained iron-deficiency anemia

Diagnosis (of exclusion)

Exclude ischemia, diverticulosis, colon cancer, inflammatory bowel disease by physical exam and testing (colonoscopy, CT scan, or small-bowel series). Do not repeat CT unless major changes in clinical findings.[CW]

Management

Improvement of Global Symptoms

- Reassurance; not life threatening; focus on relief of physical and emotional symptoms
- Dietary modification
  - Avoid foods that trigger symptoms or produce excess gas or bloating (eg, apples, onions, garlic, high-fructose corn syrup, wheat, milk, yogurt); consider a trial of a lactose-free diet.
- Behavioral interventions: hypnosis, biofeedback, CBT have been shown to be more effective than placebo.
- Exercise or increase physical activity
- Peppermint oil for relief of abdominal pain and postprandial symptoms
- Probiotics may relieve abdominal pain. *Escherichia* spp and *Streptococcus* spp have shown benefit.
- TCAs and SSRIs may be beneficial for patients with moderate to severe abdominal pain. See Depression chapter, p 92, for dosing.

IBS-Constipation *(IBS-C)*

Fiber (soluble) supplements **(Table 66)**

- Synthetic: polycarbophil
- Natural: psyllium, oat bran
- Avoid insoluble fiber (eg, wheat bran, whole grains)

Laxatives for IBS-C

- Linaclotide 290 mcg q24h on empty stomach (F)
- Plecanatide 3 mg q24h (F)
- Lubiprostone (women only) 8 mg q12h (L)
- Tenapanor 50 mg po q12h (K, L)
- Tegaserod (approved for women aged <65) 6 mg po q12h; D/C if inadequate response after 4–6 wk (F, L, K)

IBS-Diarrhea *(IBS-D)*

Antispasmodics: limited data do not support their use; harm is much greater than benefit.

Antidiarrheals: may be helpful for diarrhea but not for global IBS symptoms, abdominal pain, or constipation

- Loperamide 4 mg × 1, then 2 mg after each loose bowel movement; max 16 mg/24 h (L, F)
- Eluxadoline (opioid agonist/antagonist) 100 mg q12h; 75 mg q12h if 100 mg not tolerated due to anticholinergic activity (F)

Antibiotic

- Rifaximin *(Xifaxan)* 550 mg po q8h ×14 d; repeat × 2 if needed (F)

Serotonin antagonist

- Alosetron *(Lotronex)*: Tx of women with severe IBS-D who have not responded to conventional tx (restricted distribution in the US); 0.5 mg po q12h × 4 wk, increase to 1 mg po q12h × 4 wk, stop if no response (K, L)

CONSTIPATION

Definition

Frequency of bowel movements <2–3×/wk, straining at defecation, hard feces, or feeling of incomplete evacuation. Clinically, large amount of feces in rectum on digital exam and/or colonic fecal loading on abdominal radiograph.

Medications That Constipate

- Analgesics—opioids
- Antacids with aluminum or calcium
- Anticholinergic drugs
- Antidepressants, lithium
- Antihypertensives
- Antipsychotics
- Barium sulfate
- Bismuth
- CCBs
- Diuretics
- Iron

Management of Non–opioid-related Chronic Constipation

Step 1: Stop all constipating medications, when possible.

Step 2: Increase dietary fiber to 20–35 g/d, increase fluid intake to ≥1500 mL/d, and increase physical activity; or add bulk laxative (**Table 66**), provided fluid intake is ≥1500 mL/d. Titrate fiber by 5 g/wk to avoid flatulence and bloating. If fiber exacerbates symptoms or is not tolerated, or patient has limited mobility, go to Step 3.

Step 3: Add an osmotic (eg, 70% sorbitol sol, polyethylene glycol *[MiraLAX]).*

Step 4: Add stimulant laxative (eg, senna, bisacodyl) 2–3×/wk. (Alternative: saline laxative, but avoid if CrCl <30 mL/min.)

Step 5: Consider chronic secretagogue/guanylyl cyclase-C receptor agonists (**Table 66**).

Step 6: Use tap water enema or saline enema 2×/wk.

Step 7: Use oil-retention enema for refractory constipation.

Management of Opioid-induced Constipation

Avoid bulk-forming laxatives if insufficient oral intake.

Step 1: Use stimulant laxatives (eg, bisacodyl, senna).

Step 2: Use lubiprostone, linaclotide, plecanatide, or prucalopride if idiopathic constipation; use alvimopan, methylnaltrexone, naldemedine, or naloxegol if OIC.

Table 66. **Medications That May Relieve Constipation**

Medication	Onset of Action	Site and Mechanism of Action (Elimination)
Bulk laxatives—not useful in managing OIC		
Methylcellulose[OTC]	12–24 h (up to 72 h)	Small and large intestine; holds water in feces; mechanical distention
Psyllium[OTC,1]	12–24 h (up to 72 h)	Small and large intestine; holds water in feces; mechanical distention
Polycarbophil[1]	12–24 h (up to 72 h)	Small and large intestine; holds water in feces; mechanical distention
Wheat dextrin[OTC]	24–28 h	Small and large intestine; holds water in feces; mechanical distention

(cont.)

Table 66. Medications That May Relieve Constipation (cont.)		
Medication	**Onset of Action**	**Site and Mechanism of Action (Elimination)**
Chronic secretagogues/Guanylyl cyclase-C receptor agonists		
Lubiprostone *(Amitiza)*	24–28 h	Enhances chloride-ion intestinal fluid secretion; does not affect serum Na+ or K^+ concentrations. For idiopathic chronic constipation. (L)
Linaclotide *(Linzess)*		Guanylate cyclase-C agonist, which increases intracellular cGMP, which stimulates intraluminal secretion of chloride and bicarbonate increasing intestinal fluid and transit (F)
Plecanatide *(Trulance)*	NA	Guanylate cyclase-C agonist, which increases intracellular cGMP, which stimulates intraluminal secretion of chloride and bicarbonate increasing intestinal fluid and transit (F)
5-HT4 partial agonist		
Prucalopride *(Motegrity)*	NA	Stimulates colonic peristalsis; no affinity for 5-HT1 receptors (K, F)
Opioid antagonists		
Alvimopan *(Entereg)*	NA	Hospital use only; for accelerating time to recovery after partial large- or small-bowel resection with primary anastomosis; contraindicated if >7 consecutive d of tx opioids (L, K, F)
Methylnaltrexone *(Relistor)*	30–60 min	Peripheral-acting opioid antagonist for the tx of OIC in palliative-care patients who have not responded to conventional laxatives. Weigh-based dosing. If CrCl <30, decrease dose by 50% (L, K, F)
Naloxegol *(Movantik)*		µ-opioid receptor antagonist. Composed of naloxone conjugated with a polyethylene glycol polymer, limits its ability to cross the blood-brain barrier. Functions peripherally in tissues such as the GI tract at recommended doses. (L, F, K)
Naldemedine *(Symproic)*		Peripheral-acting opioid antagonist for the tx of OIC in adults with chronic noncancer pain (L, K, F)
Osmotic laxatives		
Lactulose	24–48 h	Colon; osmotic effect
Polyethylene glycol[OTC]	48–96 h	GI tract; osmotic effect
Sorbitol 70%[OTC]	24–48 h	Colon; delivers osmotically active molecules to colon
Glycerin Sp[OTC]	15–30 min	Colon; local irritation; hyperosmotic
Saline laxatives		
Magnesium citrate[OTC]	30 min–3 h	Small and large intestine; attracts, retains water in intestinal lumen; potential hypermagnesemia in patients with renal insufficiency or a low-salt diet
Magnesium hydroxide[OTC]	30 min–3 h	Osmotic effect and increased peristalsis in colon; potential hypermagnesemia in patients with renal insufficiency

(cont.)

Table 66. Medications That May Relieve Constipation (cont.)		
Medication	**Onset of Action**	**Site and Mechanism of Action (Elimination)**
Stimulant laxatives		
Bisacodyl tablet[OTC]	6–10 h	Colon; increases peristalsis
Bisacodyl suppository[OTC]	15 min–1 h	Colon; increases peristalsis
Senna[OTC]	6–10 h	Colon; direct action on intestine; stimulates myenteric plexus; alters water and electrolyte secretion
Surfactant laxative (fecal softener)		
Docusate[OTC]	24–72 h	Small and large intestine; detergent activity; facilitates admixture of fat and water to soften feces (effectiveness questionable); does not increase frequency of bowel movements

CrCl unit = mL/min

[1] Psyllium caplets and packets contain ≥3 g dietary fiber and 2–3 g soluble fiber each. A teaspoonful contains ~3.8 g dietary fiber and 3 g soluble fiber.

NAUSEA AND VOMITING

Causes

- CNS disorders (eg, motion sickness, intracranial lesions)
- Drugs (eg, chemotherapy, NSAIDs, opioid analgesics, antibiotics, digoxin)
- GI disorders (eg, mechanical obstruction; inflammation of stomach, intestine, acute pancreatitis, or gallbladder; pseudo-obstruction; motility disorders; dyspepsia; gastroparesis)
- Infections (eg, viral or bacterial gastroenteritis, hepatitis, otitis, meningitis)
- Metabolic conditions (eg, uremia, acidosis, hyperparathyroidism, adrenal insufficiency)
- Psychiatric disorders

Evaluation

- If patient is not seriously ill or dehydrated, can probably wait 24–48 h to see if symptoms resolve spontaneously.
- If patient is seriously ill, dehydrated, or has other signs of acute illness, hospitalize for further evaluation.
- If symptoms persist, evaluate on the basis of the most likely causes.

Pharmacotherapy

- If analgesic drug is suspected, decrease dosage, consider adding antiemetic until tolerance develops, or change to a different analgesic drug.
- Avoid[BC] haloperidol, metoclopramide, prochlorperazine, dimenhydrinate, meclizine, scopolamine.
- Drugs that are useful in the management of non–chemotherapy induced nausea and vomiting are listed in **Table 67**.

Table 67. Antiemetic Therapy	
Class/Site of Action	**Dosage (Metabolism)**
Metoclopramide[BC]	PONV: 5–10 mg IM, IV near the end of surgery Chemotherapy (IV): 1–2 mg/kg 30 min before and q2–4h or q4–6h (K)
Prochlorperazine[BC]	IM, po: 5–10 mg q6–8 h, usual max 40 mg/d IV: 2.5–10 mg, max 10 mg/dose or 40 mg/d; may repeat q3–4h prn (L)
✓Ondansetron	po, IV, IM: 4 mg for severe, acute nausea and vomiting (L)
Dimenhydrinate[OTC,BC,1]	IM, IV, po: 50–100 mg q4–6h; max 400 mg/d (L) Motion sickness: 50–100 mg q4–6h; max 400 mg/d
Meclizine[OTC,BC,1]	Motion sickness: 12.5–50 mg 1 h before travel, repeat dose q24h if needed Vertigo: 25–100 mg/d in divided doses (L)
Scopolamine[BC,1]	Motion sickness: apply 1 pch behind ear ≥4 h before travel/exposure; change q3d (L)

✓ = preferred for treating older adults

[1] Avoid unless no other alternatives.[BC]

PONV, postoperative nausea and vomiting. All have potential CNS toxicity. Metoclopramide associated with EPS and TD.

DIARRHEA

Definition

- Passage of loose or watery stools ≥3× in 24 h
- Acute: ≤14 d
- Persistent: >14 d and <30 d
- Chronic: >30 d

Causes

- Drugs (eg, antibiotics [**Table 80** and below], laxatives, SSRIs, PPIs, colchicine, metformin, cholinesterase inhibitors)
- Fecal impaction
- GI disorders (eg, IBS, malabsorption, inflammatory bowel disease)
- Infections (eg, viral, bacterial, parasitic)
- Lactose intolerance

Evaluation

- Obtain a stool culture from patients who are at high risk for complications (eg, aged ≥70, inflammatory bowel disease, or CVD exacerbated by hypovolemia).
- If patient is not seriously ill or dehydrated and there is no blood in the feces, can probably wait 48 h to see if symptoms resolve spontaneously.
- If patient is seriously ill, dehydrated, or has other signs of acute illness, hospitalize for further evaluation.
- If diarrhea persists, evaluate on the basis of the most likely causes.

Pharmacotherapy

Drugs that are useful in the management of diarrhea are listed in **Table 68**.

Table 68. Antidiarrheals

Drug	Dosage (Metabolism)
✓ Bismuth subsalicylate[OTC]	2 tabs or 30 mL po q30–60 min prn up to 8 doses/24 h (L, K) Duration: diarrhea/dyspepsia 48 h
Diphenoxylate with atropine[BC,OTC,1]	15–20 mg/d of diphenoxylate po in 3–4 divided doses; maintenance 5–15 mg/d in 2–3 divided doses (L) Duration: acute symptoms 48 h; chronic 10 d
✓ Loperamide[OTC]	Initial: 4 mg po followed by 2 mg after each loose bowel movement, up to 16 mg/d (L) Duration: acute use 48 h
Rifaximin *(Xifaxan)*	Traveler's diarrhea: 200 mg po 3×/d × 3 d

✓ = preferred for treating older adults

[1] Anticholinergic, potential CNS toxicity; OTC status varies by State.

CLOSTRIDIOIDES DIFFICILE INFECTION (CDI)

Definition

A specific form of *C difficile* pseudomembranous colitis

Risk Factors

- Almost any oral or parenteral antibiotic and several antineoplastic agents, including cyclophosphamide, doxorubicin, fluorouracil, methotrexate
- Age >65 y
- Duration of hospitalization
- PPI

Probiotics

The use of probiotic products to prevent primary or recurrent infections is not recommended by the American Gastroenterological Association.

Presentation

- Abdominal pain, cramping
- Dehydration
- Diarrhea (can be bloody)
- Fecal leukocytes
- Fever (100–105°F)
- Hypoalbuminemia
- Hypovolemia
- Leukocytosis

Symptoms appear a few days after starting to 10 wk after discontinuing the offending agent.

Evaluation, Empiric Management, and Diagnosis

- D/C unnecessary antibiotics, and agents that can slow gastric motility, such as opioids and antidiarrheal agents.
- Symptomatic patients who have had ≥3 unexplained and unformed stools in 24 h should be tested for *C difficile*.
- Test for *C difficile* with either nucleic acid amplification tests (NAAT) or glutamate dehydrogenase (GDH) and confirm with enzyme immunoassay (EIA) for toxins A and B.
  - If NAAT/GDH and EIA are positive, CDI diagnosis
  - If NAAT/GDH and EIA are negative, CDI unlikely
  - If NAAT/GDH positive and EIA negative, further clinical evaluation is advised; possible colonization

- Tx should not be withheld when suspicion of CDI is high.
- Place patient in contact isolation and observe infection control procedures. Hand washing is crucial and must be done with soap and water to remove spores. Hand sanitizers do not kill or remove spores.
- Provide adequate fluid and electrolyte replacement.
- Consider starting empiric tx when a delay in lab confirmation is anticipated or if fulminant infection (**Table 69** for dosing).
- Repeated testing within 7 d during the same episode of diarrhea is not recommended.
- Testing for a cure should not be performed.

Management

Table 69. Management of Suspected or Confirmed *C difficile* Infection

Clinical Definition	Supportive Clinical Data	Management
NAAT/GDH (-) plus EIA (-)	Low to moderate suspicion of CDI	D/C contact isolation D/C metronidazole/vancomycin Begin antidiarrheal agent Evaluate other causes
Initial episode, mild or moderate	Leukocytosis (WBC ≤15,000 cells/μL), serum Cr <1.5× premorbid level	Vancomycin 125 mg po q6h × 10–14 d ***or*** Fidaxomicin[1,2] 200 mg po q12h × 10 d Alternate: Metronidazole 500 mg po q8h × 10 d
Initial episode, severe	Leukocytosis (WBC >15,000 cells/μL), which signifies colonic inflammation; serum Cr ≥1.5× premorbid level, which signifies dehydration	Vancomycin 125 mg po q6h × 10 d ***or*** Fidaxomicin[1,2] 200 mg po q12h × 10 d Fecal microbiota transplant, if refractory to antibiotic tx
Fulminant	Severe plus hypotension or shock, ileus, megacolon in the absence of abdominal distention	Vancomycin 500 mg po or nasogastric tube q6h plus metronidazole 500 mg IV q8h; if complete ileus or toxic megacolon, add vancomycin 500 mg/500 mL pr is an option.
First recurrence		If vancomycin, fidaxomicin, or metronidazole used initially: Vancomycin pulsed-taper (125 mg q6h po × 10–14 d, q12h × 7 d, q24h × 7 d, then q2–3d × 2–8 wk) ***or*** Fidaxomicin[1,2] 200 mg q12h po × 10 d or 200 mg q12h × 5 d, then q48h × 20 d. Fidaxomicin preferred if vancomycin or metronidazole used initially. Consider bezlotoxumab[2] 10 mg/kg IV 1×. Fecal microbiota transplant as prevention (controversial after first recurrence)
Second or subsequent recurrence		Vancomycin in a pulse-taper regimen ***or*** Vancomycin 125 mg q6h po × 10 d followed by rifaximin 400 mg q8h po × 20 d ***or*** Fidaxomicin[1,2] 200 mg q12h po × 10 d ***or*** 200 mg q12h x 5d, then q48h x 20 d. Consider bezlotoxumab[2] 10mg/kg IV 1x. Fecal microbiota transplant as prevention

Sources: Adapted from Johnson S et al. *Clin infect Dis* 2021;73(5):e1029-e1044. Kelly C et al. *Am J Gastroenterology* 2021;116:1124–1147. NAAT, nucleic acid amplification tests.

[1] Fidaxomicin *(Dificid)* [92% F, minimal systemic absorption]. Preferred by IDSA/SHEA for initial and first recurrence episodes. Clinical trials did not include patients with fulminant CDI.

[2] May be limited by available resources.

- Continue contact precautions for ≥48 h after diarrhea has resolved.

Prevention of Recurrence

- Bezlotoxumab *(Zinplava)*, a human monoclonal antibody that binds to *C difficile* toxin B, indicated to reduce recurrence of CDI in patients aged ≥18 y who are receiving antibacterial drug tx of CDI and are at a high risk for CDI recurrence (includes age ≥65 y).
  - Bezlotoxumab is not an antibacterial drug and is not indicated for the tx of CDI and should only be used in conjunction with antibacterial drug tx of CDI.
  - Dose: single 10 mg/kg infusion over 60 min.
- Fecal microbiota, live (*Rebyota*) for the prophylaxis of *C difficile* recurrence.
  - Dose: 150 mL per rectum ×1 24–72 h after C difficile tx.

HEMORRHOIDS

Classification

- External: distal to the dentate line and painful if thrombotic, itchy
- Internal: proximal to the dentate line without sensitivity to pain, touch, or temperature; mucous discharge; feeling of incomplete evacuation

Management

Diet and Lifestyle Changes

- High-fiber diet (20–35 g/d) or psyllium, methylcellulose, or calcium polycarbophil
- Increased fluid intake
- Avoid prolonged time on commode

Topical Treatments

- Sitz baths (40°C)
- Non–steroid-containing products: applied 4×/d
  - Pramoxine 1%^{OTC} foam, gel, crm
  - Phenylephrine oint^{OTC}
  - Pramoxine plus phenylephrine crm^{OTC}
  - Dibucaine 1% oint^{OTC}
  - Witch hazel^{OTC} liquid, pads
- Steroid-containing products
  - Hydrocortisone 1%^{OTC} crm, enema
  - Lidocaine 2% and hydrocortisone 2% crm

Office-based Procedures

- Rubber band ligation: for internal hemorrhoids
  - Contraindicated in patients who are anticoagulated
  - D/C antiplatelet drugs (including ASA) for 5–7 d before and after banding
- Sclerotherapy
- Infrared coagulation

Candidates for Surgical Hemorrhoidectomy

- Thrombosed external hemorrhoids
- External or combined internal/external hemorrhoids

HEARING IMPAIRMENT

DEFINITION

The most common sensory impairment in old age; presbycusis affects 30–47% of the population older than 65. To quantify hearing ability, the necessary intensity (decibel = dB) and frequency (Hertz) of the perceived pure-tone signal must be described.

Importance: Hearing impairment is strongly correlated with depression, decreased quality of life, poorer memory and executive dysfunction, and incident dementia.

Aural rehabilitation: significantly reduces anxiety, social isolation, depression, and stress; may help to preserve cognition.

EVALUATION

Screening and Evaluation

- Note problems during conversation.
- Ask the question: Do you feel you have hearing loss? A "yes" response should prompt referral to audiology.
- Test with handheld audioscope or whisper test. Refer patients who screen positive for audiologic evaluation.
- Whisper test: stand behind patient at arm's length from ear, cover untested ear, fully exhale, whisper a combination of 3 numbers and letters (eg, 6-K-2) and ask patient to repeat the set; if patient unable to repeat all 3, whisper a second set. Inability to repeat at least 3 of 6 is positive for impairment.
- Apps are available for both screening for hearing loss and for adjusting direct-to-consumer (OTC) hearing aids (**Table 71**).

Audiometry

- Documents the dB loss across frequencies
- Determines the pattern of loss (see Classification, below)
- Determines if loss is unilateral or bilateral and assesses speech recognition.

CLASSIFICATION

See **Table 70**. Mixed hearing disorders are quite common, particularly involving features of age-related presbycusis and conductive loss. Central auditory processing disorders become clinically important when superimposed on other ear pathology.

Table 70. Classification of Hearing Disorders

	Sensorineural Hearing Loss	Conductive Hearing Loss	Central Auditory Processing Disorder
Pathologic process	Cochlear or retrocochlear (cranial nerve VIII) pathology	Impaired transmission to inner ear from external or middle ear pathology	CNS change interfering with ability to discriminate speech, particularly when background noise is present
Weber test findings	Lateralizes away from impaired ear	Lateralizes toward impaired ear	Normal
Rinne test findings	Normal	Abnormal in impaired ear	Normal

(cont.)

Table 70. Classification of Hearing Disorders (cont.)			
	Sensorineural Hearing Loss	**Conductive Hearing Loss**	**Central Auditory Processing Disorder**
Audiogram/ Audiometry findings	Air and bone-conduction thresholds equal	Air conduction thresholds greater than bone-conduction thresholds	Normal for pure-tone audiometry; impaired for speech discrimination
Common causes	Age-related presbycusis (high-frequency loss, problems with speech discrimination); most common cause Excessive noise exposure Acoustic neuroma Ménière disease (both high- and low-frequency loss) Ototoxic drugs	Cerumen impaction Otosclerosis RA Paget disease Psoriasis Osteoma Exostosis SCC	Dementia Stroke Presbycusis Possibly normal aging

MANAGEMENT

Remove Ear Wax

Ear wax causes conductive loss and further reduces hearing. Soft wax can be flushed with a syringe, removed with a cerumen scoop, or suctioned. Dry wax should be softened before removal. Note the following:

- Water or saline are as effective as commercial preparations. Fill ear canal with 5–10 gtt water and cover with cotton q12h × ≥4 d. Liquid must stay in contact with ear for ≥15 min. Hearing may worsen as cerumen expands.
- Patients with dryness or excessive exfoliation of the ear canal skin should avoid preparations that contain hydrogen peroxide, as this may exacerbate cerumen accumulation.
- Cerumenolytics may accumulate behind ear wax, causing irritation.
- Use of any of the commercial preparations for >4 d may cause ear irritation.

Hearing Technology

Table 71. Technology for Various Levels of Hearing Loss						
	Level of Loss, dB					
Level of Loss, dB	**16–25**	**25–40**	**41–55**	**55–69**	**70–90**	**≥91**
Degree of loss	Slight	Mild	Moderate	Moderately severe	Severe	Profound
Difficulty understanding speech	None	Normal speech	Loud speech	Anything but amplified speech	Even amplified speech	Even amplified speech

(cont.)

Level of Loss, dB	16–25	25–40	41–55	55–69	70–90	≥91
Technology or device						
Hearing assistive technology	x	x	x	x	x	x
Personal sound amplification products	x	x				
Direct-to-consumer (OTC) hearing aids		x	x			
Prescription hearing aids		x	x	x		
Active middle ear implant			x	x	x	
Electric acoustic stimulation				x	x	
Cochlear implant					x	x

Table 71. Technology for Various Levels of Hearing Loss (cont.)

Hearing Aids: Digital devices enhance select frequencies for each ear.

- Amplification in both ears (binaural) provides best speech understanding; unilateral aid may be appropriate if hearing loss is asymmetrical, if hearing-aid care is challenging, or if cost is a factor.
- Features that enhance sound and speech quality include directional microphones, open-fit hearing aids, ear-to-ear wireless coordination, and in the canal extended-wear aids *(Lyric)*.
- The mean cost of 2 hearing aids in the US is about $4700. Retailers such as Walmart and Costco sell brands at roughly half the price.

Direct-to-Consumer and OTC Hearing Aids

- These devices are technologically comparable to prescription hearing aids and may be suitable for persons with mild to moderate hearing loss at much lower cost (about $400/ear). In August 2022, the FDA issued final rules for FDA approval; some states allow direct-to-consumer sales of hearing aids.
- These devices are not self-contained, and all require an interface with a computer, smart phone, tablet, or proprietary interface for fine tuning or a hearing test (at an interface or by a hearing professional). They are sold in some audiology offices.
- Persons seeking these aids should be screened for ear pathology, severe hearing loss, ear drainage, wax, unilateral tinnitus, fluctuating hearing loss, vertigo, sudden hearing loss, or worsening hearing loss. Any of these should prompt referral to an ENT first.
- Signs of mild to moderate hearing loss (where such aids are appropriate) include speech or sounds seem muffled; trouble hearing in a group, in noise, on the phone, or when the speaker is not visible; asking others to speak more slowly, more loudly, or to repeat what was said; or needing TV or radio volumes higher than other people in the room.
- Signs of severe hearing loss (where these aids are **not** appropriate) include inability to understand voice in a quiet setting; trouble hearing loud sounds like a car or truck, noisy appliances, or loud music.

Personal Sound Amplification Products (PSAPs): Not FDA regulated

By definition, these are meant for use to hear certain sounds in certain situations (eg, bird watching); some are programmable. FDA says PSAPs are for people with normal hearing. Common products include:

- Sound World Solutions CS50+: soundworldsolutions.com/product/personal-sound-amplifier-cs50/
- Tweak Focus+T: tweakhearing.com/product/tweak-focust-instrument/

- NuHeara IQ buds: nuheara.com

Caution: Very low-cost PSAPs (under $50) amplify sound to a level that may cause injury to hearing.

Active Middle Ear Implants: A fully implantable ossicular stimulator; all components (including battery) are implanted under the skin; for adults who cannot wear hearing aids for medical (eg, collapsed ear canal, inability to handle device) or personal (ie, cosmetic) reasons. Used in patients with moderate to severe hearing loss.

- **Advantages:** better amplification capabilities with greater functional gain, improved sound quality, less distortion, more differentiated speech recognition, reduced feedback
- **Disadvantages:** ossicular disruption and device longevity; for certain devices, the ossicular chain is irreversibly disrupted; limitation in the severity of hearing loss amenable to the devices; may need to convert from an implantable hearing device to a cochlear implant as hearing deficit progresses; not covered by most insurance providers

Osseointegrated Implants (OIs) are inserted into the skull where they osseointegrate and attach with a snap or magnetically hold a removable bone-conduction hearing aid. The device bypasses the external canal and middle ear.

- *Potential indications:* conductive or mixed hearing loss, single-sided deafness (eg, after removal of an acoustic neuroma or from a viral or vascular insult). The main concern is the risk of skin complication with percutaneous (snap) OIs, which is greater than with transcutaneous OIs.

Cochlear Implants: Bypass the middle ear, directly innervate the cochlear nerve. Results after age 65 are comparable to those in younger people. Benefits are greater with bilateral implants. Early failure rate <1%, in the hands of experienced surgeons. Late complications of implants include vestibular problems (3.9%), device failure (3.4%), and taste problems (2.8%). Patient selection is important.

Electric Acoustic Stimulation: Use of a cochlear implant and hearing aid in the same ear and also in the non–implanted ear. Using both maximizes the range of sounds audible in both ears, aids in localization of sound, and speech perception in both noise and reverberation. The hearing aid amplifies residual hearing at low frequencies, while the cochlear implant provides electric stimulation to the high frequencies. Users still perform well when using the implant without the hearing aid.

Hearing Assistive Technology (HAT)

Each patient should be asked if his or her needs are being met. If the prescribed hearing aids and implants do not fully meet these needs, additional technologies may be indicated. These technologies are available at various price points.

HAT benefits people at all levels of hearing, from normal to profound impairment. Even patients with hearing aids or cochlear implants who have difficulty hearing in some or many situations will benefit. (Visit hearingloss.org/hearing-help/technology/hat/.)

People have 4 basic reception or communication needs: at home, at work, in the community, and in the world at large. These include:

- Face-to-face communication (eg, restaurants)
- Electronic media (TV, radio, movie theater, concerts)
- Telephone—both land lines and cell phones
- Warning sounds (doorbells, telephone, smoke alarm)

Face-to-Face Communication, Media, Telephone

- *Pocketalker.* A personal amplifier with microphone and earphones, this device is inexpensive and useful for talking to patients with hearing loss who do not yet have hearing aids or can be used as a hearing aid for those who are not ready for hearing aids or who have situational hearing difficulties.
- Hardwired body-style amplifiers and wireless technologies (loop, FM, infrared, and digital systems). The same devices also can be used for reception of media.
- Various auditory and visual devices are also available to facilitate telecommunication (amplifiers, FaceTime, Skype, etc).
- *CaptionCall.* A free (through a Federal grant) service for hearing-impaired persons. Requires professional certification of eligibility and internet connection. A phone with high sound quality and with a caption screen is free as part of this service (captioncall.com/products)
- Alert patients to a door knock, a doorbell, a smoke alarm, or an appliance signal.
- Wireless doorbell systems allow the chimes to be placed on each floor.
- *Ring Video Doorbell.* When visitors press the doorbell or motion sensors are activated, the owner uses an app to view and speak to the visitor remotely; allows for speech-reading.
- Smoke alarm systems will shake a bed when they go off.

Apps

In addition, apps are available to convert a smart phone and a headset into a personal listening device without the use of a hearing aid.

- Jacoti *ListenApp*®, FDA registered for mild to moderate hearing loss; based on an audiogram; left and/or right programming; settings for natural sound, speech, music, and movies.
- *HearYouNow* adjusts volume per ear in 3 bands (high, medium, low frequencies); its focus feature allows honing in on a conversation.
- Other amplifier apps: *BioAid, uSound, i-Hear, EarMachine, Hearing Aid.*
- Various apps that convert the speech of the caller to text for the hearing-impaired receiver are available and reviewed at https://www.hearinglink.org/technology/useful-apps-for-hearing-loss/

Tips for Communication with People with Hearing Difficulties

- Ask the person how best to communicate
- Stand or sit 2–3 ft away
- Have the person's attention
- Have the person seated in front of a wall, which helps reflect sound
- Speak toward the better ear
- Use lower-pitched voice
- Speak slowly and distinctly; don't shout and don't exaggerate mouth movements
- Rephrase rather than repeat
- Pause at the end of phrases or ideas
- Ask the person to repeat what was heard

Tips for Approaches to Patients Resistant to Acquiring/Using Hearing Aids

Set appropriate expectations, inform the patient, and support and assist the patient during the period of adjustment.

- Hearing aids do not produce normal hearing; they are aids to hearing

- New hearing aids usually need adjustments; expect to see the audiologist a few times. A resource to empower patients to work with their audiologist efficiently and to achieve the best fitting can be found at canadianaudiologist.ca/wp-content/uploads/2015/11/HLM_JulAug2015_Compton-Conley.pdf
- Report problems: hearing or understanding speech in specific situations (eg, noisy environments); difficulty operating the hearing aid; aid-associated discomfort
- Inquire how the patient feels about hearing-aid appearance
- Recommend group audiologic visits of newly fitted patients, if available
- Include caregivers in the process of fitting hearing aids
- Regularly examine ears for cerumen or other pathology

Tips for Treating Hearing Loss in Older Adults with Frailty or Multiple Morbidities

- Include hearing evaluation in team-based geriatric assessment
- Assess, and when possible, improve visual function
- Assess and treat physical, cognitive, and affective disorders
- For patients with hearing aids and problems with manual dexterity, consider easier-to-use hearing-aid models (eg, behind-the-ear or in-the-ear types)
- For hearing-impaired patients with advanced cognitive deficits
  - Prevent loss of hearing aid by attaching a metal loop to its body and tying a thin nylon line through the loop, fasten the other end of the line to the patient's clothing
  - Educate caregivers on proper use of hearing aids
  - Consider use of personal amplifier *(Pocketalker)* or other assistive listening device if patient is unable to use a hearing aid
- Assess for hearing deficits and correct them in patients presenting with geriatric syndromes

TINNITUS

Definition

The perception of sound in the absence of external acoustic stimulus, most often nonpulsatile. Pulsatile tinnitus is rhythmic, may indicate a more serious underlying disorder. The patient's description of the sound helps in diagnosis of the cause. Some tinnitus is normal, typically last <5 min, <1×/wk. Pathologic tinnitus last >5 min, >weekly. Prevalence is 30% after age 55 y.

Evaluation

- Examine ear canals for cerumen, otitis externa or interna; treat and reassess.
- Check medications that cause or exacerbate tinnitus, eg, NSAIDs, ASA, antibiotics (especially erythromycin), loop diuretics (especially furosemide), chemotherapy, quinine.
- Assess the severity of tinnitus using the Tinnitus Handicap Inventory: https://ata.org/wp-content/uploads/2022/08/Tinnitus_Handicap_Inventory.pdf.
- Unless initial evaluation shows the likely cause to be presbycusis or a myofascial disorder, refer to otolaryngology.
- If the examiner can hear the tinnitus (objective tinnitus), refer the patient to otolaryngology.

Some of the More Common Causes of Tinnitus

- **Originating from the auditory system:** presbycusis, otosclerosis, vestibular schwannoma, Chiari malformations
- **Myofascial disorders:** temporomandibular joint (TMJ) dysfunction, whiplash injuries, craniocervical disease

- **Vascular disorders:** arterial bruits, arteriovenous shunts, paraganglioma, venous hums, high cardiac output states
- **Neurologic disorders:** tensor tympani and/or stapedius muscle spasm, palatal muscles myoclonus
- **Patulous eustachian tube**

Causes of Pulsatile Tinnitus: refer to ENT for evaluation

- Structural: neoplasm or temporal bone pathology
- Metabolic: ototoxic medications; vitamin B_6 toxicity; myoclonus; high cardiac output
- Vascular: venous or arterial

Management

- The first and often the only thing needed when tinnitus has a benign cause is patient education on the natural hx (may remit) and coping strategies.
- Also treat the underlying disorder (eg, hearing aids for hearing impairment).
- If the patient still has tinnitus that produces distress, symptom-oriented tx includes:
    - CBT: improves quality of life, reduces depression, and has the best evidence supporting its use.
    - Acoustic stimulation at levels that masks tinnitus; combination hearing aids with sound generators may be superior to aids alone for those with significant hearing loss.
    - Cochlear implants for those with moderate or greater sensorineural hearing loss may improve tinnitus in up to 75% of patients.
    - Apps are largely untested for efficacy but provide white noise, CBT directed at tinnitus, customized tone to phase out tinnitus; or combination of these.
- For more information, visit the American Tinnitus Association website (www.ata.org/managing-your-tinnitus/treatment-options)

INCONTINENCE—URINARY AND FECAL

URINARY INCONTINENCE (UI)

UI is the complaint of involuntary leakage of urine. In older adults, it is most often multifactorial and results from some combination of lower urinary tract abnormalities, changes in neurologic control of voiding, multimorbidity, and functional impairment.

Like other geriatric syndromes, effective tx requires addressing more than one factor.

Classification of UI

Transient UI and Factors Contributing to UI: UI is caused by some combinations of medications, comorbidities, functional and cognitive impairment with or without lower urinary tract abnormalities including UTI. However, UI from these sources is transient only if they are recognized and addressed. These same factors are frequent contributors to UI in patients with urge, stress, and other causes of persistent UI.

Table 72. Types of Persistent Urinary Incontinence: Characteristics and Causes

Type	Characteristic	Causes
Urge	UI with compelling and often sudden need to void	Idiopathic or associated with CNS lesions or bladder irritation from infection, stones, or tumors. In men, also see BPH (p 296); in women, see GSM (p 329).
Stress	UI with increased intra-abdominal pressure (eg, cough or sneeze)	Due to failure of sphincter mechanisms to remain closed during bladder filling; insufficient pelvic support in women; prostate surgery in men
Mixed	UI with both urgency and increases in intra-abdominal pressure	Some of the above
Overflow (chronic urinary retention)	UI is continual, and postvoid residual urine is increased (typically >500 mL)	Causes vary by gender (**Table 75**)
Detrusor hyperactivity with impaired contractility (DHIC)	UI with urge symptoms, but stress-related UI may occur; postvoid residual >50% of voided volume in the absence of obstruction	Detrusor does not contract sufficiently to empty but still has low-grade hyperactivity causing urgency.

Other (rare): Bladder-sphincter dyssynergia, fistulas, reduced detrusor compliance

Overactive Bladder: Frequency and urgency without UI (more common in men); tx is the same as for urge UI.

Evaluation

History

- Determine type of UI (**Table 72**)
- Identify "red flag" symptoms including sudden onset of UI, pelvic pain (constant, worsened, or improved with voiding), or hematuria. These suggest neoplastic or urologic disease and require prompt referral to a urologist if UTI is excluded.
- Lower urinary tract symptom review: frequency, nocturia, slow stream, hesitancy, interrupted voiding, terminal dribbling

- Medical condition status and medications used to treat them, reviewed in association with onset or worsening of UI
- Ask "How does UI affect your life?" and also ask about the presence of fecal incontinence (FI).

Physical Exam

- Functional status (eg, mobility, dexterity)
- Mental status (important for planning tx)
- Findings:
  - Bladder distention
  - Cord compression (interosseous muscle wasting, Hoffmann or Babinski signs)
  - Rectal mass or impaction
  - Sacral root integrity (anal sphincter tone, anal wink, perineal sensation)
  - Volume overload, edema

Male GU

Prostate consistency; symmetry; if uncircumcised, check phimosis, paraphimosis, balanitis

Female GU

Atrophic vaginitis (p 329); pelvic support (cystocele, rectocele, prolapse; p 366)

Testing

- **Bladder Diary:** Record time and volume of incontinent and continent voids, activities and time of sleep; knowing oral intake is sometimes helpful. Sample diary available at niddk.nih.gov/-/media/Files/Urologic-Diseases/diary_508.pdf.
- **Postvoid Residual:** If available, bladder ultrasound after voiding is preferred to catheterization. If >200 mL, repeat; still >200 mL suggests detrusor weakness, neuropathy, medications, fecal impaction, outlet obstruction, or DHIC. Even if postvoid residual is not available, begin tx steps as shown in **Figure 7**.
- **Laboratory:** UA to check for hematuria or glycosuria; urine C&S if onset of UI or worsening of UI is acute; serum glucose and calcium if polyuric; renal function tests and B_{12} if urinary retention; urine cytology if hematuria or pain.
- **Testing:** Urodynamics usually not needed; indicated before corrective surgery, when diagnosis is unclear, when empiric tx is ineffective, or if postvoid residual volume >200–300 mL (possibly lower in men).
- Don't perform cystoscopy, urodynamics, or renal and bladder ultrasound in workup of uncomplicated urge UI.[CW]
- Do not order upper tract imaging if there are only lower urinary tract symptoms.[CW]

Management in a Stepped Approach

Contributing Factors

- Environment: ensure adequate access
- Mentation: if the patient is cognitively impaired, recommend **prompted voiding** (p 167).
- Manual dexterity: compensate for deficits, eg, by adapting clothing
- Medical conditions: optimize tx for HF, COPD, or chronic cough
- Medications: eliminate or minimize those with adverse effects (**Table 73**)
- Mobility: improve mobility or adapt environment

Figure 7. Stepwise Evaluation and Management of Common UI Conditions

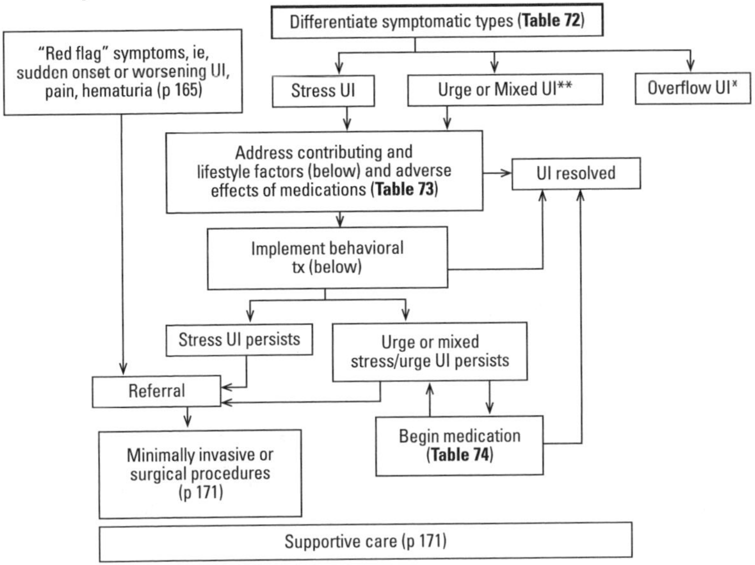

* Referral to differentiate neuropathy from obstruction (**Table 75**)

** Treat both components of Mixed UI

Lifestyle Factors

- Caffeine and diuretic (including carbonated and alcoholic) beverages produce rapid bladder filling and increase urgency; consume small volumes of liquids (mainly water) throughout the day.
- Fluid intake: avoid extremes of fluid intake (<32 oz or >64 oz), reduce fluids after supper time to minimize nocturia
- Constipation: produces urethral obstruction or places pressure on bladder
- Weight loss: 60% UI reduction with large weight loss (≥16 kg); 30% decrease in odds for stress UI with 3.5 kg loss
- Smoking: produces chronic cough, encourage patient to quit

Behavioral Therapy

- Effective in urge, stress, and mixed UI
- Efficacy for behavioral tx: >35% reduction in UI; 50% greater patient perception of cure
- Two components of bladder training for urge UI:
  1) Voiding on schedule during the day (start q2h) to keep bladder volume low. When no incontinence for 2 d, increase voiding interval by 30–60 min until voiding q3–4h.
  2) Urge suppression (**Figure 8**), which retrains the CNS and pelvic mechanisms to inhibit contractions and leakage

Figure 8. Urge Suppression

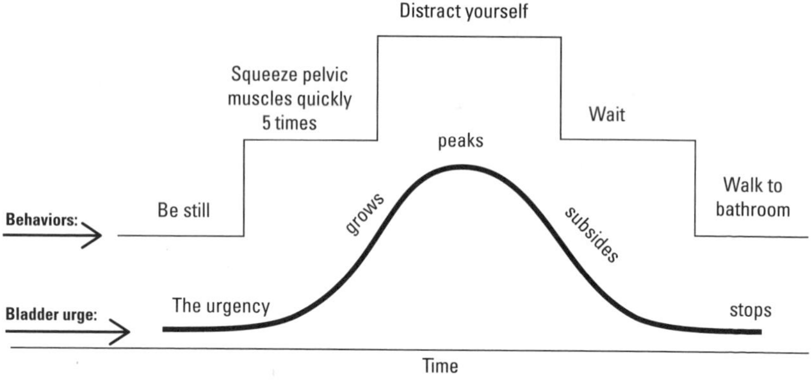

Note: Used with permission from Catherine E. DeBeau, MD

- Tx for stress UI involves timed voiding (as above) and also pelvic muscle (Kegel) exercises—isolate pelvic muscles (avoid thigh, rectal, buttocks contraction); perform slow velocity contraction, sustained for 6–8 sec. Perform 3 sets of 8–12 contractions in each set, on 3–4 d/wk (not daily) for at least 15–20 wk. An instructional booklet alone can reduce leakage by 50% (medlineplus.gov/ency/patientinstructions/000141.htm). Biofeedback can help with teaching; covered by Medicare if patient unsuccessful after 4 wk of conventional teaching (refer to continence specialist PT or advanced practice nurse).
- Tx for postprostatectomy UI
  - Urge UI occurs in 30–40% of men treated with TURP for benign disease; much less often with laser ablation, bladder lift, and aquablation (see Prostate chapter, p 296).
  - UI after radical prostatectomy for malignancy improves for up to 2 y; persistent UI more likely at greater age, high BMI, pre-existing lower urinary tract symptoms
  - Pelvic-floor electrical stimulation and biofeedback begun soon after catheter removal in postprostatectomy patients improves early recovery of continence.
  - Even for those with UI ≥1 y after prostatectomy, pelvic-floor exercises and urge control (**Figure 8**) reduces the number of incontinence episodes by more than half. Send patients to an experienced continence specialist for training (nurse practitioner or PT).
- Behavioral tx is at least as effective for overactive bladder symptoms in men on α blocker tx as antimuscarinic tx. For benefit, patients should not have outlet obstruction (ie, postvoid residual urine <200 mL) (also Prostate, p 296).
- DHIC is first treated with behavioral methods; may add detrusor muscle-relaxing medications but follow postvoid residual; clean intermittent self-catheterization if needed.

Pharmacotherapy

- First eliminate medications causing/exacerbating UI if possible (**Table 73**).

Table 73. Medications Commonly Associated with UI

Medication/Class	Adverse Effects/Comments
ACEIs	Cough (stress UI) or cough-induced urge UI
Alcohol	Frequency, urgency, sedation, immobility
α-Adrenergic agonists	Outlet obstruction (men)
α-Adrenergic blockers (Avoid[BC])	Stress leakage (women)
Anticholinergics (Avoid[BC])	Impaired emptying, delirium, fecal impaction
Cholinesterase inhibitors	Increased uninhibited contractions and urgency
CCBs	Impaired detrusor contraction, edema with nocturnal diuresis
Estrogen (oral, transdermal)[BC]	Stress and mixed UI (women), avoid systemic estrogens in women with UI
GABA-ergics (gabapentin, pregabalin)	Edema, nocturnal diuresis
Loop diuretics	Polyuria, frequency, urgency
NSAIDs/thiazolidinediones	Edema, nocturnal diuresis
Sedative-hypnotics	Sedation, delirium, immobility
SGLT2 inhibitors	Diuresis, polyuria
Opioid analgesics	Constipation, sedation, delirium
TCAs and antipsychotics (Avoid[BC])	Anticholinergic effects, sedation, immobility

General Principles

- Topical vaginal estrogen is effective for tx of dysuria, urgency, urge UI, and recurrent UTI; evidence is less certain for an effect on nocturia or frequency or stress UI. Experts recommend at least a 3-mo trial of topical estrogen for postmenopausal women with either urge or stress UI.
- All vaginal estrogen preparations are equally effective (**Table 127**). See also GSM, p 329.
- Oral estrogens appear to worsen UI and may not effectively treat symptoms of GSM.
- See **Table 74** for pharmacotherapy for urge and mixed UI. All show efficacy in RCTs.
- Pharmacotherapy should be offered based on frailty, not age. Frail people should have remediable factors for UI addressed before pharmacotherapy for urge UI is started.

Urge UI

- β-3 agonists
  - Have similar effectiveness to antimuscarinics; head-to-head trials are very limited.
  - Are preferred tx for UI in patients who also take cholinesterase inhibitors and those with cognitive impairment
- Antimuscarinics
  - IR formulations are associated with greater side effects (ie, dry mouth, constipation, cognitive dysfunction).
  - Longitudinal cohort studies suggest long-term use is associated with cognitive dysfunction, altered CNS metabolism, and brain atrophy.
  - Before prescribing, consider the total anticholinergic burden (eg, anticholinergic risk scale); >50% of patients stop antimuscarinic tx by the end of 1 y. Avoid use of anticholinergic agents.[BC]

- Chronic antimuscarinic use is associated with tooth loss and caries; routine dental care is important.
- Combining antimuscarinics and cholinesterase inhibitors should be avoided..

- Select among alternative medications based on ADRs (harms) (**Table 74**).
- Reevaluate use of these agents regularly after they are prescribed for lack of efficacy. D/C medication if not effective.

Stress UI

- Consider a 3-mo trial of topical vaginal estrogen.
- Duloxetin is recommended for women only when there is also an indication to treat depression.

Table 74. Pharmacotherapy for Urge or Mixed Urinary Incontinence

Medication	**Adverse Events/Other (RR for cure; NNT for cure)**
Antimuscarinics	*Class AEs:* dry mouth, blurry vision, dry eyes, delirium/confusion/dementia, constipation. All metabolized by L, CYP2D6, CYP3A4
Oxybutynin *(IR,* Oxybutynin *XL, Gelnique)*	Dry mouth and constipation less with XL and pch than immediate-release; doses above 10 mg/d not recommended. RR 1.7; NNT 9
(Oxytrol Women[OTC])	pch: rotate sites to reduce skin irritation (L); OTC *Oxytrol* is less expensive
Tolterodine, Tolterodine LA	P450 interactions RR 1.2; NNT 12
Trospium	Dyspepsia, headache; caution in liver dysfunction; dose 1×/d hs in patients aged ≥75 or with CrCl <30; XR formulation not recommended if CrCl <30 (L, K) RR 1.2; NNT 12
Darifenacin	Gastric retention; not recommended in severe liver impairment. Withdrawal from tx trials for ADRs not different from placebo RR 1.3, NNT 9
Solifenacin	Same as darifenacin; max dose 5 mg if CrCl <30 or moderate liver impairment. Women with urge UI who have taken other antimuscarinics that have failed may benefit from a trial dose of the 5-mg dose (no additional benefit at the 10-mg dose) RR 1.5; NNT 9
Fesoterodine	Max dose 4 mg if CrCl <30. RR 1.3, NNT 8
β-3 agonists	
Mirabegron *(Myrbetriq)*	HTN (monitor BP), nausea, headache, dizziness, tachycardia, AF; max dose 25 mg if CrCl <30; not recommended in severe kidney or severe liver impairment; raises venlafaxine, dextromethorphan, digoxin, TCAs, and reduces metoprolol levels (L, CYP2D6). Combination with antimuscarinics should be done with caution while monitoring postvoid residual urine.
Vibegron *(Gemtesa)*	No effect on BP. Headache, nausea, constipation, diarrhea; no dose titration (L, not CYP2D6, 20% unchanged in urine)

NNT, number needed to treat for the effect according to 2017 guidelines of the European Urological Association; RR, risk ratio for substantial improvement; CrCl unit = mL/min.

Note: For prostate obstruction UI, see Benign Prostatic Hyperplasia, p 296.

Procedures-based and Surgical Treatment for Urge UI

- Botulinum toxin is the tx of choice for refractory urge UI, risk of retention and need for self-catheterization is low. Cure rates for overactive bladder and urge UI may be higher than with pharmacotherapy.
  - >50% reduction in UI with first tx is expected; nonresponders often improve with a second series of injections; duration of effect 8–12 mo; repeat tx is equally effective.
  - Greater risk of UTI, use with caution in patients with recurrent UTI.
- Neuromodulation
  - Sacral nerve neuromodulation is preferred tx for refractory urge UI when both UI and FI are present. Reduces frequency, urinary retention (both idiopathic and neurogenic), and FI. Electrode is implanted to stimulate S3; done as a trial before permanent device. Safety and effectiveness are similar in older as in younger patients.
  - Percutaneous posterior tibial nerve stimulation through a fine needle in the tibial nerve around the ankle simulates stimulation of the pudendal nerve. Tx weekly for 30 min for 6–12 wk, then as needed:
    - 60–80% of patients have at least a 50% reduction in urge UI episodes in sham control trials after ≥6 weekly tx; effects may last up to 24 mo.
    - Insufficient data that electrical stimulation is better for urge UI than pelvic-floor muscle exercises
- Both neuromodulation and botulinum toxin are safe and effective in frail men and women.

Surgical and Other Therapy for Stress UI

- Consider surgery for the 50% of women whose stress UI does not respond adequately to behavioral tx and exercise; provides the highest cure rates. Older women have more persistent postop urgency.
- Type of surgery depends on type of urethral function impairment, patient-related factors, and coexisting conditions (eg, prolapse).
- Only effective tx for intrinsic sphincter insufficiency
- Men with postprostatectomy stress UI who do not improve after watchful waiting and bladder training can be referred for transurethral bulking agents, urethral sling, or artificial sphincter; candidate selection determines outcome. Studies suggest that these procedures are underused in men.
- Pessaries
  - Benefit women with vaginal or uterine prolapse (p 366) who experience retention and stress or urge UI that is exacerbated by bladder or uterine prolapse.
  - Should be fit by an experienced urogynecologist or advanced practice nurse.
  - *Poise Impressa* is an OTC bladder support in 3 sizes; starter pack has all 3; worn for up to 12 h, replaced daily.

Supportive Care

- Incontinence products
  - Is the most prevalent strategy used among adults to manage UI and FI.
  - Should be chosen based on gender and volume of urine loss.
  - The Wound, Ostomy, and Continence Nurses Society (WOCN) has an evidence- and consensus-based online algorithm for selecting optimal products (https://bwap.wocn.org/#start-screen)
  - Medicaid (some states) covers pads; Medicare does not.
- Because of the expense, patients may not change pads frequently enough.

- Incontinence-associated dermatitis prevention and tx (see also Dermatology, p 99).
  - Gentle cleansing (no vigorous rubbing) of the genital, perianal, and groin areas with soap-free cleanser (restores normal acidic skin pH); pat dry; hydrate with a barrier cream, not ointment.

Causes of Nocturnal Frequency

Defined as >2 voiding episodes/night, is a common, troublesome, and often treatable problem

- Consider these more common causes first:

Cause	Characteristics	Therapy
Overactive bladder	Day- and nighttime frequency	**Table 74**
BPH	Elevated AUA symptom score (p 296)	Tx for BPH (p 297)
Sleep disorders	Complaints of poor sleep	p 342
Stasis edema	Edema accumulates through the day	Compression stockings during the day
Uncontrolled DM	Elevated A1c	p 115
Excess PM fluid intake	Especially alcohol after supper	Restrict fluids 4 h before bedtime

- Then consider these causes of nocturnal polyuria defined as >1/3 of 24-h urine output between bedtime and waking; use bladder diary with measured voided volumes.

Sleep apnea	Snoring or observed apnea	p 346
Heart failure	Consistent hx and exam	p 64
Autonomic dysfunction	Orthostatic hypotension; Parkinson disease and Parkinson plus syndromes; little voiding when upright, diuresis when supine; often hypotensive in the AM	Desmopressin[BC] 0.83, 1.66 mcg intranasal or 27.7, 55.3 mcg sl 1 h before bedtime; monitor for hyponatremia 7 d and 30 d after initiation and with dose increase; contraindicated if hyponatremic (or hx of hyponatremia) and with liver, renal (eGFR <50 mL/min), or HF; many drug interactions.
Reversal of diurnal fluid excretion	Patient often describes putting out more urine through the night than during the day	Trial short-acting potent diuretic after supper (eg, bumetanide 0.5–1.5 mg) to induce a brisk diuresis; if no response consider a trial of desmopressin[BC] (as above). May cause severe hyponatremia.

CHRONIC URINARY RETENTION (CUR)

Definition: PVR >300 mL urine on 2 occasions over 6 mo

Symptoms: patients still voiding urine but with hesitancy, straining, poor or intermittent stream, nocturnal enuresis; not painful

History: UTI, hematuria, stones, previous bladder instrumentation, catheter, prostate surgery, constipation, DM

Physical: distended bladder on exam; rectal for impaction and prostate size, consistency, nodularity

Medication review: anticholinergics, sympathomimetics, muscle relaxants, antipsychotics, narcotics

Red flag: abnormal renal function or hydronephrosis signals high-pressure CUR and should prompt immediate referral for evaluation; low-pressure CUR can be managed outpatient.

Causes

- Detrusor underactivity (DU) from aging, DM, neurologic disorders, and medications
- Anatomic causes vary by gender (see **Table 75**)
- Functional obstruction dysfunctional voiding, detrusor sphincter dyssynergia

Management: see **Table 75**

Table 75. Treatment of Chronic Urinary Retention by Cause

Cause	Treatment[1]	Other Treatment Options	Notes
Anatomic in men: BPH, urethral stricture	Prostate surgery, dilation of stricture	Intermittent clean catheterization	Bladder tone may not be restored after surgery
Anatomic in women: prolapse, urethral stricture, mass tumor, or foreign body	Surgical correction, urethral dilation	Intermittent clean catheterization	
Detrusor underactivity	Careful medication review; intermittent clean catheterization	Neuromodulation; intraurethral valve-pump for women	Intraurethral valve-pump is changed monthly; only 40% tolerate (discomfort, leakage)
Functional bladder outlet obstruction (BOO) dysfunctional voiding	Pelvic-floor muscle training	Selective α-1a blockers, sacral neuromodulation	Least studied intervention: intraurethral botulinum toxin, may result in UI
Detrusor sphincter dyssynergia	No first-line tx; selective α-1a blockers	Intermittent clean catheterization; limited success with botulinum toxin and bladder-neck incision	Cause is neurologic; may be transient if associated with stroke

[1] Credé maneuver (suprapubic pressure in an effort to increase intravesical pressure and expel urine) is not recommended; may increase intraurethral pressure by closure of external sphincter and bladder floor.

UI in Special Populations

Nursing-Home Residents and People with Cognitive Impairment

- Rather than bladder diaries, observe voiding patterns and UI episodes over several days.
- Trial of prompted voiding in patients who are able to state their name and transfer with assist of no more than one, who void ≤4× during daytime, and who accept and follow the prompt to void. Continue prompted schedule; if able to void at least 75% of the time during a 3-d trial which is considered a success.
- **Prompted voiding** consists of:
  - Asking if patient needs to void, and taking him or her to toilet starting at 2- to 3-h intervals during day; encourage patients to report continence status; praise patient when continent and responds to toileting.
  - Simply asking the patient if they need to void or use of a fixed voiding schedule will **not** improve UI.

- Consider use of mirabegron in patients with urge UI who succeed with prompted voiding and still have UI episodes.
- 1/3 will have bladder outlet problems, stress UI, or obstruction. Evaluate based on patient and family preference.

UI in Patients with Heart Failure

- 50% of HF patients have lower urinary tract symptoms
- If complaint is stress UI due to cough, check to see if patient is taking an ACEI; if so switch to ARB
- If complaint is urge UI or nocturia:
  - Rule out HF exacerbation and treat if needed
- If pedal edema is present, reduce or eliminate CCBs and other edema-causing drugs **(Table 73)**; use compression stockings if HF is stable and elevate legs at the level of the heart in late afternoon or evening
- Reduce/taper diuretics with careful follow-up of patient; avoid hs dosing
- Keep fluid intake at about 1.5 L/d and <2 L/d
- See Lifestyle and Behavioral Therapy p 167
- Caution in the use of antimuscarinics, which can cause dry mouth, increase fluid intake, and exacerbate HF

Catheter Care

- Use catheter **only** for CUR not amenable to tx (**Table 75**), to protect pressure ulcers, and when requested by patients or families to promote comfort (eg, at end of life).[CW]
- Clean intermittent catheterization is a safe and effective alternative for many patients.
  - Sterile technique not needed for self-catherization. Good handwashing and regular decontamination of the catheter are needed. Sterile technique for those who are frail or institutionalized.
  - Adjust frequency of catheterization to keep bladder volume <400 mL.
- Leakage around catheter can be caused by large Foley balloon, too large catheter diameter, constipation, impaction.
- Bacteriuria is universal; treat only if symptoms (eg, fever, inanition, anorexia, delirium) or if bacteriuria persists after catheter removal.
- Suprapubic catheters reduce meatal and penile trauma but not infection. Condom catheters are less painful and have a somewhat lower complication rate.
- Replace catheter if symptomatic bacteriuria develops, then culture urine from new catheter.
- Nursing-facility patients with catheters should reside in separate rooms.
- For acute retention, catheterize for 7–10 d, then do voiding trial after catheter removal.

Replacing Catheters: Routine replacement is not necessary. Changing q4–6wk is reasonable to prevent blockage. Patients with recurrent blockage need increased fluid intake, possibly acidification of urine, or change of catheter q7–10d.

FECAL INCONTINENCE (FI)

Definition

"Involuntary loss of liquid or solid stool that is a social or hygienic problem" (International Continence Society). Major FI is loss of feces; minor FI is staining with liquid feces. Some definitions include involuntary flatus.

Prevalence

After age 65: 6–10% of men and 15% of community-dwelling women, 14% of hospitalized, 45% of nursing-home residents

Risk Factors

Constipation, diarrhea, age >80, female sex, UI, impaired mobility, dementia, neurologic disease

Age-related Factors

Decreased strength of external sphincter and weak anal squeeze, increased rectal compliance, decreased resting tone in internal sphincter, and impaired anal sensation

Causes: FI is commonly multifactorial.

- Overflow: from colonic distention by excessive feces, causing continuous soiling
- Loose feces: caused by medications, neoplasia, colitis, lactose intolerance
- Functional incontinence: associated with poor mobility
- Dementia related: uninhibited rectal contraction, often have UI
- Anorectal incontinence: weak external sphincter (surgery, multiparity, etc)
- Comorbidity: stroke, DM (autonomic neuropathy), sacral cord dysfunction

Evaluation

History

- Ask about "red flag" symptoms or signs that signal serious disease and require prompt referral to a gastroenterologist (ie, hematochezia, anemia, unexplained weight loss, refractory constipation, new-onset constipation or diarrhea, and positive family hx of colon cancer or inflammatory bowel disease)
- Description of FI (eg, diarrhea, hard feces), including usual bowel habit, change in habit, usual fecal consistency.
- Because hx is critical, clinicians are encouraged to use the Bristol Stool Form Scale (https://www.gundersenhealth.org/document/20176) to aid patients in accurate description of stools.
- Frequency, urgency, ability to delay, difficulty wiping, postdefecation soiling, ability to distinguish feces and flatus
- Evacuation difficulties: straining, incomplete emptying, rectal prolapse or pain
- Functional: communication of needs, need for assistance, toilet access
- Other: bowel medications, UI, prior tx (eg, pads)

Medication Review

- Medications causing constipation (p 150)
- Medications causing diarrhea (p 154)

Examination

- Examine/palpate abdomen for colonic distention (consider checking abdominal x-ray), and visually inspect anus for fissures and hemorrhoids.
- Pelvic and rectal exams for:
  - Rectal prolapse while patient seated on commode; check for rectocele in women.
  - Perform rectal exam for resting tone (perceived tone around the examiner's finger after a Valsalva maneuver; is mainly from the internal sphincter) and during squeeze around the examiner's finger (requires both internal and external sphincter). Weakness in either internal or external sphincter can result in FI.

- ◦ Volume and consistency of feces; perform fecal immunochemical test.
- Observe gait, mobility, dressing, hygiene, mental status.

Laboratory

- TSH, electrolytes, calcium

Bowel investigations

- Abdominal radiograph: may identify colonic distention by excessive feces
- Colonoscopy: only when pathology suspected (unexplained loose feces, bleeding)
- Anorectal manometry and endorectal ultrasound: not generally needed for tx and are reserved for patients who do not respond to usual tx. Defecography not indicated unless surgery is planned.

Management: Multiple interventions may be required. Tx approaches based on symptoms and condition are effective, and significant improvement is maintained for up to 12 mo.

Main approach is to simulate the patient's usual bowel pattern.

- Use rectal evacuants to stimulate evacuation and to establish a bowel pattern.
- Use evacuants in the following order: glycerine Sp, bisacodyl Sp, microenemas (eg, *Enemeez,* docusate 5 mL), phosphate or tap-water enemas; digital stimulation.
- Use antidiarrheals to slow an overactive bowel or to enable planned evacuation with rectal preparations.

Constipation (p 150): often plays a role; evaluate (if needed) and treat

Modify fecal consistency to achieve soft, formed feces.

- Loose feces: use fiber or loperamide titrated to effect, sometimes as little as q48h.
- Increase fiber gradually by 5 g q1–2wk to 20–30 g/d (see Constipation, p 150)
- Hard feces: modify diet; add stimulant (eg, *Senokot*) or osmotic (eg, polyethylene glycol) at low dosages. In poorly mobile people, bran and fiber may exacerbate constipation.
- Optimal stool consistency/form for continence is type 3 or 4 on the Bristol Stool Form Scale (staging.continence.org.au/sites/default/files/2021-08/Bristol_Stool_Chart_PDF-compressed.pdf).

Patient education

- Respond promptly on urge to defecate.
- Take loperamide 2–4 mg 45 min before meal or social event to prevent evacuation.
- Use coffee to stimulate the gut.
- Position on toilet with back support, foot stool to achieve squat position.
- Exercise to improve bowel motility.

Rectal evacuation and toilet training: basic approach for most patients

- Following a routine improves bowel control.
- When no spontaneous bowel action, stimulate with suppositories or enemas (**Table 66**); those with incompetent sphincters may need microenemas.
- Bedpans should not be used; bedside commodes are not as good as toilets.

Exercise and other therapy

- Those who are able may be taught rectal sphincter exercises (tighten rectal sphincter for 10 sec 50× 2–3 d/wk) or may train using biofeedback (refer to PT).
- Biofeedback improves FI by strengthening pelvic-floor muscles, improving the ability to sense rectal distension, and improving coordination of sensory and strength components.

- Eclipse System: an inflatable balloon inserted into the vagina places pressure on the rectum and reduces episodes of FI.
- Anal electrical stimulation of the anal sphincter a few minutes/d over 8–12 wk has modest benefit.
- Sacral nerve stimulation for patients with both intact and defective rectal sphincters is FDA approved for chronic FI in patients who cannot tolerate more conservative tx or in whom such tx has not been effective. Patients must show appropriate response to a trial of stimulation and must be able to operate the device.
- A perianal bulking agent *(Solesta)* is available for patients in whom other tx has failed. Gel is injected into the tissue below the anal lining to promote tissue growth. In turn, the anal opening narrows, and patients may have better bowel control; benefit declines with time. Tx is contraindicated in active inflammatory bowel disease, immunodeficiency disorders, previous pelvic radiation, and significant rectal prolapse.

Nursing-home residents and very disabled older adults: FI is most often due to colonic loading and overflow. Treat as follows:

- Daily enemas (or suppositories) until no more results.
- Add a daily osmotic laxative (**Table 66**) and follow bowel training (above).
- Fecal transit can be stimulated with abdominal massage in the direction of colonic transit.

Other therapies

- Manual evacuation may be appropriate in some patients.
- Skin care: Wet wipes better than dry; soap-free cleansers are better than soap and water; to protect skin, use pads that fit between the folds of the buttocks.
- Toilet tongs and bottom wipers help those with shoulder disease.
- Surgery:
  - Full-thickness rectal prolapse usually requires surgery using a transanal or intra-abdominal approach.
  - When FI is the result of sphincter injury (eg, obstetrical or fistula repair), surgical repair is often successful.
  - Sphincter dysfunction without an identifiable cause has a lower surgical cure rate, but may approach 50%.
  - Division of the external anal sphincter or anal fissure can be repaired, but long-term results are less than satisfactory.
- Selected patients have improved quality of life through the creation of a stoma.

ANTIMICROBIAL STEWARDSHIP: PRINCIPLES FOR PRESCRIBERS

- Collaborate with local antimicrobial stewardship teams and efforts.
- Be familiar with formulary restrictions and preauthorization requirements.
- Participate in educational offerings on antimicrobials and antimicrobial stewardship.
- In long-term care facilities, review antibiotic prescriptions upon admission, return from the hospital, or emergency department started by the covering provider, during monthly medication review.
- Streamline or deescalate empirical antimicrobial tx based on C&S results.
- Optimize and individualize antimicrobial dose and duration of tx.
- Avoid duplicative, redundant, or overlaps in tx (eg, piperacillin/tazobactam with metronidazole or another β-lactam).
- Switch eligible patients from IV to oral antimicrobials.
- Use AHRQ minimum criteria toolkits on whether to treat UTI, skin and soft-tissue infection, or URI: ahrq.gov/nhguide/toolkits/determine-whether-to-treat/index.html
- CMS mandates that long-term care facilities develop, promote, and implement an antibiotic stewardship program (F881): cms.gov/Regulations-and-Guidance/Guidance/Manuals/downloads/som107ap_pp_guidelines_ltcf.pdf
- CDC Core Elements of Antibiotic Stewardship by setting: www.cdc.gov/antibiotic-use/core-elements/index.html
- CDC Antibiotic Prescribing and Use: www.cdc.gov/antibiotic-use/

METHICILLIN-RESISTANT STAPHYLOCOCCUS AUREUS (MRSA)

See digital text.

PNEUMONIA

Presentation

Can range from subtle signs such as lethargy, anorexia, dizziness, falls, and delirium to septic shock or acute respiratory distress syndrome. Pleuritic chest pain, dyspnea, productive cough, fever, chills, or rigors are not consistently present in older adults.

Evaluation and Assessment

- Physical exam: RR >25 breaths/min; low BP; chest sounds may be minimal, absent, or consistent with HF; 20% are afebrile.
- Imaging: infiltrates may not be present on the initial on CXR if the patient is dehydrated. CT scan may be indicated when CXR is inconclusive or compromised by other lung pathology.
- Sputum: Gram stain and culture in hospitalized patients or for severe CAP
- CBC with differential: Up to 50% of patients have a normal WBC count, but 95% have a left shift.
- BUN, Cr, electrolytes, glucose
- Blood culture × 2 in hospitalized patients or for severe CAP
- Oxygenation: ABG or oximetry <90% suggestive of pneumonia
- CRP >61 mg/L is associated with pneumonia.
- Test for *Mycobacterium tuberculosis* with acid-fast bacilli stain and culture in selected patients.

- Urinary antigen test for *Streptococcus* pneumonia and *Legionella* pneumophila in hospitalized patients or patients who cannot produce a sputum sample. Not routinely recommended for CAP unless severe. Legionella pneumophila urinary antigen test may be appropriate in residents of long-term care facilities when outbreaks are suspected or setting is optimal. Urinary antigen testing is highly specific for serotype 1 but lacks specificity for other serotypes. Value and use vary by geographic region.
- Thoracentesis (if moderate to large effusion)

Severe CAP per ATS and IDSA Guidelines

Major criteria (1 or more)

- Septic shock with need for vasopressors
- Respiratory failure requiring mechanical ventilation

Minor criteria (3 or more)

- RR ≥30 breaths/min
- PaO_2/FiO_2 ratio ≤250
- Multilobar infiltrates
- BUN ≥20 mg/dL
- WBC <4000 cells/µL
- Platelets <100,000/µL
- Core temperature <36°C
- Hypotension requiring aggressive fluid resuscitation

CURB-65 Pneumonia Severity Scale (recommendation based on mortality probability)

Score each of the follow as 1 = Present and 0 = Absent: Confusion, BUN ≥19 mg/dL, RR ≥30, SBP <90 mm Hg or DBP <60 mm Hg, and age ≥65.

Interpretation: 1 = outpatient tx, 2 = consider hospitalization or outpatient tx, 3 = hospitalize, 4–5 = hospitalize consider ICU assessment

Aggravating Factors († indicates modifiable)

- Age-related changes in pulmonary reserve
- Alcoholism
- Altered mental status
- Aspiration
- Comorbid conditions that alter gag reflexes or ciliary transport
- COPD or other lung disease
- Dysphagia, including esophageal strictures and motility disorders
- Head, neck, and esophageal cancers
- Heart disease
- Heavy sedation† or paralytic agents
- Hyperglycemia†
- Intubation, mechanical ventilation (orotracheal intubation and orogastric intubation preferred)
- Malnutrition
- Medications†: immunosuppressants, sedatives, antipsychotics, inhaled corticosteroids, anticholinergic or other agents that dry secretions, agents that increase gastric pH (eg, PPIs, H2RAs)
- Nasogastric tubes and tube feeding
- Neurologic diseases (seizures, MS, parkinsonism, stroke, dementia)
- Oral care† (manual brushing plus rinse with fluoride/chlorhexidine 0.12% × 30 sec/d)
- Poor compliance with infection control† (eg, hand disinfection)
- Supine positioning† (semirecumbent, 30–45° preferred)

- Swallowing† (eat/feed upright at 90° over 15–20 min)

Predominant Three Organisms by Setting

Community acquired:

- *Streptococcus pneumoniae*
- *Haemophilus influenzae*
- respiratory viruses

Nursing home acquired:

- *Streptococcus pneumoniae*
- *Haemophilus influenzae*
- *Staphylococcus aureus* (including MRSA)

Hospital acquired:

- gram-negative bacteria
- anaerobes
- gram-positive bacteria

Supportive Management

- Short-acting inhaled β-adrenergic agonists
- Mechanical ventilation (if indicated)
- Oxygen as indicated
- Rehydration

Table 76. Treatment of Community-acquired Pneumonia by Clinical Circumstances or Setting[1]

Clinical Circumstances or Setting	Treatment Options
Outpatient, no comorbidities or risk factors for MRSA or Pseudomonas and no antibiotic tx in past 3 mo	Amoxicillin or doxycycline or a macrolide (ie, azithromycin or clarithromycin), if local pneumococcal resistance <25%
Outpatient, with comorbidities[2]	Combination tx with amoxicillin-clavulanate or cephalosporin (cefpodoxime or cefuroxime) plus a macrolide or doxycycline or fluoroquinolone[3,4] monotx
Hospitalized patient, nonsevere	Ampicillin + sulbactam, cefotaxime, ceftriaxone, or ceftaroline plus a macrolide or a fluoroquinolone[3,4] monotx
Hospitalized patient, severe	
No prior isolation of MRSA or Pseudomonas	Ampicillin + sulbactam, cefotaxime, ceftriaxone, or ceftaroline plus a macrolide or ampicillin + sulbactam, cefotaxime, ceftriaxone, or ceftaroline plus a fluoroquinolone[3,4]
Prior MRSA isolation	Add vancomycin or linezolid
Prior Pseudomonas isolation	Add piperacillin-tazobactam, cefepime, ceftazidime, imipenem, meropenem, or aztreonam
Recent hospitalization and parenteral antibiotics and MRSA risk factors	Add vancomycin or linezolid
Recent hospitalization and parenteral antibiotics and *Pseudomonas* risk factors	Add piperacillin-tazobactam, cefepime, ceftazidime, imipenem, meropenem, or aztreonam

[1] Because of the geographical variability in antimicrobial resistance patterns, refer to local tx recommendations.

[2] Comorbidities: chronic heart, lung, liver, or kidney disease; DM; alcoholism; malignancies; or asplenia

[3] Fluoroquinolones (respiratory): moxifloxacin, or levofloxacin

[4] Avoid fluoroquinolones in patients with a hx of existing aortic aneurysm or increased risk of developing an aortic aneurysm.

Nursing-home or Hospital-acquired Pneumonia Requiring Parenteral Treatment: Alternative Recommendations

Antibiotics are indicated if:

- Temperature ≥102°F (38.9°C) + RR >25 or productive cough
- Temperature ≥100°F (37.8°C) + <102°F (38.9°C) + RR >25, pulse >100, rigors or new-onset delirium

- Afebrile with COPD + new or increased cough with purulent sputum
- Afebrile without COPD + new or increased cough + RR >25 or new-onset delirium

Duration of Treatment

- Community-acquired pneumonia (CAP)
  - A minimum of 5 d; before stopping antibiotics, patients should be afebrile **and** have no more than 1 CAP–associated sign of clinical instability:
    - HR >100 bpm
    - RR ≥25/min
    - SBP <90 mm Hg

Require supplemental O_2 (unless required for a pre-existing condition)

- Hospital-acquired pneumonia

Tx courses average 7–8 d for clinically improving hospital-acquired pneumonia not caused by *Pseudomonas* spp or other nonfermenting gram-negative bacilli.

- Long-term care facility

5–7 d is usually sufficient if stable 48–72 h before stopping antibiotics.

Switch from parenteral to oral antibiotics when patient is hemodynamically stable, shows clinical improvement, is afebrile for 16 h, and can tolerate oral medications.

Note: The empiric use of vancomycin should be reserved for patients with a serious allergy to β-lactam antibiotics or when MRSA is known to be a problem pathogen.

URINARY TRACT INFECTION OR UROSEPSIS

See Prostate Disorders for prostatitis.

Definition

Bacteriuria is the presence of a significant number of bacteria in the urine without reference to symptoms.

- **Symptomatic bacteriuria** usually has signs of acute dysuria and new or increased frequency or urgency of urination or incontinence; fever, chills, nausea may be present; >10^5 cfu/mL of a single organism from a single specimen supports the diagnosis of UTI, counts ≥10^3 cfu/mL are diagnostic for specimens obtained by in and out catheterization.
  - Nursing-home residents without an indwelling catheter, ≥3 of the following: fever (>38°C) or chills, new or increased burning pain on urination, frequency or urgency, new or increased incontinence, new flank or suprapubic pain or tenderness, change in character of urine, or worsening of mental or functional status
  - Nursing-home residents with an indwelling catheter, >2 of the following: fever (>38°C) or chills, new flank or suprapubic pain or tenderness, change in character of urine, or worsening of mental or functional status
- **Asymptomatic bacteriuria** (ASB) is seen when there is an absence of symptoms, including absence of fever (<100.4°F [38°C]) plus:
  - the same organism(s) (≥10^5 cfu/mL) is found on 2 consecutive cultures in women
  - one bacterial species (≥10^5 cfu/mL) in a single clean-catch specimen in men
  - one bacterial species (≥10^2 cfu/mL) in a catheterized specimen in men and women
  - change in urine color, odor, or turbidity by themselves are not suggestive of UTI and do not warrant a urine culture
  - asymptomatic bacteria in the presence of delirium do not merit immediate antibiotic tx; first address hydration and other contributing factors and causes

- **Complicated UTI in women** affecting the lower or upper urinary tract and associated with underlying condition that increases risk of infection and of tx failure (eg, obstruction, anatomical abnormality, resistant organisms, or urologic dysfunction)
- **Recurrent UTIs in postmenopausal women:** culture-proven UTIs that have occurred at least 2× within 6 mo or 3× within 12 mo.

Risk Factors

- Abnormalities in function or anatomy of the urinary tract
- Catheterization or recent instrumentation
- Comorbid conditions (eg, DM, BPH)
- Female sex
- Limited functional status

Assessment and Evaluation

- Screening for ASB is not recommended in older adults residing in the community or long-term care facilities, regardless of cognitive or functional status, or the presence of a long-term indwelling catheter.
- Screening for ASB and tx is recommended before a urologic procedure anticipated to result in mucosal bleeding, prosthesis implantation, and UTI symptoms. However, prophylactic tx before a procedure remains controversial for other than outright UTI. Tx of asymptomatic bacteriuria yields no difference in outcomes.
- Choice is based on presenting symptoms and severity of illness.
  - UA with culture (do not obtain sample from catheter bag)
  - Blood culture × 2
  - BUN, Cr, electrolytes
  - CBC with differential

Expected Organisms

Noncatheterized Patients: Most common: *Escherichia coli, Proteus* spp, *Klebsiella* spp, *Providencia* spp, *Citrobacter* spp, *Enterobacter* spp, coagulase-negative staphylococci, *Gardnerella vaginalis*, group B streptococci, and *Pseudomonas aeruginosa* if recent antibiotic exposure, known colonization, or known institutional flora

Nursing-Home–Catheterized Patients: All of the above plus enterococci, *staphylococcus aureus*, and fungus (eg, candida)

Empiric Antibiotic Treatment

- Routine tx of asymptomatic bacteriuria is not recommended.[CW]
  - Asymptomatic bacteriuria has not been associated with adverse outcomes.
- Empiric regimens should be changed based on C&S results, patient factors (eg, previous microbiology), and tx costs.
- Tx duration should be at least 3–7 d for women with uncomplicated UTI; 7–12 d for complicated UTI; and 7 d (if afebrile) to 14 d and up to 6 wk for men if prostatitis present (see Prostate Disorders for prostatitis).

First-line Treatment of Uncomplicated UTI (outpatient, oral)

- Cephalosporin (eg, cefpodoxime or cefdinir) or amoxicillin/clavulanate × 7 d
- Nitrofurantoin[BC] 50–100 mg q6h × 7 d if CrCl >30 mL/min
- Trimethoprim/Sulfamethoxazole[BC] 160/800 mg 2×/d (if local resistance rate <20%) × 3–5 d if female and no catheter, × 7 d if catheter or male. Trimethoprim, alone or in combination with sulfamethoxazole, is associated with increased risk for AKI and hyperkalemia. This risk appears to be magnified when used concurrently with an ACEI, ARB, or potassium-sparing diuretic.
- Fosfomycin (second-line): 3 g po × 1 d (K, F)

The FDA is advising that the serious ADRs associated with systemic fluoroquinolone antibacterial drugs generally outweigh the benefits for patients with these conditions. Fluoroquinolones should only be used in patients who do not have alternative tx options. Serious ADRs associated with fluoroquinolones include hypo- and hyperglycemia (in people with DM); delirium; agitation; disturbances in attention, memory, and orientation; tendonitis and tendon rupture; CDI; and QTc-interval prolongation and torsades de pointes (except delafloxacin). Avoid fluoroquinolones in patients with a hx of existing aortic aneurysm or increased risk of developing an aortic aneurysm.

Empiric Treatment of Complicated UTI (Inpatient)

Not septic: Low risk of extended-spectrum β-lactamase (ESBL): ceftriaxone; moderate- to high-risk ESBL: piperacillin/tazobactam, cefepime, or carbapenem

Suspected urosepsis (IV route): Low risk of carbapenem-resistant enterobacteriaceae (CRE): carbapenem ± vancomycin or piperacillin/tazobactam or third-generation cephalosporin if ESBL risk is low; moderate- to high-risk CRE: ceftazidime-avibactam or ceftolozane-tazobactam.

Vancomycin should be reserved for patients with a serious allergy to β-lactam antibiotics.

UTI Prophylaxis

- Leads to antibiotic resistance regardless of patient's catheter status or duration of catheterization; generally not recommended. Vaginal atrophy due to estrogen depletion may predispose women to recurrent UTIs.
- Meta-analyses have reached mixed conclusions on the benefit of cranberry products for reducing UTIs in women with recurrent UTIs. All meta-analyses were derived from studies with methodological problems.
- Local topical estrogen replacement may be indicated (**Table 127**). May take 2 to 3 mo to take effect.

SEPSIS AND SYSTEMIC INFLAMMATORY RESPONSE SYNDROME (SIRS)

Definition

Life-threatening organ dysfunction due to sepsis, a consequence of a dysregulated inflammatory response to an infection

Septic shock: subset of sepsis

- Serum lactate >2 mmol/L (18.2 mg/mL) plus fluid resuscitation
- Hypotension requiring vasopressors to maintain mean BP ≥65 mm Hg

Diagnostic Criteria

Outside the ICU (quick Sequential Oxygen Failure Assessment [qSOFA], www.mdcalc.com/qsofa-quick-sofa-score-sepsis):

1 point for each; used to predict mortality risk; >2 high risk

ICU (SOFA, https://www.mdcalc.com/calc/691/sequential-organ-failure-assessment-sofa-score): estimates ICU mortality risk

Risk Factors

- Bacteremia
- Age ≥65
- ICU admission or previous hospitalization
- Immunosuppression
- DM or obesity
- Cancer
- CAP
- Genetic factors

Management

Supportive Care

- Respiratory: Oxygen and ventilator assistance as needed
- Goal-directed tx (if needed)
  - Rapidly infused bolus IV fluids defined by volume status; assess before and after each bolus
  - Use pressors when IV fluids are not sufficient or lead to cardiogenic pulmonary edema
  - Reserve inotropics (eg, dobutamine) for refractory patients with decreased cardiac output
  - RBC transfusion if Hb <7 g/dL, hemorrhagic shock, or myocardial ischemia

Early Goals of Treatment

- MAP >65 mm Hg
- Urine output >0.5 mL/kg/h
- Central venous pressure 8–12 mm Hg
- Central venous oxygen saturation ($ScvO_2$) ≥70% or SvO_2 ≥65%

Infection

- Identify and remove (when possible) infection loci
- IV antibiotics started promptly after diagnosis
- Empiric: Broad-spectrum coverage of gram-negative and gram-positive bacteria. If MRSA is suspected, include vancomycin (or daptomycin for nonpulmonary MRSA, or linezolid). If fungal infections are suspected, include antifungal agent.
- Glucocorticoids if SBP <90 mm Hg persists ×1 h after fluids and vasopressors (refractory shock)

HERPES ZOSTER ("SHINGLES")

Definition

Cutaneous vesicular eruptions followed by radicular pain secondary to the recrudescence of varicella zoster virus. Recurrence may occur but rare in immunocompetent older people.

Prevention

- A recombinant, adjuvanted zoster vaccine *(RZV, Shingrix)* is approved for individuals aged ≥50. Vaccination requires 2 doses given 2–6 mo apart. ACIP recommended vaccination of immunocompetent persons ≥50, including those who previously received the live vaccine or who had a prior episode of herpes zoster. Inform patients of potential ADRs ranging from injection-site reactions (pain, redness, swelling), headache, myalgia, fever, shivering and fatigue. Flu-like symptoms can affect 1 in 6 patients and last 2–3 d. Reaction to the first dose is not predictive of reaction to the second. A single dose does not convey maximum immune protection. ACIP does recommend vaccinating immunocompetent persons with *RZV* previously vaccinated with live vaccine *(Zostavax)*.(**Table 107**).

Clinical Manifestations

- Abrupt onset of pruritus or pain along a specific dermatome
- Macular, erythematous rash that becomes vesicular and pustular (Tzanck cell test positive) after ~3 d, crusts over and clears in 10–14 d
- Complications: postherpetic neuralgia, visual loss or blindness if ophthalmic involvement

Pharmacotherapy

When started within 72 h of the rash's appearance, antiviral tx (**Table 77**) decreases the severity and duration of the acute illness and possibly shortens the duration and reduces the risk of postherpetic neuralgias. (See p 245 for tx of postherpetic neuralgia.)

Table 77. Antiviral Treatments for Herpes Zoster

Medication	Dosage	Reduce dosage when CrCl[1] is
Acyclovir	800 mg po 5 ×/d for 7–10 d 10 mg/kg IV[2] q8h for 7 d	<25 <50
Famciclovir	500 mg po q8h for 7 d	<60
Valacyclovir[3]	1000 mg po q8h for 7 d	<50

[1] The CrCl listed is the threshold below which the dosage (amount or frequency) should be reduced. See package insert for detailed dosing guidelines. CrCl unit = mL/min.

[2] Use IV for serious illness, ophthalmic infection, or patients who cannot take oral medication.

[3] Preferred to po acyclovir; prodrug of acyclovir with serum concentrations equal to those achieved with IV administration.

INFLUENZA

Vaccine Prevention (ACIP Guidelines)

Yearly vaccination is recommended for all adults aged ≥65, all residents and staff of nursing homes or residential or long-term care facilities, and all healthcare providers. Nursing-home residents admitted during the winter months after the vaccination program has been completed should be vaccinated at admission if they have not already been vaccinated. The influenza vaccine is contraindicated in people who have a severe allergic reaction to any of the components of the vaccine. Persons aged ≥65 may receive any age-appropriate inactivated influenza vaccine (IIV) (standard- or high-dose, trivalent or quadrivalent, adjuvanted or unadjuvanted) or recombinant influenza vaccine (RIV4). High-dose IIV3 exhibited superior efficacy over a comparator standard-dose IIV3 in a large RCT and may provide better protection than standard-dose IIV3 for this age group. Dose: 0.5 mL IM 1× in the fall for those living in the northern hemisphere. For more information, see CDC guidance released each autumn.

Table 78. Diagnostic Tests for Influenza[1]

Method	Test Time	Acceptable Specimens, Detection and Differentiation
Rapid influenza diagnostic tests	<30 min	NP swab (throat swab), nasal wash, nasal aspirate Antigen (EIA) detects and differentiates between A and B, and detection of Type B varies with EIA
Reverse-transcriptase-polymerase chain reaction (RT-PCR)	1–6 h	Includes subtypes NP swab, throat swab, NP or bronchial wash, nasal or endotracheal aspirate, sputum; detects and differentiates Types A and B, including H1N1 and avian H5N1 subtypes
Immunofluorescence, direct (DFA) or indirect (IFA) antibody staining	1–4 h	NP swab or wash, bronchial wash, nasal or endotracheal aspirate Detect and differentiate between Types A and B, between A/B, and other respiratory viruses

[1] Testing indicated early in the season or during outbreaks

EIA, enzyme immunoassay; NP, nasopharyngeal.

Pharmacologic Prophylaxis and Treatment with Antiviral Agents

Indications

- Prevention (during an influenza outbreak): people who are not vaccinated, are immunodeficient, or may spread the virus
- Prophylaxis: during 2 wk required to develop antibodies for people vaccinated after an outbreak of influenza A
- Reduction of symptoms, duration of illness when started within the first 48 h of symptoms
- During epidemic outbreaks in nursing homes
- Resistance to antivirals and the emergence of specific strains of influenza (eg, H1N1) have led to frequent updates of recommendations for prophylaxis and tx. Check the CDC website for the most current information and guidance (cdc.gov/flu/professionals/antivirals/).

Duration

Treatment of symptoms: 3–5 d or for 24–48 h after symptoms resolve.

Prophylaxis during outbreak: minimum 2 wk or until ~1 wk after outbreak ends.

Table 79. Antiviral Treatment of Influenza

Agent	Dosage
✓ Oseltamivir[1]	Tx: 75 mg po q12h × 5 d; 30 mg po q12h× 5 d if CrCl >30–60; 30 mg po q24h × 5 d if CrCl = 10–30; 30 mg q24h; Hemodialysis: 30 mg immediately and 30 mg after every hemodialysis cycle for ESRD patients on hemodialysis, not to exceed 5 d; ESRD patients on CAPD: a single 30-mg dose immediately.
	Prophylaxis of influenza: 75 mg po q24h for 7–10 d
	Community outbreak: 75 mg po q24h for up to 6 wk for immunocompetent patients and 12 wk for immunocompromised patients
	Institutional outbreak: continue for ≥2 wk until >7 d after onset in last patient
Baloxavir marboxil *(Xofluza)*	Tx: 40 kg to <80 kg: 40 mg po × 1 within 48 h of symptom onset
	≥80 kg: 80 mg po × 1 within 48 h of symptom onset
Zanamivir *(Relenza)*[1,2]	Tx: 2 × 5-mg inhalations q12h × 5 d
	Give doses on first d ≥2 h apart
	Prophylaxis: 2 × 5-mg inhalations q24h
	Household setting: start 36 h after onset of signs and symptoms of initial case, duration 10 d
	Community: begin within 5 d of outbreak, duration 30 d or until ~7 d after onset in last patient
Peramivir *(Rapivab)*	Tx: 600 mg IV × 1 CrCl 30–49: 200 mg × 1 CrCl 10–29: 100 mg × 1 ESRD requiring hemodialysis: 100 mg × 1, administered after dialysis

✓ = preferred for treating older adults; CAPD, continuous ambulatory peritoneal dialysis; CrCl unit = mL/min

[1] Must be started within 2 d of symptom onset or of contact with an infected individual.

[2] Do not use in patients with COPD or asthma.

OTHER RESPIRATORY VIRUSES

Coronavirus (COVID-19)

Seasonality: Year round

Presentation: Respiratory symptoms; influenza-like illness, acute exacerbation of chronic bronchitis and pneumonia; fever, chills, cough, shortness of breath, fatigue, myalgia, headache, delirium, new loss of taste or smell, sore throat, congestion, runny nose, nausea, vomiting, diarrhea. Atypical presentation is common in older adults, including afebrile temperature or delirium.

Diagnosis: Nasopharyngeal or oral swab, or saliva sample; RT-PCR; at home rapid-antigen tests

Treatment: Recommendations are updated frequently, for the most recent vaccine and pharmacotherapy guidelines see the NIH and CDC webpages: covid19treatmentguidelines.nih.gov/therapeutic-management/ and cdc.gov

- Vaccination, including booster shots, are recommended for the prevention of COVID-19 for all older adults, including those previously diagnosed with COVID-19.
- Outpatient, mild to moderate symptoms: nirmatrelvir-ritonavir *(Paxlovid)* po for symptomatic patients at risk for progression to severe disease; start within 5 d of onset (CPY3A4 inhibitor). Alternative: remdesivir *(Veklury)* IV; start within 7 d of onset.
- Monitor oxygenation using home pulse oxygen.
- Repeat testing only if symptomatic after ≥5 d.

Human Metapneumovirus

Seasonality in the US: Late winter, early spring

Presentation: Respiratory, especially wheezing; may exacerbate asthma, pneumonia

Diagnosis: Nasopharyngeal sample

Treatment: Supportive; ribavirin is active in vitro but has not been tested.

Parainfluenza Virus (PIV)

Seasonality in the US:
PIV-1: Fall of odd number years
PIV-2: Fall, annual
PIV-3: Spring, less predictable
PIV-4: Not yet characterized

Presentation: Mild URI to pneumonia (in immunocompromised patients)

Diagnosis: Viral culture of nasal washing preferred with PCR for PIV detection

Treatment: Supportive; reduce immunosuppression if possible (eg, lower dose of corticosteroids); no known antiviral agent

Respiratory Syncytial Virus (RSV)

Seasonality:
Northern hemisphere: November–April
Southern hemisphere: May–September

Risk factors: Immunocompromised, significant asthma, cardiopulmonary disease, functional disability, institutionalization, residence in altitude >2500 m

Diagnosis: Isolation of human epithelial type 2 (HEp-2) cells

Treatment:

- Supportive (oxygen, bronchodilators, corticosteroids)
- Ribavirin + passive immunotherapy or corticosteroids

TUBERCULOSIS (TB)

TB in older adults may be the reactivation of old disease or a new infection due to exposure to an infected individual. If a new infection is suspected or if the patient has risk factors for resistant organisms, bacterial sensitivities must be determined.

Risk or Reactivating Factors

- Chronic institutionalization
- Corticosteroid use
- DM
- Malignancy
- Malnutrition
- Kidney failure

Diagnosis

- Mantoux tuberculin skin test (TST): 0.1 mL of tuberculin PPD intradermal injection into the inner surface of the forearm
  - Read 48–72 h after injection (see CDC TB guidelines for interpretation www.cdc.gov/tb/publications/guidelines/default.htm).
  - Repeat ("booster") 1–2 wk after initial skin testing can be useful for nursing-home residents, healthcare workers, and others who are retested periodically to reduce the likelihood of misinterpreting a boosted reaction to subsequent TSTs.
- Interferon-gamma release assays (IGRAs)
  - QuantiFERON = TB Gold In-Tube test (QFT-GIT)
  - T-SPOT

  (+) Patient has been infected; additional tests if latent TB or tubercular disease

  (–) Latent TB or tubercular disease not likely

Treatment of Latent and Active Infection

Refer to the CDC-IDSA-ATS guidelines at www.atsjournals.org/doi/10.1164/rccm.201909-1874ST and www.idsociety.org/practice-guideline/treatment-of-drug-resistant-tb/

HUMAN IMMUNODEFICIENCY VIRUS (HIV)

Presentation

Many symptoms that are common in older adults may delay diagnosis:

- Anorexia
- Arthralgias
- Earlier, more symptomatic menopause
- Fatigue
- Flu-like symptoms
- Forgetfulness
- Hypogonadism
- Insomnia
- Myalgias
- Pain in hands or feet (neuropathy)
- Recurrent pneumonia
- Sexual disorders
- Weight loss

Comorbidities common in older adults that can occur earlier in people with HIV:

- Cancers (eg, anal, liver, lung)
- Cirrhosis
- Cognitive deficits
- CAD
- DM
- Dyslipidemia
- HTN
- Obstructive lung disease
- Osteoporosis
- Vascular disease
- Visual impairment (cataracts, macular degeneration)
- Presbycusis
- Olfactory dysfunction
- Chronic pain

Lab Abnormalities

- Anemia
- Leukopenia
- Low cholesterol
- Persons aged ≥65 have a lower CD4 count at diagnosis
- Transaminitis

Screening

Routine screening of adults aged ≥65 is not recommended.

Screening is recommended regardless of age if:

- Starting tx for TB
- Treating a sexually transmitted disease
- Other HIV risk factors are present: unprotected sex and multiple partners, hazardous alcohol or illicit drug use
- Unexplained anemia
- Peripheral neuropathy
- Oral candidiasis
- Herpes zoster (widespread infection)
- Recurrent bacterial pneumonia
- Unexplained weight loss or pronounced fatigue
- Hx of monkeypox

Pharmacotherapy

Antiretroviral tx is recommended in patients aged >50, regardless of CD4 count.

- Viral load suppression greatest in patients aged ≥60 after initiating antiretroviral tx
- HIV-1 RNA suppression old > young
- CD4 response to tx young > old

For complete guidelines on antiretroviral regimens, see https://clinicalinfo.hiv.gov/en/guidelines/hiv-clinical-guidelines-adult-and-adolescent-arv/whats-new-guidelines.

Pre-exposure Prophylaxis

The combination of emtricitabine and tenofovir (*Truvada*; 200 mg/300 mg po q24h; [K] not recommended if CrCl <60 mL/min; *Descovy*; 200 mg/25 mg po q24h; [K] not recommended if CrCl <30 mL/min) in combination with safer sex practices is approved for pre-exposure prophylaxis to reduce the risk of sexually acquired HIV-1 in adults at high risk.

Complications of Pharmacotherapy

- Increased cholesterol (accelerated atherosclerosis)
- Glucose intolerance
- Drug-drug interactions (hiv-druginteractions.org)
- Drug toxicity
- Little data on the effects of age on drug pharmacokinetics in HIV-positive patients
- Increased pill burden

Monitor

- BMD
- Kidney function
- Liver function

Table 80. Antibiotics

Antimicrobial Class, *Subclass*	**Route of Administration**	**Adjust When CrCl[1] Is: (Elimination)**
β-Lactams Penicillins		
Amoxicillin	po	<30 (K)
Ampicillin	po, IM, IV	≤50 (K)
Penicillin G	IM, IV	[2] (K, L)
Penicillin VK	po	[2] (K, L)
Antistaphylococcal Penicillins		
Dicloxacillin	po	NA (K)
Nafcillin	IV	NA (L)
Oxacillin	IV	<10 (K)
Monobactam (antipseudomonal)		
Aztreonam	IM, IV	<30 (K)
Carbapenems		
Ertapenem *(Invanz)*	IM, IV	≤30 (K, F)
Imipenem-cilastatin	IV	60 (K)
Imipenem-cilastatin-relebactam *(Recarbrio)*	IV	<60 (K)
Meropenem	IV	≤50 (K, L)
Meropenem-vaborbactam *(Vabomere)*	IV	eGFR <50 (K)
Penicillinase-resistant Penicillins		
Amoxicillin-clavulanate	po	<30 (K, L)
Ampicillin-sulbactam	IM, IV	<30 (K)
Penicillinase-resistant and Antipseudomonal Penicillins		
Ceftazidime-avibactam *(Avycaz)*	IV	<50 (K)
Ceftolozane-tazobactam *(Zerbaxa)*	IV	<50 (K)
Piperacillin-tazobactam	IV	<40 (K, F)
First-generation Cephalosporins		
Cefadroxil	po	≤50 (K)
Cefazolin	IV	<50 (K)
Cephalexin	po	<30 (K)
Second-generation Cephalosporins		
Cefaclor	po	NA (K)
Cefotetan	IM, IV	≤30 (K)
Cefoxitin	IV	≤50 (K)
Cefprozil	po	<30 (K)
Cefuroxime axetil	po, IV	<30 (K)
Third-generation Cephalosporins		
Cefdinir	po	<30 (K)
Cefixime	po	<60 (K)
Cefotaxime	IV	<50 (K)
Cefpodoxime	po	<30 (K)
Ceftazidime	IV	≤50 (K)
Ceftriaxone	IM, IV	NA (K)

(cont.)

Table 80. Antibiotics (cont.)		
Antimicrobial Class, *Subclass*	**Route of Administration**	**Adjust When CrCl[1] Is: (Elimination)**
Fourth-generation Cephalosporins		
Cefepime	IV	≤60 (K)
Fifth-generation Cephalosporin		
Ceftaroline fosamil *(Teflaro)*	IV	≤50 (K)
Aminoglycosides		
Amikacin	IM, IV	<60, TDM (K)
Gentamicin	IM, IV	<60, TDM (K)
Plazomicin *(Zemdri)*	IV	<60, TDM (K)
Streptomycin	IM, IV	<50 (K)
Tobramycin	IM, IV	<60, TDM (K)
Macrolides		
Azithromycin	po, IV	NA (L)
Clarithromycin[BC]	po	<30 (L, K)
Erythromycin[BC]	po, IV	NA (L)
Fidaxomicin *(Dificid)*	po	NA (F)
Quinolones		
Ciprofloxacin[BC]	po, IV	≤50 (L, K)
Delafloxacin *(Baxdela)*	po, IV	IV: eGFR<30 (K)
Levofloxacin	po, IV	<50 (K)
Moxifloxacin	po, IV	NA (L, F, K)
Ofloxacin	po	≤50 (K)
Tetracyclines		
Doxycycline	po, IV	NA (K)
Eravacycline *(Xerava)*	IV	NA (L, K, F)
Minocycline	po, IV	NA (K)
Omadacycline *(Nuzyra)*	po, IV	NA (K, F)
Sarecycline *(Seysara)*	po	NA (K, F, L)
Tetracycline	po	<50 (K)
Glycylcycline		
Tigecycline	IV	NA (K, F, L)
Other Antibiotics		
Chloramphenicol	IV	NA (L)
Clindamycin	po, IM, IV	NA (L)
Trimethoprim-sulfamethoxazole[BC]	po, IV	≤30 (K, L)
Dalbavancin *(Dalvance)*	IV	<30 (K, F)
Daptomycin	IV	<30 (K, L)
Fosfomycin *(Monurol)*	po, IV	<40 (K, F)
Lefamulin *(Xenleta)*	po, IV	NA (L, F, K)
Linezolid	po, IV	NA (K, L)
Metronidazole	po, IV	≤10 (L, K, F)
Nitrofurantoin[BC]	po	Do not use if <30 (L, K)
Oritavancin *(Orbactiv)*	IV	NA (K, F)
Quinupristin-dalfopristin *(Synercid)*	IV	NA (L, B, F, K)

(cont.)

Table 80. Antibiotics (cont.)		
Antimicrobial Class, *Subclass*	**Route of Administration**	**Adjust When CrCl[1] Is: (Elimination)**
Tedizolid *(Sivextro)*	po, IV	NA (L)
Telavancin *(Vibativ)*	IV	≤50 (K)
Vancomycin	po, IV, pr	<90 (K)
Antifungals (also **Table 46**)		
Amphotericin		
Amphotericin B	IV	[3] NA (K)
Amphotericin B Lipid Complex *(Abelcet)*	IV	[3] NA (K)
Amphotericin B Liposomal *(AmBisome)*	IV	[3] NA (K)
Azoles		
Fluconazole	po, IV	≤50 (K)
Isavuconazonium *(Cresemba)*	po, IV	NA (L, F)
Itraconazole	po	NA (L)
Ketoconazole	po	NA (L, F)
Miconazole *(Oravig)*	po	NA (L, F)
Oteseconazole (Vivjoa)	po	Do not use if <30 (F, K)
Posaconazole	po, IV	NA (F, K)
Voriconazole	po, IV	NA (L)
Echinocandins		
Anidulafungin *(Eraxis)*	IV	NA (L, F)
Caspofungin	IV	NA (L, F)
Micafungin	IV	NA (L, F, K)
Other Antifungals		
Flucytosine	po	≤40 (K)
Griseofulvin	po	NA (L)
Terbinafine	po	<50 (L, K)

NA, not applicable; TDM, adjust dose on basis of therapeutic drug monitoring principles and institutional protocols.

[1] The CrCl (mL/min) listed is the threshold below which the dosage (amount or frequency) should be adjusted. See package insert for detailed dosing guidelines.

[2] Dosage should not exceed 250 mg q6h in kidney impairment.

[3] Adjust dosage if decreased kidney function is due to the medication or give every other day.

[BC]Avoid.

KIDNEY DISORDERS

HEMATURIA

Definition

Microscopic: ≥3 RBCs per high-power field; Gross: red or brown urine visible to the naked eye; may be transient.

Common causes in older persons

- Bladder cancer (more common in older persons)
- UTI
- Stones
- AKI
- Glomerulonephritis
- Interstitial disease (eg, analgesic nephropathy)
- BPH or prostate cancer
- Vigorous exercise
- Excessive anticoagulant tx
- No cause identified (may be up to 60%)

Evaluation

- Dipstick and microscopic analysis
- If microscopic only, assess for other causes including UTI or recent urologic procedures and treat appropriately. Repeat UA.[CW] If negative, no further workup. If positive, renal function testing, cystoscopy, and imaging with either CT urography or ultrasound and selective CT. Ultrasound plus cystoscopy is most cost efficient to exclude malignancy. If proteinuria, RBC or WBC casts, worsened KFTs or edema, refer to nephrology for glomerular evaluation.
- If gross, and visible clots, CT and urgent urology referral. If no clots, renal function testing, cystoscopy, and imaging with either CT urography or ultrasound and selective CT. If proteinuria, RBC or WBC casts, worsened KFTs or edema, refer to nephrology for glomerular evaluation.
- Don't perform urine cytology for routine hematuria investigation.[CW]
- If due to UTI, repeat UA 6 wk after completing tx.
- Women may need pelvic exam to exclude vaginal bleeding.

ACUTE KIDNEY INJURY

Definition

An acute deterioration defined by increased values of kidney function tests (eg, increase in Cr of ≥0.3 mg/dL within 48 h or by >50% within 7 d, or decreased urine volume (<0.5 mL/kg/h for 6 h). May present with edema, HTN, decreased urine output, or without symptoms. Oliguria (<500 mL urine output/d) has worse prognosis.

Precipitating and Aggravating Factors *(Italicized type indicates most common.)*

- *Acute tubular necrosis* due to hypoperfusion or nephrotoxins
- Medications (eg, aminoglycosides, NSAIDs, ACEIs), including those causing allergic interstitial nephritis (eg, NSAIDs, penicillins and cephalosporins, sulfonamides, fluoroquinolones, allopurinol, rifampin, PPIs). Less evidence for IV radiocontrast administration-induced AKI with newer agents.
- Multiple myeloma
- Obstruction (eg, BPH)
- CVD (cardiorenal syndrome, thromboembolic, atheroembolic)
- *Volume depletion* (prerenal) or redistribution of ECF (eg, cirrhosis, burns)

Evaluation

- Review medication list
- Catheterize bladder or determine postvoid residual by ultrasound.
- UA (**Table 82** for likely diagnoses) and urine albumin:Cr ratio (predicts progression of kidney disease)
- If patient is not on diuretics, determine fractional excretion of sodium (FENa). If on diuretics, determine fractional excretion of urea (FEUrea) **(Table 81)**.

Table 81. Urine Tests for Acute Kidney Injury

	Prerenal	Acute Tubular Necrosis	Nondiagnostic
FENa (Fractional Excretion of Sodium)	<1%	>2%	1–2%
FEUrea (Fractional Excretion of Urea)	<35%	>50%	36–50%

Table 82. Likely Diagnoses Based on UA Findings

Findings	Diagnoses
Hematuria, RBC casts, heavy proteinuria	Glomerular disease or vasculitis
Granular and epithelial cell casts, free epithelial cells	Acute tubular necrosis
Pyuria, WBC casts, granular or waxy casts, little or no proteinuria	Acute interstitial nephritis, glomerulitis, vasculitis, obstruction, renal infarction
Normal UA	Prerenal disease, obstruction, hypercalcemia, myeloma, acute tubular necrosis

Note: Urinary eosinophils are neither sensitive nor specific for acute interstitial nephritis but may be helpful in some cases.

- Renal ultrasonography
- Renal biopsy in selected cases

Management of Acute Kidney Injury

- D/C medications that are possible precipitants
- Renally dose medications.
- Crystalloid (eg, Ringers solution or *PlasmaLyte*) rather than saline fluid replacement.
- If prerenal pattern, hemodynamically stable, and not anuric, treat HF (p 64), if present, with furosemide IV 80–200 mg. Otherwise, volume repletion. Begin with fluid challenge 500–1000 mL over 30–60 min. If urine output does not increase in response, give furosemide 100–400 mg IV.
- If obstructed, leave urinary catheter in place during evaluation and while specific tx is implemented.
- If acute tubular necrosis, monitor weight daily, record intake and output, and monitor electrolytes frequently. Fluid replacement should be equal to urinary output plus other drainage plus 500 mL/d for insensible losses.
- If acute interstitial nephritis (except if NSAID-induced) and does not resolve with 3–7 d, glucocorticoids (eg, prednisone 1 mg/kg/d po or IV) for a minimum 1–2 wk and gradual taper when Cr has returned near baseline for a total duration of 2–3 mo.
- Dialysis is indicated when exposure to certain toxins (eg, methanol, ethylene glycol, lithium, metformin) severe hyperkalemia, acidosis (pH <7.1), or volume overload cannot be managed with other tx or when uremic symptoms (eg, pericarditis, coagulopathy, seizures, or encephalopathy) are present.

ACUTE AND CHRONIC KIDNEY DISEASE

Definition

Kidney damage as evidenced by urinary albumin excretion of >30 mg/d or eGFR <60 mL/min for <3 mo (acute) or 3 mo or more (chronic) irrespective of the cause.

Classification (Kidney Disease Outcomes Quality Initiative)

- *Stage G1:* GFR >90 mL/min and persistent albuminuria
- *Stage G2:* GFR 60–89 mL/min and persistent albuminuria
- *Stage G3a:* GFR 45–59 mL/min
- *Stage G3b:* GFR 30–44 mL/min
- *Stage G4:* GFR 15–29 mL/min
- *Stage G5:* GFR <15 mL/min or ESRD

Albumin (a marker of kidney damage)

A1: Daily albumin excretion rate <30 mg/dL

A2: Daily albumin excretion rate 30–300 mg/dL

A3: Daily albumin excretion rate >300 mg/dL

- Cause of CKD also has prognostic value for kidney outcomes and other complications.
- Refer to a nephrologist for co-management if stages G3A3, G4, G5, or CKD complications (see below).

Evaluation

- Hx and physical exam: assess for DM, HTN, obesity, vascular disease, HF, NSAIDs, angiographic procedures with possible cholesterol embolization, glomerulonephritis, myeloma, BPH or obstructive cancers, current or previous tx with a nephrotoxic drug, hereditary kidney disease (eg, polycystic)
- Blood tests (CBC, comprehensive metabolic profile, phosphorus, cholesterol, ESR, serum protein immunoelectrophoresis). Cystatin C to measure eGFR is not affected by race but is more expensive. Using both creatinine and cystatin C ($eGFR_{cr\text{-}cys}$) may be preferable in assessing kidney failure and mortality risk among Black persons.
- Older people with eGFR 45–59 mL/min may have normal kidney function for their age and are less likely to progress to kidney failure compared younger persons. Rates of kidney failure or death are similar to older persons with normal eGFR, except for mild increased risk of kidney failure in persons ages 65–69 and risk of death in persons aged 65–74. An age-adapted threshold of eGFR <45 mL/min may be more appropriate but has not yet been endorsed.
- If GFR 15–59 mL/min, measure iPTH; if iPTH >100 pg/mL, measure serum 25(OH)D.
- UA and spot (early morning sample is preferred) quantitative urine protein (albumin:Cr ratio [abnormal if ≥30 mg/g] or 24-h urine for protein and Cr); urine immunoelectrophoresis, if indicated; at all stages, heavier proteinuria is predictive of mortality, ESRD, and doubling of serum Cr.
- Renal ultrasound (large kidneys suggest tumors, infiltrating disease, cystic disease; small kidneys suggest CKD; can also identify cysts, stones, masses, and hydronephrosis)
- If acute rise in Cr shortly after beginning tx with ACEI or ARB, exclude renal artery stenosis with MRI angiography, CT angiography, or duplex Doppler ultrasound.
- Renal biopsy in selected cases

Management

- Progression to kidney failure can be predicted by age, sex, eGFR, urine albumin:Cr ratio, serum calcium, serum phosphate, serum bicarbonate, and serum albumin using an equation: qxmd.com/calculate/calculator_125/kidney-failure-risk-equation-8-variable
- Attempt to slow progression of kidney failure by:
  - Controlling BP *most important* (target <120 SBP [KDIGO]) though less evidence if >90 y
    - Limit sodium intake to <2 g/d
    - Physical activity of ≥150 min/wk, can be moderate intensity
    - Renin-angiotensin-system inhibitors (ACEI or ARB) (**Table 25**) if A3 with or without DM and if A2 without DM
  - Avoid potassium-sparing diuretics and NSAIDs[CW] in Stages 4 and 5 CKD.[BC]
  - If DM2 and K+ <5 and CKD, consider finerenone (20 mg/d if eGFR ≥60 and 10 mg/d if eGFR ≥25 to < 60) to prevent CKD progression, HF hospitalization, and CVD death.
  - Consider SGLT2 inhibitor (**Table 50**), if proteinuria, with or without DM.
  - Smoking cessation
  - Diet: if eGFR <60 mL/min
    - Restrict dietary caloric intake to 30–35 kcal/kg/d, with <30% as fat with saturated fat <10%
    - Restrict dietary protein to 0.8 g/kg/d
    - Restrict dietary sodium to <2 g/d if HTN, volume overload, or increased protein excretion, and to <2.3 g/d if none of these comorbidities
    - Restrict total dietary calcium to 1000–1500 mg/d
    - Restrict phosphorus intake to 0.8–1 g/d
    - Restrict dietary potassium if serum potassium is high
  - Treat hyperlipidemia (p 51).
  - Treat chronic acidosis: Sodium bicarbonate (daily dosage of 0.5–1 mEq/kg) tx to maintain serum bicarbonate concentration ≥23 mEq/L
  - Control blood sugar if patient has DM2. Consider SGLT2 inhibitors but not if eGFR <45 (**Table 50**).

Prevent and Treat Symptoms and Complications

- Hyperkalemia: if present (p 202); low-potassium diet <40–70 mEq/d; avoid NSAIDs, potassium-sparing diuretics, ACEIs, ARBs.
- Mineral and bone complications:
  - Avoid aluminum and magnesium phosphate binders.
  - Normalize serum calcium with calcium carbonate (500 mg po elemental calcium q6–24h) or calcium acetate *(Phoslo)* (3 or 4 tabs q8h with meals); if hypocalcemia is refractory, consider calcitriol *(Rocaltrol)* 0.25 mcg/d po.
  - Normalize serum phosphate (2.7–4.6 g/dL) if not on dialysis and maintain between 3.5 and 5.5 mg/dL if on dialysis; restrict dairy products and cola to phosphate intake <900 mg/d. When hyperphosphatemia is refractory, begin:
    - If serum calcium is low, calcium carbonate (1250–1500 mg po q8h with meals) or calcium acetate *(Phoslo)* (3 or 4 tabs q8h with meals).
    - If serum calcium is normal or calcium supplementation is ineffective:
      - Sevelamer hydrochloride *(Renagel)* or sevelamer carbonate *(Renvela)*, which does not increase the risk of metabolic acidosis; doses for both are 800–1600 mg po q8h with each meal. Might not have lower risk of atherosclerotic cardiovascular disease (ASCVD) compared to calcium carbonate if ESRD on dialysis. Does not reduce proteinuria if receiving maximal ACEI or ARB tx.
      - Lanthanum carbonate *(Fosrenol)* at initial dosage of 250–500 mg po q8h with each meal, then titrate in increments of 750 mg/d at intervals of 2–3 wk to max of 3750 mg/d.

- Patients on dialysis with hyperparathyroidism should be treated with the phosphate binders, vitamin D tx, and possibly calcimimetics.
- Anemia: Monitor Hb yearly if Stage G3, q6mo if Stages G4 or G5, and q3mo if on dialysis. Treat anemia with iron (if iron deficient) to maintain transferrin saturation >20% and serum ferritin >100 ng/L and, if necessary, erythropoietin-darbepoetin to maintain a target Hb goal of ≤11 g/dL. Don't administer erythropoiesis-stimulating agents to patients with CKD with Hb ≥10 g/dL without signs or symptoms.[CW]
- Cardiovascular (as noted above): Can use loop diuretic to manage volume if Stage G4. If on dialysis, titrate medications based on BP readings not obtained during dialysis.
- Prevention: Immunize with *Pneumovax, Prevnar 20* (if not previously vaccinated with *Prevnar 13*), and, if Stage G4 or G5 CKD, hepatitis B vaccines if hepatitis B surface antigen and antibody are negative.
- Elicit the patient's goals of care, including discussions with family. Educate patients regarding options of hemodialysis, peritoneal dialysis, kidney transplantation, conservative medical tx, and hospice.
- If preferred by patient, prepare for dialysis or transplant. If eGFR <25 mL/min, recommend referral for arteriovenous fistula access, which takes months before it is ready to be used.
- If eGFR <20 mL/min, patients can be listed for cadaveric kidney transplant. Patients aged >65 can be considered for transplantation if substantial life expectancy.
- Dialysis is medically indicated when severe hyperkalemia, acidosis, HTN, or volume overload cannot be managed with other tx or when uremic symptoms (eg, pericarditis or pleuritis, coagulopathy, persistent nausea and vomiting, severe malnutrition, or encephalopathy) are present. Relative indications included decreased alertness and cognition, depression, persistent pruritus, or RLS.
- Other than transplantation, renal replacement therapy (RRT) can be by hemodialysis or peritoneal dialysis (continuous or automated, which uses short dwells and automated technology to operate at near maximum solute clearance rates). Although more older persons select hemodialysis and few switch from hemodialysis to peritoneal dialysis, differences in survival between approaches have not been demonstrated.
- Because life expectancy is limited in ESRD in older persons, shared decision-making about whether to initiate RRT, which approach to use, and when to stop that considers personal preferences and challenges to life with RRT is essential. Benefits are less in persons with severe cognitive impairment or terminal illness.
- Don't perform routine cancer screening for dialysis patients with limited life expectancies without signs or symptoms.[CW]
- Avoid respiratory fluoroquinolones if on hemodialysis (increased risk of sudden cardiac death)
- If quality of life on dialysis is unsatisfactory or medical conditions have progressed, discuss discontinuing dialysis.

VOLUME DEPLETION (DEHYDRATION)

Definition

Losses of sodium and water that may be isotonic (eg, loss of blood) or hypotonic (eg, nasogastric suctioning)

Precipitating Factors

- Blood loss
- Diuretics
- GI losses
- Skin losses
- Kidney or adrenal disease (eg, renal sodium wasting)
- Sequestration of fluid (eg, ileus, burns, peritonitis, acute pancreatitis)

- Age-related changes (impaired thirst, sodium wasting due to hyporeninemic hypoaldosteronism, and free water wasting due to renal insensitivity to antidiuretic hormone)

Evaluation

Clinical Symptoms

- Anorexia
- Nausea and vomiting
- Orthostatic lightheadedness
- Delirium
- Weakness
- Acute weight loss

Clinical Signs

- Dry tongue and axillae
- Oliguria
- Orthostatic hypotension
- Elevated HR
- Weight loss (most specific)

Laboratory Tests

- Serum electrolytes
- Urine sodium (usually <10 mEq/L) and FENa (usually <1% but may be higher because of age-related sodium wasting, diuretics, renal ischemia, situations with high rates of water reabsorption, metabolic alkalosis due to vomiting)
- Serum BUN and Cr (BUN:Cr ratio often >20)
- Urine osmolality (often >450 mOsmol/kg)
- Point-of-care ultrasound measurement of internal jugular venous pressure, if available

Management

- Weigh daily; monitor fluid losses and serum electrolytes, BUN, Cr.
- If mild, oral rehydration of 2–4 L of water/d and 4–8 g Na diet; if poor oral intake, give IV D5W 1/2 NS with potassium as needed.
- If hemodynamically unstable, give packed RBCs or blood substitutes if actively bleeding. If not, give IV balanced crystalloids (Ringer's lactate, Plasma-Lyte A) if patient is in ICU. Balanced crystalloids and 0.9% saline are equally effective in ICU and non–ICU settings. Give 1–2 L as quickly as possible until SBP ≥100 mm Hg and no longer orthostatic. Then switch to D5W 1/2 NS. Monitor closely in patients with a hx of HF. Albumin is second-line tx. Avoid hyperoncotic starch solutions, which are associated with AKI and increased mortality.

HYPERNATREMIA

Causes

- Pure water loss
  - Insensible losses due to sweating and respiration
  - Impaired thirst (eg, delirious or intubated) or access to water (eg, functionally dependent) may sustain hypernatremia
  - Central (eg, posttraumatic, CNS tumors, meningitis) diabetes insipidus or nephrogenic (eg, hypercalcemia, lithium) diabetes insipidus
- Hypotonic sodium loss
  - Renal causes: osmotic diuresis (eg, due to hyperglycemia), postobstructive diuresis, polyuric phase of acute tubular necrosis, diabetes insipidus, diuretics
  - GI causes: vomiting and diarrhea, nasogastric drainage, osmotic cathartic agents (eg, lactulose)
- Hypertonic sodium gain (eg, massive salt ingestion, tx with hypertonic saline)
- Hypothalamic disease impairing thirst or osmoreceptor function

Evaluation

- Measure intake and output.
- Obtain urine osmolality:
  - >600 mOsm/kg suggests extrarenal (eg, water loss and volume depletion) if urine Na <25 mEq/L) or remote renal water loss or administration of hypertonic Na+ salt solutions (if urine Na >100 mEq/L).
  - 300–600 mOsm/kg suggests osmotic diuresis or diabetes insipidus. If total solute excretion (urine osmolality × urine daily volume) >1000 mOsm/d, suggests osmotic diuresis.
  - <300 mOsm/kg and polyuria suggest diabetes insipidus.

Management

- Treat underlying causes.
- If acute (eg, developing over hours), correct using D5W at a rate of 3–6 mL/kg/h with a goal of correcting by no more than 1–2 mEq/L/h and to near normal within 24 h. Monitor q2–3h and reduce to 1 mL/kg/h when Na <145 mEq/L. When target correction rate has been achieved, can reduce monitoring to q12–24 h unless continued large ongoing water losses.
- If chronic (present for >48 h), correct over 48–72 h using oral (can use pure water), nasogastric (can use pure water), or IV (D5W, 1/2 or 1/4 NS) fluids at 1.35 mL/h × body weight in kg (approximately 70 mL/h for a 50-kg person and 100 mL/h for a 70-kg person) with correction goal of ~10 mmol/L/d.
- If central diabetes insipidus, will also need desmopressin tx.
- Correct with NS only in cases of severe volume depletion with hemodynamic compromise; once stable, switch to hypotonic solution.

HYPONATREMIA

Classifications

Acuity: hyperacute (within hours), acute (within 48 h), chronic (at least 48 h or unknown)

Severity: mild (130–134 mEq/L), moderate (121–129 mEq/L), severe (≤120 mEq/L)

Symptoms: absent, mild to moderate (eg, headache, nausea, vomiting, fatigue, gait disturbances, confusion), severe (eg, seizures, obtundation, coma, respiratory arrest)

Causes

- With increased plasma osmolality: hyperglycemia (~2 mEq/L decrement for each 100 mg/dL increase in plasma glucose)
- With normal plasma osmolality (pseudohyponatremia): severe hyperlipidemia, obstructive jaundice, hyperproteinemia (eg, multiple myeloma)
- With decreased plasma osmolality:
  - With ECF excess: kidney failure, HF, hepatic cirrhosis, nephrotic syndrome
  - With decreased ECF volume: renal loss from salt-losing nephropathies, diuretics, cerebral salt wasting, osmotic diuresis; extrarenal loss due to vomiting, diarrhea, skin losses, and third-spacing (usually urine Na <20 mEq/L, FENa <1%, and uric acid >4 mg/dL)
  - With normal ECF volume: primary polydipsia (urine osmolarity <100 mOsm/kg), hypothyroidism, adrenal insufficiency, SIADH (urine Na >40 mEq/L and uric acid <4 mg/dL), reset osmostat (urine Na< 25 mEq/L and urine osmolarity <100 mOsm/kg if measured after water ingested and similar to SIADH if water intake is restricted), which has moderately reduced Na that is stable on multiple measurements

Management

Treat underlying cause. General measures include discontinuing contributing medications, reducing free water intake, and increasing dietary salt intake. Specific tx only if symptomatic (eg, altered mental status, seizures), severe (<120 mEq/L), or acute (<48 h) hyponatremia.

- If initial volume estimate is equivocal, give fluid challenge of 0.5–1 L of isotonic (0.9%) saline.
- If volume depletion, give saline IV (corrects ~1 mEq/L for every liter given) or oral salt tablets.
- If edematous states, SIADH, or CKD, fluid restriction to below the level of urine output is the primary tx.
- Hypovolemic hyponatremia is almost always chronic (except for cerebral salt wasting and after diuretic initiation), and hypertonic saline is seldom indicated.
- If acute, patients are typically hospitalized.
  - If asymptomatic, treat with 3% hypertonic saline 50 mL bolus or slow infusion 15–30 mL/h.
  - If any symptoms of increased intracranial pressure, treat with hypertonic (3%) saline initially with 100 mL bolus over 10–15 min; may repeat 2× if symptoms persist. Risk of overcorrection is similar whether rapid intermittent bolus or slow continuous infusion, but bolus has less need for relowering tx and more likely to achieve target correction rate within 1 h. Goal is to increase Na by 4–6 mEq/L) over a few hours. Concurrent desmopressin (1–2 mcg IV or SC q6–8h for 24–48 h) may help prevent overly rapid correction but is usually not used if HF or cirrhosis. Monitor sodium q2h.
- If chronic, hospitalize if severe symptoms, severe hyponatremia, or known intracranial pathology.
  - If severe symptoms or known intracranial pathology, treat with 3% saline initially with 100 mL bolus over 10–15 min; may repeat 2× if symptoms persist.
- If no or mild to moderate symptoms and severe hyponatremia, treat with 3% saline at 15–30 mL/h. May need to add furosemide if edematous. Monitor Na closely and taper tx when >120 mEq/L or symptoms resolve.
  - If no or mild to moderate symptoms and moderate hyponatremia (120–129 mEq/L), treat underlying causes and free water restriction.
  - Goal is <4–6 mEq/L Na rise during first 24 h and no more than 8 mEq/L in any 24 h (more rapid correction can result in central pontine myelinolysis).
- Arginine vasopressin receptor antagonists; uncommonly used in acute hyponatremia
  - Conivaptan *(Vaprisol)* is effective in euvolemic hyponatremia in hospitalized patients; 20 mg IV over 30 min 1×, followed by continuous infusion of 20–40 mg over 24 h for 4 d max (L) (CYP3A4 interactions).
  - Tolvaptan 15–60 mg/d po: initiate in hospital and monitor blood sodium concentration closely. Not to be given to patients with liver disease and not to be used for ≥30 d.

SYNDROME OF INAPPROPRIATE SECRETION OF ANTIDIURETIC HORMONE (SIADH)

Definition

Hypotonic hyponatremia (<280 mOsm/kg) with:

- Less than maximally dilute urine (usually >100 mOsm/kg)
- Elevated urine sodium (usually >40 mEq/L)
- Normal volume status
- Normal kidney, adrenal, and thyroid function

Precipitating Factors, Causes

- Medications (eg, SSRIs [typically occurs between week 1 and 13 of tx] and SNRIs, especially if borderline low Na; carbamazepine; oxcarbazepine; NSAIDs; barbiturates; antipsychotics; mirtazapine, sodium valproate, amiodarone, ciprofloxacin. Use with caution.[BC])
- Neuropsychiatric factors (eg, neoplasm, subarachnoid hemorrhage, psychosis, meningitis)
- Postprocedure (eg, cardiac catheterization) and postoperative state, especially if pain or nausea
- Pulmonary disease (eg, pneumonia, tuberculosis, acute asthma)
- Tumors (eg, small-cell lung cancer, pancreas, thymus, olfactory neuroblastoma)
- Reset osmostat (mild hyponatremia stable over days despite variations in Na and water intake)

Evaluation

- BUN, Cr, serum cortisol, TSH
- CXR
- Review of medications
- Neurologic tests as indicated
- Urine sodium and osmolality
- If osmostat reset is suspected, give water load (10–15 mL/kg po or IV); if reset osmostat, will excrete water load within 4 h.

Management

Acute Management: See euvolemic hyponatremia management, p 199. Also urea in patients with cancer (see below).

Chronic Management:

- D/C offending medication or treat precipitating illness.
- Goal is Na ≥130 mEq/L.
- No tx is needed for reset osmostat.
- Restrict water intake (unless due to subarachnoid hemorrhage) to <800 mL/d with goal of Na ≥130 mEq/L. Rate of correction should be <8 mEq/L/d. Increase Na by 3 mEq/L at 3 d, but little improvement after.
- Liberalize salt intake or give salt tablets. Can also give IV saline but the electrolyte concentration of the fluid must be greater than the electrolyte concentration of urine. Usually, hypertonic saline, if given.
- If urinary osmolality is twice the plasma osmolality, loop diuretics (eg, furosemide 20 mg po q12h) may help facilitate excess water excretion.
- If symptomatic and above steps do not work:
  - Demeclocycline 150–300 mg po q12h (may be nephrotoxic in patients with liver disease).
  - Tolvaptan 15–60 mg/d po: initiate in hospital and monitor blood sodium concentration closely only if symptomatic and above steps do not work. Risk of hepatotoxicity. Do not use for >30 d, and do not use in patients with chronic liver diseases.
  - Oral urea (medical food with urea 15 g/pck) usual dose 15–30 g/d. Not studied in placebo-controlled trials, but a study of patients previously treated with vasopressin tolvaptan or satavaptan showed comparable effectiveness as the vaptans. Also has been used as first-line tx in patients with cancer.

HYPERKALEMIA

Persistent hyperkalemia only occurs if impaired urinary potassium excretion.

Causes

- Kidney failure
- Addison disease
- Hyporeninemic hypoaldosteronism
- Renal tubular acidosis
- Metabolic acidosis
- Diabetic hyperglycemia
- Hemolysis, tumor lysis, rhabdomyolysis
- Reduced distal sodium and water delivery to distal nephron due to volume depletion, HF, or cirrhosis
- Transfusions of stored blood
- Constipation
- Medications (potassium-sparing diuretics, ACEIs, trimethoprim-sulfamethoxazole, β blockers, NSAIDs, cyclosporine, tacrolimus, pentamidine, calcineurin inhibitors, heparin, digoxin toxicity)
- Pseudohyperkalemia from extreme thrombocytosis or leukocytosis or improper blood drawing (betadine antiseptic, mechanical trauma, repeated fist clenching, prolonged tourniquet application) or handling (not centrifuged within 30 min of drawing)

Evaluation

- If not extremely high, consider repeating to confirm
- ECG; peaked T waves typically occur when K^+ exceeds 6.5 mEq/L. ECG changes are more likely with acute increases of K^+ than with chronic increases.

Management

- K^+ <6 mEq/L without ECG changes:
  - Low-potassium diet (restrict orange juice, bananas, potatoes, cantaloupe, honeydew, tomatoes)
  - May be stable and not need medical tx
  - Oral diuretics (eg, oral torsemide or bumetanide, combined oral loop and thiazide-like diuretics; metolazone is the most K^+ wasting); avoid hypovolemia
  - Oral sodium bicarbonate (650–1300 mg po q12h); not recommended as a single agent
  - Reduce or D/C medications that increase K^+
- K^+ 6–6.5 mEq/L without ECG changes: above tx plus potassium binder:
  - Patiromer *(Veltassa)* 8.4 g/d po with food and may be titrated up each wk to max 25.2 g. If taking ciprofloxacin, levothyroxine, or metformin, separate administration of patiromer and other drug by 3 h.
  - Sodium zirconium cyclosilicate *(Lokelma)* 10 g po 3×/d for 48 h; adjust dose by 5 g/d po at 1-wk intervals; effective in those receiving maintenance dialysis. More rapid onset of action compared to patiromer.
  - Sodium polystyrene sulfonate: Some experts recommend against using because of potential AEs. If taken orally, can bind to other drugs, and when given rectally, can cause intestinal necrosis if bowel dysfunction or recent GI surgery.
- K^+ 6.5 mEq/L with peaked T waves but no other ECG changes: hospitalization is decided case-by-case based on acuteness of onset, cause, and other patient factors.

Absolute indications for hospitalization

- K^+ >8 mEq/L
- Symptoms of muscle weakness or paralysis, GI bleeding, concurrent tissue breakdown (eg, rhabdomyolysis)
- ECG changes other than peaked T waves (eg, prolonged PR, loss of P waves, widened QRS)
- Acute deterioration of kidney function

Inpatient Management of Hyperkalemia

- Antagonism of cardiac effects of hyperkalemia (most rapid-acting acute tx; use only for severe hyperkalemia with significant ECG changes when too dangerous to wait for redistribution tx to take effect)
  - 10% calcium gluconate IV infused over 2–3 min (20–30 min if on digoxin) with ECG monitoring; effect lasts 30–60 min, may repeat if needed
- Reduction of serum K^+ by redistribution into cells (acute tx; can be used in combination with calcium gluconate, and different redistribution tx can be combined depending on severity of hyperkalemia)
  - Insulin (regular) 10 U in 500 mL of 10% dextrose over 30–60 min or bolus insulin (regular) 10 U IV followed by 50 mL of 50% dextrose. Can drop serum K^+ by 0.5–1.2 mEq/L, even with CKD.
  - Albuterol 0.5 mg in 100 mL of 5% dextrose given over 10–15 min or nebulized 10–20 mg in 4 mL of NS over 10 min (should not be used as single agent)
  - Sodium bicarbonate if significant metabolic acidosis, but should not be used as single agent.
- Removal of potassium from body (definitive tx; work more slowly)
  - Diuretics (eg, oral torsemide or bumetanide, IV furosemide, combined oral loop and thiazide-like diuretics; metolazone is the most K^+ wasting). Avoid hypovolemia.
  - Fludrocortisone 0.1–0.3 mg/d po
  - Potassium binders (see K^+ 6–6.5 mEq/L without ECG changes p 202). Patiromer and zirconium cyclosilicate are preferred over sodium polystyrene sulfonate.
  - Dialysis (most effective, can normalize within 4 h)

REQUIREMENTS, DIET, AND SUPPLEMENTS

Calculating Basic Energy (Caloric), Protein, and Fluid Requirements

- WHO energy estimates for adults aged 60 and older:
  - Women (10.5) (weight in kg) + 596
  - Men (13.5) (weight in kg) + 487
  - Depending on activity and physiologic stress levels, these basic requirements may need to be increased (eg, 25% for sedentary or mild, 50% for moderate, and 100% for intense or severe activity or stress).
  - Based on observational data that associated lower protein intake with increased incident mobility limitation, protein intake of ≥1 g/kg body weight/d may be optimal.
- Fluid requirements for older adults without heart or kidney disease are ~30 mL/kg/d.
- US Department of Agriculture guidelines recommend for all above age 14:
  - Added sugars: <10% of calories
  - Saturated fat: <10% of calories
  - Sodium: < 2300 mg/d
  - Calcium 1200 mg/d (for women age ≥51 and men age ≥71)
  - Vitamin D 800 IU (for women and men age ≥71)

Mediterranean and Related Diets

- Observational data indicate improved health status and reductions in CVD, cancer, DM2, and overall and cardiovascular mortality, as well as lower incidences of Parkinson disease and Alzheimer disease (AD).
- Clinical trial data demonstrate reduction in stroke and cognitive decline but not overall or cardiovascular mortality with Mediterranean diet supplemented by either extra-virgin olive oil or mixed nuts.
- In observational studies, DASH and Mediterranean-DASH Intervention for Neurodegenerative Delay (MIND) diets have also been associated with slowed cognitive decline and reduced incidence of AD.

Vitamins and Supplements

Vitamin D and Calcium (see Osteoporosis chapter)

- All older adults should receive calcium 1200 mg/d and vitamin D 800–1000 IU/d. Each 8 oz glass of milk or fortified orange juice has approximately 100 IU vitamin D. D_3 (cholecalciferol) is the preferred form of supplementation. The USPSTF concluded that there is insufficient evidence to recommend screening for vitamin D deficiency and recommends against vitamin D to prevent falls. Don't routinely measure 1,25(OH)2D or 25(OH)D unless the patient has hypercalcemia or decreased kidney function.[CW]
- Calcium supplements probably do not increase the risk of CVD. Data on risk of dementia and stroke-related dementia remain inconclusive. Risk of kidney stones is increased.

Multivitamins and Other Supplements

- Most older persons who eat a balanced diet do not need multivitamins.
- Supplementation in doses of 50–200% of the Recommended Daily Allowance (RDA) is probably safe.
- Observational data in postmenopausal women indicate no effect of multivitamins on breast, colorectal, endometrial, lung, or ovarian cancers, MI, stroke, VTE, or mortality.

- In clinical trials, multivitamins have shown:
  - No decrease CVD or mortality, but a small reduction in total cancer risk among middle-aged men.
  - No benefit on immune function or in reducing infections in outpatient and nursing-home settings.
  - Improved vitamin C and zinc status and self-reported health (days ill × severity) among older adults (mean age 64 y).
  - No benefit of fatty acids (docosahexaenoic acid [DHA]/eicosapentaenoic acid [EPA]), antioxidants (lutein/zeaxanthin), or zinc supplements on cognitive decline.
- USPSTF recommends against use of beta-carotene or vitamin E supplements to prevent CVD or cancer.
- Treat specific vitamin (eg, vitamin B_{12}, folate) or micronutrient deficiencies if there are medical indications (see Hematologic Disorders, p 29, Neurologic Disorders, p 234). Don't routinely use vitamin B supplements for tx of polyneuropathy or neuropathic pain unless a deficiency exists.[CW]

UNDERNUTRITION

Definition

There is no uniformly accepted definition of undernutrition in older adults. Some commonly used definitions include those listed below.

Community-dwelling Older Adults

- American Society for Parenteral and Enteral Nutrition (ASPEN; 2012) criteria for adult malnutrition (2 of the following):
  - Insufficient energy intake
  - Loss of muscle mass
  - Fluid accumulation (eg, edema)
  - Weight loss
  - Loss of subcutaneous fat
  - Diminished function by handgrip strength
- Global Leadership Initiative on Malnutrition (GLIM; 2018) requires:
  - 1 etiologic criterion
    - reduced food intake or assimilation
    - inflammation or disease burden
  - and ≥1 phenotypic criteria
    - nonvolitional weight loss
    - low BMI
    - reduced muscle mass

Table 83. Severity Grading of Malnutrition into Stage 1 (Moderate) and Stage 2 (Severe) Malnutrition

	Phenotypic Criteria		
	Weight Loss, %	**Low BMI, kg/m²**	**Reduced Muscle Mass**[1]
Stage 1 (moderate malnutrition) requires 1 phenotypic criterion that meets this grade	5–10% within the past 6 mo or 10–20% beyond 6 mo	<20 if aged <70, <22 if aged ≥70	Mild-to-moderate deficit
Stage 2 (severe malnutrition) requires 1 phenotypic criterion that meets this grade	>10% within the past 6 mo or >20% beyond 6 mo	<18.5 if aged <70, <20 if aged ≥70	Severe deficit

[1] Measurement by dual-energy absorptiometry, bioelectrical impedance, ultrasound, CT, or MRI. Calf or arm muscle circumference are alternatives.

- Cancer-related anorexia/cachexia syndrome: a hypercatabolic state (increased resting energy expenditure) with high levels of tumor-activated or host-produced immune responses (eg, proinflammatory cytokines) to the tumor
- Sarcopenia age-related loss of muscle mass (eg, 2 SDs below mean for young healthy adults) with loss of strength and performance; contributors include decreased sex hormones, increased insulin resistance, increased inflammatory cytokines, decreased physical activity, inadequate protein intake, and spinal cord changes (decreased motor units)

Hospitalized Patients

- Dietary intake (eg, <50% of estimated needed caloric intake)
- Hypoalbuminemia (eg, <3.5 g/dL)
- Refeeding syndrome caused by the glucose-induced acute transcellular shift of phosphate typically occurs in malnourished patients (low BMI, unintentional weight loss) who have had poor oral intake for >5 d and then receive either IV glucose-containing fluids or enteral or parenteral nutrition. Symptoms occur most commonly within 2–4 d of refeeding and include hypophosphatemia, hyperglycemia, and hyperinsulinemia, which may be accompanied by hypokalemia, hypomagnesemia, fluid retention (edema, HF), rhabdomyolysis, seizures, and hemolysis. Prevention includes correcting baseline electrolyte abnormalities, reducing energy intake (eg, 10–15 kcal/kg/d for high risk), replacing fluids to maintain zero balance, and restricting sodium and gradually increasing these over 5–10 d. Thiamine 200–300 mg/d po or IV is given days 1–5 and multivitamins on days 1–10.

Nursing-home Patients (triggered by the CMS Minimum Data Set)

- Weight loss of ≥5% in past 30 d; ≥10% in 180 d
- Dietary intake <75% of most meals

Screening

Proposed screening instruments have not been adequately validated or do not demonstrate sufficient sensitivity and specificity to warrant use in clinical practice.

Multidimensional Assessment

In the absence of valid nutrition screening instruments, clinicians should focus on whether the following issues may be affecting nutritional status:

- Economic barriers to securing food
- Social isolation (eg, eating alone)
- Availability of sufficiently high-quality food
- Dental problems that preclude ingesting food
- Medical illnesses that:
    - interfere with ingestion (eg, dysphagia), digestion, or absorption of food
    - increase nutritional requirements or cause cachexia (especially cancer)
    - require dietary restrictions (eg, low-sodium diet or npo)
    - are treated with digoxin, cholinesterase inhibitors, SSRIs, amiodarone, topiramate
- Functional disability that interferes with shopping, preparing meals, or feeding
- Food preferences or cultural beliefs that interfere with adequate food intake
- Poor appetite
- Depressive symptoms (most common cause)

Anthropometrics

Weight on each visit and yearly height

Evaluation for Comorbid Medical Conditions

- CBC, ESR, and comprehensive metabolic panel (if none abnormal, likelihood ratio for cancer is 0.2)
- CXR
- TSH

Biochemical Markers

Serum Proteins: All may drop precipitously because of trauma, sepsis, or major infection.

- Albumin (half-life 18–20 d) has prognostic value in all settings.
- Transferrin (half-life 7 d)
- Prealbumin (half-life 48 h) may be valuable in monitoring nutritional recovery.

Nonpharmacologic Interventions

- If possible, remove disease-specific (eg, for hypercholesterolemia) dietary restrictions.
- If needed, help arrange shopping, cooking, and feeding assistance, including home-delivered meals and between-meal snacks.
- Increase caloric density of foods.
- Posthospitalization home visits by a dietitian may be valuable.
- Congregate Nutrition Program provides meals and related nutrition in congregate settings
- Supplemental Nutrition Assistance Program (SNAP) offers temporary benefits to purchase food for those on limited income
- Commodity Supplemental Food Program provides packaged food to low-income older adults
- Home-delivered nutrition services for those who have difficulty leaving the home
- Child and Adult Care Food Program (CACFP): a federal program that provides reimbursement for meals to older adults enrolled in daycare facilities

Pharmacotherapy: Appetite Stimulants

- No medications are FDA approved to promote weight gain in older adults. Avoid using prescription appetite stimulants.[CW]
- Dronabinol and megestrol acetate (not covered by Medicare Part D) have been effective in promoting weight gain in younger adults with specific conditions (eg, AIDS, cancer). Avoid megestrol; may increase risk of thrombosis and death.[BC]
- A minority of patients receiving mirtazapine report appetite stimulation and weight gain.
- All medications used for appetite have substantial potential AEs.

Nutritional Supplements

- Protein and energy supplements in older adults at risk of malnutrition appear to have beneficial effects on weight gain, chair rise time, handgrip strength, and mortality, and shorten length of stay in hospitalized patients. Among those who are well nourished at baseline, the benefit is less clear. Supplements should be given between rather than with meals.
- In malnourished or at-risk hospitalized patients, nutritional support reduces mortality for up to 6 mo and readmission rates, and is associated with weight gain.
- For ICU patients, enteral nutrition is preferred over parenteral nutrition and should be started within the first 24–48 h after admission. Absence of bowel sounds and evidence of bowel function (eg, passing flatus or feces) are not contraindications to beginning tube feeding.

- Many formulas are available. Read the content labels and choose on the basis of calories/mL, protein, fiber, lactose, and fluid load. (See digital text for nutrition tables.)
  - Oral (not covered by Medicare): Many (eg, *Resource Health Shake, Carnation Breakfast Essentials*) are milk-based and provide ~1–1.5 calories/mL.
  - Enteral (covered by Medicare Part B): Commercial preparations have between 0.5 and 2 calories/mL; most contain no milk (lactose) products. For patients who need fluid restriction, the higher concentrated formulas may be valuable, but they may cause diarrhea. Because of reduced kidney function with aging, some recommend that protein should contribute no more than 20% of the formula's total calories. If the formula is the sole source of nutrition, consider one that contains fiber (25 g/d is optimal).

Important Drug-Enteral Interactions

- Soybean formulas increase fecal elimination of levothyroxine; time the administration of levothyroxine and enteral nutrition as far apart as possible.
- Enteral feedings reduce absorption of phenytoin, L-DOPA, levofloxacin, and ciprofloxacin; administer these medications at least 2 h after a feeding and delay feeding at least 2 h after medication is administered; monitor levels (if taking phenytoin) and adjust dosages, as necessary.
- Check with pharmacy about suitability and best way to administer SR, enteric-coated, and microencapsulated products (eg, omeprazole, lansoprazole, diltiazem, fluoxetine, verapamil).

Gastrostomy/Jejunostomy Tube Feeding

- Chronic artificial nutrition and hydration is not a basic intervention and is associated with uncertain benefit and considerable risks and discomfort.
- Do not insert percutaneous feeding tubes if advanced dementia; instead offer oral assisted feedings.[CW]
- Artificial nutrition and hydration should be used only for specific medical indications, not to increase patient comfort.
- Some evidence supports the use of gastrostomy tubes in patients with head and neck cancer, brain injury, and neurodegenerative disorders (eg, ALS), and stroke patients with dysphagia, particularly within 30 d to 6 mo of stroke.
- For dysphagia and aspiration, the evidence for gastronomy tubes is conflicting and there are no RCTs.

Tips for Successful Tube Feeding

- Tube management
  - Polyurethane tubes have less dysfunction than silicone tubes.
  - Bolster should be positioned to allow 1–2 cm movement.
  - Gauze pads should be placed over, not underneath, the external bolster.
  - Tubes removed inadvertently during the first 4 wk should not be reinserted blindly. Rather, they should be endoscopically, radiologically, or surgically reinserted, which can usually occur through the same site.
- Using the tube
  - Tube feeding can begin 4 h after placement, though early feeding may result in increased gastric residual volumes.
  - Gastrostomy tube feeding may be either intermittent or continuous.

- Check gastric residual volume before each bolus feeding. Gastric residual volumes in the range of 200–500 mL should raise concern and lead to the implementation of measures to reduce the risk of aspiration, but automatic cessation of feeding should not occur for gastric residual volumes <500 mL in the absence of other signs of intolerance. If needed, naloxone *(Narcan)* 8 mg q6h per nasogastric tube, metoclopramide 10 mg, per nasogastric tube or IV, or erythromycin 250 mg IV [5 mg/5 mL] q6h may be useful for problems with high gastric residual volume after mechanical obstruction has been excluded.
- During daily care, the gastrostomy tube should be pushed forward into the wound slightly and rotated to ensure that the internal bumper does not become buried into the gastric mucosa. After rotation, the gastrostomy should be returned to its original position.
- Jejunostomy tube feedings must be continuous. Rapid feeding may cause "dumping syndrome" with fainting, palpitations, sweating, tachycardia, rebound hypoglycemia, and diarrhea.
- Continuous tube feeding is associated with less frequent diarrhea but with higher rates of tube clogging.

• Preventing complications
  - To help prevent aspiration, maintain a 30–45° elevation of the head of the bed during continuous feeding and for at least 2 h after bolus feedings.
  - To prevent clogging and to provide additional free water, flushing with at least 30–60 mL of water q4–6h is recommended. Do not allow formula bags to run dry. Administer only liquid or crushed and dissolved medication through tubes. (See Appropriate Prescribing, p 18.)
  - Do not give more than one medication at a time; flush with 20 mL of water before and after medication administration and with 5–10 mL between medications. Do not mix medications directly into the enteral feeding formula.
  - Do not administer bulk-forming laxatives (eg, methylcellulose or psyllium) or resins (eg, cholestyramine) through feeding tubes.

• Treating complications
  - If clogged, first attach a 30- to 60-mL syringe and pull back plunger to help dislodge clog. Then gently flush with warm water with 30- to 60-mL syringe. Allow water to sit for up to 20 min and repeat. Pancrelipase *(Viokase)* mixed with a bicarbonate 650-mg tab or 1/8 tsp baking soda in warm water may be helpful. Papain and chymopapain are more effective at clearing clogged tubes than sugar-free carbonated beverages or cranberry juice. If these fail, an endoscopic cytology brush, dedicated gastrostomy tube brush, or commercial devices (eg, *Clog Zapper*) may be effective.
  - Diarrhea, which develops in 5–30% of people receiving enteral feeding, may be related to the osmolality of the formula, the rate of delivery, high sorbitol content in liquid medications (eg, APAP, lithium, oxybutynin, furosemide), or other patient-related factors such as antibiotic use or impaired absorption.
  - Hypergranulation at tube sites may be treated with silver nitrate, sprinkled salt, or steroid cream.

Parenteral Nutrition

- Indicated in those with digestive dysfunction precluding enteral feeding.
- In ICU settings, if enteral nutrition is not feasible, should wait 8 d to begin parenteral nutrition.
- Delivers protein as amino acids, carbohydrate as dextrose (D5 = 170 kcal/L; D10 = 340 kcal/L), and fat as lipid emulsions (10% = 1100 kcal/L; 20% = 2200 kcal/L).
- Usually administered as total parenteral nutrition through a central catheter, which may be inserted peripherally.

OBESITY AND OVERWEIGHT

Definitions

- Overweight (BMI 25–29.9 kg/m²); not associated with increased mortality if aged >70
- Obesity (BMI ≥30 kg/m²)

Overview

- Overweight probably does not increase mortality risk; however, weight loss in obese older adults may decrease mortality risk and is associated with health benefits; 5–7% is a good initial weight loss goal.
- Assess and treat obesity-related comorbidities (eg, CVD, HTN, DM, dyslipidemia, sleep apnea).
- If BMI >30 or 25 to <30 and at least 1 comorbidity and patient seems ready to make lifestyle changes, begin comprehensive lifestyle intervention (diet, exercise, and behavioral modification) +/ pharmacotherapy (especially if patient has failed to achieve >5% weight loss at 3–6 mo). If BMI >40 or >35 with at least 1 comorbidity, consider bariatric surgery.
- After weight loss, counterregulatory hormones attempt to re-establish higher weight (may be less after bariatric surgery or long-term drug tx), and reduced energy expenditure as a result of weight loss make maintenance difficult.

Nonpharmacologic Interventions

- Combinations of weight management (eg, low-calorie diet with deficit of 500–750 calories/d) plus moderate exercise (90 min/3×/wk, preferably combined aerobic and resistance) has resulted in weight loss of 10% and improved functional status in younger (mean age 70) obese older persons.
- Goal of dietary tx is to reduce total number of calories consumed; no single diet fits all patients' needs.
- Various macronutrient composition low-calorie diets are equally effective.
- Very low–calorie programs with intake <800 calories/d (Health Management Resources, *Medifast*, and OPTIFAST) are no more effective than low-calorie diets and require medical supervision. Severe energy restriction (65–75% energy restriction) results in greater weight loss and proportional lean body mass loss and lower BMD compared to moderate energy restriction (25–35%).
- Patients on diet tx tend to lose weight over initial 6 mo and regain it over next 2–3 y. Lower energy-density diet (fewer calories per volume of food) and high-protein, low-glycemic index may be more effective in reducing weight regain after loss. Behavioral interventions (up to 52 mo) may be helpful in maintaining weight loss.
- mHealth (mobile and wireless technologies) behavioral change lifestyle interventions (eg, *Noom*) have demonstrated weight loss, including in older persons.
- Intensive lifestyle interventions aimed at eating and physical activity delivered in primary care by health coaches were successful in achieving clinically significant weight loss at 24 mo primarily in underserved patients <75 y.
- No commercial weight-loss programs have been evaluated in older persons. In younger patients:
  - Weight Watchers is more effective than education alone.
  - Jenny Craig is more effective than education or behavioral counseling, more expensive than Weight Watchers.
  - Self-directed programs (Atkins) are more effective than education or counseling. Internet-based (The Biggest Loser Club, eDiets, Lose It!) appear more effective than education alone but are comparable to counseling.

Devices and Endoscopic or Embolization Procedures

BMI indications vary by device. EWL indicates excess weight loss above BMI 25.

- **Hydrogels**. 2.25-g cellulose and citric acid hydrogel taken orally before lunch and dinner that expand to create satiety results in weight loss (6.4% vs 4.4%) compared to placebo at 24 wk.
- **Endoscopic sleeve gastroplasty**. 56–62% EWL, with 2% serious AEs: at 5 y; mean total weight loss 15.9%.
- **Gastric balloon device** endoscopically placed and left in place for up to 6 mo; 25–30% EWL
- **Endoscopic gastrointestinal bypass devices** (*EndoBarrier*, 60 cm long from proximal duodenum to mid-jejunum;) prevent luminal contents from being absorbed in proximal small intestine; 23–40% EWL but high rates of removal due to pain.
- **Maestro Rechargeable System** uses high-frequency electric pulses to block vagus signals; 25% EWL.
- ***AspireAssist*** (similar to PEG feeding tube) allows patients to partially drain stomach contents after meal, reducing absorbed calories by 30%; 32–49% EWL.
- **Bariatric arterial embolization to left gastric artery**. 11–17% EWL at 1 y; less effective than bariatric surgery but favorable safety profile.

Bariatric Surgery

- Most are performed laparoscopically. In younger patients, increased remissions from DM and lower incidence of micro- and macrovascular complications. Reduced obesity-related cancer and cancer-related, cardiovascular, and all-cause mortality.
  - Adjustable gastric banding placed laparoscopically: 47% EWL at 15 y; safest but least effective procedure
  - Sleeve gastrectomy with most of greater curvature removed: 59% EWL; less effective than gastric bypass or Roux-en-Y but lower rate of complications
  - Roux-en-Y gastric bypass creating pouch of stomach anastomosing jejunum: 54–74% EWL but more interventions, operations, and hospitalizations over 5 y compared to sleeve gastrectomy
  - Biliopancreatic diversion with duodenal switch combines restrictive procedure similar to sleeve with bypass about 3/4 small intestine; 70–80% EWL but higher complications and mortality.
  - Single-anastomosis duodeno-ileal bypass with sleeve gastrectomy: 67–91% EWL; fewer anastomotic complications, bowel obstructions, internal hernias, volvulus compared to Roux-en-Y or sleeve gastrectomy but greater risk of chronic diarrhea.

Pharmacotherapy

- Drugs to treat obesity have not been studied extensively in older persons; the information below is based on studies of younger persons. GLP-1 receptor agonists, especially weekly injectable semaglutide, may be preferred agent.
- When using pharmacologic management, weight loss of 10–15% is considered a good response and >15% is considered excellent. If ≥5% weight loss is not achieved in 12 wk, stop or taper depending on the specific drug.
- Based on a meta-analysis, 23% of placebo recipients achieved 5% weight loss; 5% loss rates for individual drugs are listed in **Table 84**.

Table 84. Drugs for Weight Loss in Older Persons (in approximate order of effectiveness)

Drug	Average Weight Loss, kg	Percentage Losing ≥5%	Conditions for Which Drug Is a Preferred Tx	Adverse Effects
Orlistat *(Xenical)* (120 mg)	2.5–3.4	35–73%	DM2, high BP, CAD, arrhythmia, CKD (mild or moderate), depression, anxiety, glaucoma, seizure disorder	Abdominal discomfort, flatus; may increase risk of calcium oxalate renal stones; rare reports of liver injury
(Alli)[OTC] (60 mg)	2.6	40%		
Naltrexone-*bupropion (Contrave)*	3.7–5.2	39–66%	DM2, CKD (mild or moderate, lower max dose), anxiety	Nausea, vomiting, headache, constipation, dizziness, dry mouth, lowered seizure threshold, abnormal LFTs
Liraglutide *(Saxenda)*[2]	3.7–5.8	44–62%	DM2, high BP (monitor HR), CAD, arrhythmia, CKD (mild or moderate), depression, anxiety, glaucoma, seizure disorder	Nausea, vomiting, constipation, diarrhea; contraindicated if MTC or family hx or MEN 2
Phentermine-topiramate ER *(Qsymia)*	6–13	45–70%	DM2, high BP (monitor HR), CKD (mild or moderate, lower max dose), depression, anxiety,[1] seizure disorder	Dry mouth, paresthesia, constipation, dysgeusia, cognitive changes. Higher dose should not be used if CVD or HTN.
Semaglutide *(Wegovy)*[2]	9.7–16.8	86%	DM2, weight loss	Nausea, vomiting, constipation, diarrhea; contraindicated if MTC (or family hx) or MEN 2
Tirzepatide *(Mounjaro)*[3]	12.6–24.7 depending upon dose	14–80% depending on dose	DM2	Thyroid C-cell tumors; contraindicated in patients with a personal or family hx of MTC or in patients with MEN 2

MEN 2, multiple endocrine neoplasia type 2; MTC, medullary thyroid carcinoma.

[1] Avoid max dose.

[2] Weekly semaglutide is more effective than daily liraglutide for weight loss.

[3] At higher doses, tirzepatide is more effective in achieving weight loss than semaglutide midrange dose, but has no FDA indication for weight loss.

Note: Other drugs have limited effectiveness or high potential for ADRs or abuse.

MUSCULOSKELETAL DISORDERS

NECK PAIN: DIFFERENTIAL DIAGNOSIS AND MANAGEMENT

Cervical Stenosis/Radiculopathy

May present with weakness or atrophy in arms, legs, or both; sensory loss; neck or shoulder pain; gait disorder; bladder or rectal sphincter dysfunction. MRI and electromyography (EMG) are the most useful diagnostic tests.

Noncompressive: Herpes zoster, Lyme disease, lymphoma, carcinomatosis, demyelination

Compressive: Cervical spondylosis, disk herniation; MRI abnormalities are common in asymptomatic older persons; must have correlation between findings and clinical symptoms.

Management: Most patients improve without tx. If radicular pain, paresthesias, numbness, or nonprogressive neurologic deficits, prescribe oral analgesics and avoid aggravating movements. If severe, prescribe a short course of oral prednisone. PT when pain is tolerable. Trigger-point injections with an anesthetic agent may be helpful for isolated neck spasm or chronic neck pain. If persistent severe or disabling symptoms, epidural steroids may reduce ≥50% pain for ~50% of patients at 1–3 mo. Acute deterioration or sudden presentation with myelopathy warrants IV corticosteroids and urgent surgical consultation. Surgery is also indicated if symptoms, neurologic signs, documented nerve root compression by MRI or CT, persistence of pain for 6–12 wk, or progressive motor weakness. Anterior cervical discectomy and fusion is the most common procedure, but cervical disc arthroplasty may have better success and lower rates of implant or surgery-related serious AEs.

SHOULDER PAIN: DIFFERENTIAL DIAGNOSIS AND MANAGEMENT

Rotator Cuff Tendonopathy, Subacromial Bursitis, or Rotator Tendon Impingement on Clavicle

May cause shoulder impingement syndrome (insidious onset of anterolateral acromial pain radiating to lateral midhumerus). Pain is worse with overhead activity and at night, exacerbated by lying on the involved shoulder or sleeping with the arm overhead. Active and passive ranges of motion are normal. Use lidocaine injection to differentiate shoulder pain syndromes. Insert a 1½-inch, 22-gauge needle 1½ inches below the midpoint of the acromion 1–1½ inches deep. The angle of entry parallels the acromion. Inject 1 mL of lidocaine into the deltoid and 1–2 mL into the subacromial bursa. Dramatic relief of pain and improvement of function by injection into subacromial bursa excludes glenohumeral joint process. Lidocaine injection results in normal strength and temporary pain relief.

Most accurate bedside tests are (muscle being tested):

- Painful arc test: pain on abduction 60–120° and external rotation suggests impingement or rotator cuff disorder due to compression
- Drop arm test (supraspinatus): inability to maintain the arm in an abducted 90° position indicates tear
- External rotation resistance test (infraspinatus): elbows flexed, thumbs up with examiner's hands outside patient's elbows; patient is asked to resist inward pressure; pain or weakness indicates tendonitis or tear
- External rotation lag test (supraspinatus and infraspinatus): elbow at 90° flexion and 20° abduction, examiner passively rotates patient's arm into full external rotation; inability to maintain this position indicates tear
- Internal rotation lag test (subscapularis): elbow at 90° flexion, dorsum of hand on back; hand is lifted off back by examiner; inability to maintain position indicates tear

• Imaging, if indicated, with ultrasound or MRI; plain x-ray is of limited value

Management: Identify and eliminate provocative, repetitive injury (eg, avoid overhead reaching). Brief rest and immobilization with a sling may help. Kinesio tape may provide small benefit on immediate pain and mobility, but lacks evidence. Pain control with APAP or a short course of NSAIDs (**Table 87**), home exercises or PT in 3 phases: (1) mobility to recover full range of motion by stretching the posterior and anterior joint capsule; (2) strength using elastic bands and light weights; and (3) shoulder function using exercises that stimulate joint reactivation. Corticosteroid injection (p 224) may be useful but repeat injections may be harmful. Surgical tx as a last resort if symptoms last >6 mo with worsening function and persistent pain.

Rotator Cuff Tears

Mild to complete; characterized by diminished shoulder movement. Chronic full-thickness tear may not have pain but have loss of range of active or passive motion. After lidocaine injection of shoulder (see above), weakness persists despite pain relief. Consider evaluating with ultrasound first.[CW] MRI or MR arthrography establishes diagnosis.

Management: If due to injury, brief rest and immobilization with a sling may be helpful. Manage as above (Rotator Cuff Tendinopathy). Subacromial glucocorticoid injections may provide short-term pain relief, but multiple injections may be deleterious to healthy tendons. If no improvement after 6–8 wk of conservative measures, consider surgical repair, which may improve long-term (5 y) pain but not function.

Bicipital Tendonopathy (Tendonitis)

Pain felt on anterior lateral aspect of shoulder, tenderness in the groove between greater and lesser tuberosities of the humerus. Pain is elicited on resisted flexion of shoulder, flexion of the elbow, or supination (external rotation) of the hand and wrist with the elbow flexed at the side.

Management: Identify and eliminate provocative, repetitive activities (eg, avoid overhead reaching). Rest (≥7 d with no lifting), local or oral NSAIDs, subacromial or tendon sheath injection, and corticosteroid injections (p 224) are major components of tx. After rest period, PT should focus on range of motion and stretching biceps tendon (eg, putting arm on doorframe and hyperextending shoulder, with some external rotation).

Frozen Shoulder (Adhesive Capsulitis)

Loss of passive external (lateral) rotation, abduction, and internal rotation of the shoulder to <90°. Often follows 3 phases: painful (freezing) phase lasting weeks to a few months; adhesive (stiffening) phase lasting 4–12 mo; resolution phase lasting 6–24 mo. Lidocaine injection (see above) does not restore range of motion. Ultrasound can identify accompanying soft-tissue changes and assess rotator cuff.

Management: Avoid rest and begin with gentle home exercises for shoulder mobility (eg, stretching the arm in flexion, horizontal adduction, and internal and external rotation). Transition to PT when patient begins to improve. Low-dose (eg, 20 mg triamcinolone) intra-articular or subacromial corticosteroid injections (p 224) given early reduces pain and improves range of motion for as long as 6 mo. Intra-articular injection of saline and anesthetic (hydrodilatation) may provide modest 8–12 wk benefit on pain. PT provides best 4–6 mo outcomes. If no response after 6–12 mo, consider surgical manipulation under anesthesia or arthroscopic capsular release.

BACK PAIN: DIFFERENTIAL DIAGNOSIS AND MANAGEMENT OF COMMON CAUSES IN OLDER PERSONS

Acute (<4 wk) Back Pain

Do not perform imaging for low-back pain within the first 6 wk unless red flags are present (severe or progressive neurologic deficits or when serious underlying conditions are present).[CW] Red flags include:

- trauma
- fever
- incontinence
- unexplained weight loss
- GU symptoms
- anticoagulation
- cancer hx
- long-term steroid use
- parenteral drug abuse
- recent surgery or spinal injection
- abnormal neurologic exam
- intense localized pain
- inability to get into a comfortable position

Acute Lumbar Strain (Low-Back Pain Syndrome)

Acute pain is often precipitated by heavy lifting or exercise. Pain may be central or more prominent on one side and may radiate to sacroiliac region and buttocks. Pain is aggravated by motion, standing, and prolonged sitting, and relieved by rest. Sciatic pain may be present even when neurologic exam is normal. In sciatica, pain radiating below the knee is more likely to represent true radiculopathy (typically L5 or S1) than proximal leg pain. Avoid imaging in the emergency department if nontraumatic back pain unless severe or progressive neurologic deficits or severe underlying condition is suspected.[CW] See *Red flags* above.

Management: Most can continue normal activities. Patients should remain as active as possible.[CW] If symptoms are relieved from bed rest, 1–2 d lying in a semi-Fowler position or on the side with hips and knees flexed with pillow between legs will suffice. Do not recommend bedrest without completing an evaluation or for more than 2 d.[CW] Treat muscle spasm with ice, applied by massage over the muscles in spasm. A short course of NSAIDs (**Table 87**) can be used to control pain. Spinal manipulation, including high-thrust osteopathic manipulation, is also effective for uncomplicated low-back pain. Non–benzodiazepine antispasmodics reduce pain intensity at 2 wk, but are associated with increased risk of AEs. If severe refractory symptoms, consider systemic or epidural glucocorticoids. Gabapentin and pregabalin are not effective. Do not prescribe opioids for acute disabling low-back pain before evaluation and trial of other alternatives.[CW] As pain diminishes, encourage patient to begin isometric abdominal and lower-extremity exercises. Symptoms often recur. Educate on back posture, lifting precautions, and abdominal muscle strengthening to prevent recurrence. In younger patients with acute back pain with sciatica, PT results in less disability at 6 mo.

Acute Disk Herniation

Over 90% of cases have herniation at L4–L5 or L5–S1 levels, resulting in unilateral impairment of ankle reflex, toe and ankle dorsiflexion, and pain (commonly sciatic) on straight leg raising (can be tested from sitting position by leg extension). Pain is acute in onset and varies considerably with changes in position. If progressive or severe motor deficit, suspected neoplasm or epidural abscess, urinary retention, saddle anesthesia, or bilateral symptoms, order urgent MRI, CT, or CT myelography.

Management: Initially the same as acute lumbar strain (above). The value of epidural injections and surgery for pain without neurologic signs remains controversial. Epidural injection of a long-acting corticosteroid with an epidural anesthetic may provide modest, transient relief and results in less surgery at 1 y if symptoms unresponsive to conservative tx. Consider surgery if recurrence or neurologic signs persist beyond 6–8 wk after conservative tx. Gabapentin and pregabalin are not effective. Surgery for persistent sciatica (4–12 mo) provides greater pain relief at 6 mo and improvement on some measures of disability at 1 y compared with conservative tx.

Vertebral Compression Fracture

Immediate onset of severe pain; worse with sitting or standing; sometimes relieved by lying down. CT scan can help determine instability and MRI (bone scan if MRI contraindicated) can determine acuity of fracture.

Management: See Osteoporosis, p 246. Bed rest, analgesia (APAP, NSAIDs, if mild; opioids, if severe), and mobilization as tolerated. May require hospitalization to control symptoms. Bracing is unproved except for traumatic vertebral fractures and may cause core muscle atrophy if prolonged use. Nasal calcitonin (for ≤2–4 wk) may provide symptomatic improvement but is not effective immediately. Mixed evidence for bisphosphonates and teriparatide. Mixed evidence on using percutaneous vertebral augmentation (vertebroplasty, if no loss of vertebral height, and kyphoplasty, which partially restores height but is more expensive and technically difficult) for acute or subacute osteoporotic vertebral fractures. AAOS and NICE recommend augmentation for severe ongoing pain from a known fracture. Avoid muscle relaxants. Pain may persist for ≥1 y. As pain diminishes, exercise (eg, aquatic-based) should be initiated.

Subacute (4–12 wk) and Chronic (>12 wk) Low-Back Pain

Osteoarthritis and Chronic Disk Degeneration

Characterized by aching pain aggravated by motion and relieved by rest. Occasionally, hypertrophic spurring in a facet joint may cause unilateral radiculopathy with sciatica.

- Management: Identify and eliminate provocative activities. Education on back posture, lifting precautions, and abdominal muscle strengthening. APAP or a short course of NSAIDs, including topicals (**Table 87**). Duloxetine may be helpful. Corticosteroid inj (p 224), acupuncture, and sham acupuncture may provide benefit.
- Nondrug tx (mostly studied in younger patients) for chronic low-back pain include exercise (PT, OT, walking, tai chi, yoga), chiropractic tx, acupuncture (covered by Medicare), TENS, qi gong, massage, heat, spinal manipulation, CBT, acceptance and commitment tx, guided imagery with progressive muscle relaxation, music, mindfulness-based meditation, self-management, education, and hypnosis.
- Motor skill training to replace long-standing, pain-provoking movements with pain-free versions resulted in less disability at 1 y, compared to strength and flexibility exercises.
- Psychological tx aimed at changing beliefs about causes of and threat value of pain has shown benefit at 1 y.
- Closed-loop (measuring evoked compound action potentials) spinal-cord stimulation is more effective than open-loop stimulation in reducing overall pain at 3, 12, and 24 mo.

Little evidence supports intradiscal injection of corticosteroids, anti-TNF, or methylene blue; facet joint injections; medial branch blocks, sacroiliac joint injections, intradiscal electrothermal tx; radiofrequency denervation; prolotherapy; botulinum toxin injection; gabapentin or pregabalin.

For persistent symptoms >3 mo of sciatica from disk herniation, diskectomy provides more pain relief at 6 mo compared to medical tx. Do not prescribe lumbar supports or braces for long-term tx of low-back pain.[CW]

Lumbar Spinal Stenosis

Symptoms increase with spinal extension (eg, prolonged standing, walking downhill, lying prone) and decrease with spinal flexion (eg, sitting, bending forward while walking, lying in a flexed position). The only symptoms may be fatigue or pain in buttocks, thighs, and legs when walking (pseudoclaudication). May have immobility of lumbar spine, pain with straight leg raises, weakness of muscles innervated by L4 through S1. Over 4 y, 15% improve, 15% deteriorate, and 70% remain stable.

Management: APAP or a short course of NSAIDs (**Table 87**), PT, and exercises to reduce lumbar lordosis (eg, bicycling) are sometimes beneficial. Gabapentin and pregabalin are not effective. Corticosteroid injections show no advantage over lidocaine-only injections. If cauda equina or conus medullaris syndrome, urgent surgical consultation.

Despite mixed evidence, surgical decompression (laminectomy and partial facetectomy) may be more effective than conservative tx (eg, PT) in relieving moderate to severe symptoms. If no spondylolisthesis; interspinous spacer insertion (distraction) may be effective and is less invasive. If spinal instability is confirmed on flexion-extension radiographs, vertebral destruction, or spinal deformities (eg, scoliosis), fusion may be better than simple decompression. Both simple and complex fusion have more complications and cost more than decompression alone. Pain can recur several years after surgery and reoperation rates are high.

Depression, comorbidity influencing walking capacity, cardiovascular comorbidity, and scoliosis predict worse surgical outcomes. Male sex, younger age, better walking ability and self-rated health, less comorbidity, and more pronounced canal stenosis predict better surgical outcomes.

Piriformis Syndrome

Gradual-onset buttock pain due to entrapment of sciatic nerve, which passes inferior to the piriformis muscle. "Wallet sign" when patient cannot sit with wallet in back pocket due to pain. Freiberg test places hip in extension and internal rotation. Pain or sciatica when resisting external rotation is a positive test. Ultrasound of muscle thickness may help.

Management: PT strengthening of pelvic and hip region and stretching of piriformis. Ultrasound-guided corticosteroid and botulinum toxin injections may be helpful; surgery (piriformis tenotomy) if disabling and persistent.

Nonrheumatic Pain (eg, tumors, aneurysms)

Gradual onset, steadily expanding, often unrelated to position, not relieved by lying down. Night pain when lying down is characteristic. Upper motor neuron signs may be present. Typically involves thoracic and upper lumbar spine.

HIP PAIN: DIFFERENTIAL DIAGNOSIS AND MANAGEMENT

Greater Trochanteric Pain Syndrome (Trochanteric Bursitis)

Pain in lateral aspect of the hip due to gluteus medius or minimus tendinopathy that worsens when patient sits on a hard chair, lies on the affected side, or rises from a chair or bed (within 30 sec); pain may improve with walking. Local tenderness over greater trochanter is often present, and pain is often reproduced on resisted abduction of the leg or internal rotation of the hip. However, trochanteric pain does not limit range of motion or cause pain on range of motion, pain in the groin, or radicular signs. Pelvic x-rays and ultrasound may be helpful. MRI if suspected muscle tear, suspicion of tumor, or persistent symptoms.

Management: Identify and eliminate provocative activities. Position pillow posterolaterally behind the involved side to avoid lying on bursae while sleeping. Check for leg length discrepancy, prescribe orthotics if appropriate. Trial of ≤2 wk of APAP and, if persistent, 2 wk of NSAIDs. PT for isometric loading of gluteus medius, gluteus minimus, and quadriceps, and calf-strengthening. If no improvement, inject a long-acting corticosteroid with an anesthetic. Refer to surgery if gluteus medius tear on MRI or refractory symptoms for ≥12 mo. Limited evidence on short-term effectiveness of platelet-rich plasma injections.

Osteoarthritis

"Boring" quality pain in the hip, often in the groin, and sometimes referred to the back or knee with stiffness after rest. Passive motion is restricted in all directions if disease is fairly advanced. In early disease, pain in the groin on internal rotation of the hip is characteristic.

Management: See also Osteoarthritis, p 221, and ACR recommendations (**Table 85**). Elective total hip replacement is indicated for patients who have radiographic evidence of joint damage and moderate to severe persistent pain, disability, or both, that is not substantially relieved by an extended course of nonsurgical tx. Anterior approach has a small increased risk of surgical complications compared to posterior or lateral approaches.

Hip Fracture

Sudden onset, typically after a fall, with inability to walk or bear weight, frequently radiating to groin or knee. If hip radiograph (anterior-posterior with maximal internal rotation and lateral view) is negative and index of suspicion is high, obtain MRI or CT. Up to 39% can be occult. Fractures are 45% femoral neck, 45% intertrochanteric, and 10% subtrochanteric.

Management: For most patients, tx is surgical with ORIF, hemiarthroplasty, or total hip replacement, depending on site of fracture and amount of displacement. For patients who were nonambulatory before the fracture and have mild pain, conservative tx is an option. Frail, institutionalized patients may be offered nonoperative management, which has similar quality of life and fewer AEs but much higher 30-d mortality compared to operative tx. Sliding hip screws may have lower complication rates than intramedullary nails for extracapsular fractures. Displaced femoral neck fractures are typically treated with hemiarthroplasty or total hip replacement. Cemented fixation is associated with lower risk for aseptic revisions, better quality of life, and lower risk of periprosthetic fracture compared to uncemented fixation. Subtrochanteric fractures can be treated with intramedullary nails.

Perioperative Care

Comanagement of hip fracture by geriatrics and orthopedic surgery improves patient outcomes, including risk of delirium. Features of a comanagement service typically include:

- Placing patient on orthopedic ward with daily visits by orthopedic and geriatrics services
- Clearly delineating who writes orders for managing fluids, pain, anticoagulation, catheter care, and antibiotics
- 24-h/d availability of geriatrics services
- Standardized order sets
- Frequent daily communication between orthopedic and geriatrics services (eg, co-rounding)

Care Related to Procedure and Prevention of Complications

- Timing of surgery: Early surgery (within 24 h) is associated with better outcomes, but that may relate more to comorbidity in those with delayed surgery. Compared to surgery within 24 h, surgery within 6 h results in fewer strokes and infections without sepsis, less delirium, and shorter lengths of stay, but with no difference in mortality or major complications.
- Treat comorbid conditions (eg, anemia, volume depletion, metabolic abnormalities, infections, HF, CAD).
- Preoperative traction has no demonstrated benefit.
- Adequate pre- and postoperative analgesia (eg, 3-in-1 femoral nerve block, intrathecal morphine); ultrasound-guided femoral nerve block administered in the emergency department improves pain and functional outcomes compared to conventional analgesics. Strong opioids (oxycodone) are not superior to weaker opioids (APAP and codeine).
- Regional anesthesia does not reduce the risk of delirium.

- Spinal anesthesia is not superior to general anesthesia with respect to delirium, survival, and recovery of ambulation at 60 d.
- Antibiotics: Perioperative antibiotics (cefazolin or, if allergic, clindamycin or vancomycin) should be given beginning within 1 h of surgery.
- DVT prophylaxis: Give preoperatively if >48 h surgery delay is expected; otherwise begin 12–24 h after surgery. First choices are enoxaparin, UFH, and dalteparin but other agents can be used (Antithrombotic Therapy and Thromboembolic Disease, p 39). ASA may be as effective. Recommended for up to 35 d but at least 10 d and probably 1 mo if patient is inactive or has comorbidities.

Postoperative Care

- Pressure-reducing rather than standard mattress; if high risk of pressure sore, use large cell, alternating pressure air mattress.
- Oximetry for at least 48 h with supplemental oxygen prn
- Graduated compression stockings do not add benefit beyond DVT prophylaxis medications.
- Intermittent pneumatic leg compression is recommended for the duration of the hospital stay.
- Monitor for the development of delirium, malnutrition, and pressure sores.
- Hip precautions: No adduction past midline; no hip flexion beyond 90%; no internal rotation (toes upright in bed)
- Begin assisted ambulation within 48 h.
- Weightbearing: Typically as tolerated for hemiarthroplasty or total hip replacement; toe-touch if ORIF or intertrochanteric fracture
- Treat osteoporosis regardless of BMD: Wait 2 wk before starting parenteral bisphosphonates; ensure vitamin D is replete (Osteoporosis, p 246).
- Fall prevention: See Fall Prevention, p 136.

Nonrheumatic Pain

Referred pain from viscera, radicular pain from the lower spine, avascular necrosis, Paget disease, metastasis. Tx based on identified etiology.

KNEE PAIN: DIFFERENTIAL DIAGNOSIS AND MANAGEMENT

Osteoarthritis

Pain typically related to activity (eg, climbing stairs, arising from chair, walking long distances). Morning stiffness lasts <30 min. Crepitation is common. Exam should rule out other causes of knee pain: hip arthritis with referred knee pain (decreased hip range of motion), chondromalacia patellae (tenderness only over patellofemoral joint), iliotibial band syndrome (tenderness lateral to the knee at site of insertion in fibular head or where courses over lateral femoral condyle), anserine bursitis (tenderness distal to knee over medial tibia). Also determine malalignment varus (bowlegged) or valgus (knock-kneed). Avoid routinely performing arthroscopy with lavage or debridement.[CW]

Management: See Osteoarthritis, p 221, and ACR recommendations (**Table 85**), including APAP, NSAIDs, and duloxetine. Modest evidence supports curcumin supplements and Boswellia serrata extract, but trials were of low quality with small effect sizes. Don't use glucosamine and chondroitin to treat patients with symptomatic OA of the knee.[CW] Stable supportive shoes reduce pain more than flat flexible shoes. Biomechanical footwear (convex adjustable rubber pods screwed to the outsole at the heel and forefoot) reduces some pain and functional decline. Use medially wedged insoles if knee lateral compartment OA. Don't use lateral wedge insoles if medial compartment knee OA.[CW] Correcting malalignment with bracing (eg, neoprene sleeves over the knee, valgus brace) often helps.

PT reduces pain and improves function more than corticosteroid injections. Walking and home-based quadriceps strengthening have comparable effectiveness on pain and disability. High-intensity strength training is no more effective than low-intensity strength training. Video-based telehealth exercise and weight loss programs can improve pain and function at 6 and 12 mo. PT, OT, PT-prescribed, internet-delivered, home exercise and pain coping skills training may help. In mild to moderate knee OA, intra-articular platelet-rich plasma is ineffective. In moderate to severe knee OA, surgery is more effective than medical tx but has more complications (ie, DVT and stiffness requiring brisement forcé). Avoid recommending knee arthroscopy as initial tx.[CW] Don't use needle lavage for long-term relief.[CW]

HAND AND WRIST PAIN AND RELATED CONDITIONS: DIFFERENTIAL DIAGNOSIS AND MANAGEMENT (see digital text for common foot disorders)

Osteoarthritis

Hand pain (including hand aching or stiffness) plus ≥3 of the following 4 features (ACR):

(1) hard tissue enlargement of 2 of the following: second and third distal interphalangeal (DIP) joints, the second and third proximal interphalangeal (PIP) joints, and the first carpometacarpal (CMC) of both hands

(2) hard enlargement of 2 or more DIP joints

(3) fewer than 3 swollen metacarpophalangeal (MCP) joints

(4) deformity of at least 1 of the 10 joints above

X-ray confirmation is not necessary.

Management: See Osteoarthritis, p 221, and ACR recommendations (**Table 85**). For base-of-thumb OA, using a custom-made neoprene splint worn only at night decreases pain and disability at 12 mo. Combining splints, hand exercises, and topical NSAIDs led to small improvements in function at 6 wk compared to education alone.

Inflammatory (Rheumatoid and Psoriatic) Arthritis

Typically MCP and PIP joints with morning stiffness often lasting >1 h

Management: See Rheumatoid Arthritis.

Wrist Fracture

ORIF with volar-locking plate is no more effective than closed reduction and cast immobilization on pain, function, and quality of life.

De Quervain Tendinopathy

Pain or tenderness at radial side of wrist

Management: Forearm-based thumb splint, NSAIDs, and, if refractory, glucocorticoid injections. If no improvement after injections, consider surgery

Stenosing Flexor Tenosynovitis (Trigger Finger)

Painless (initially) catching, snapping, or locking during flexion due to disparity in the size of flexor tendons and retinacular pulley system overlying the metacarpal-phalangeal joint; may affect multiple fingers

Management: Modify activity, splint to keep metacarpal-phalangeal joint in slight flexion, short-term NSAIDs if mild; glucocorticoid injections if severe or pain; may repeat in 6 wk if not improved by 50%; surgery if refractory (at 6–12 mo)

Dupuytren Contracture

Loss of full extension of the finger at the metacarpal-phalangeal joint, which is fixed and chronic and is characterized by painless nodular lesions that progress to form a fibrous cord from the palm to the digit

Management: Modification of hand tools to increase padding or using glove for mild symptoms; glucocorticoid and lidocaine injections if more severe symptoms of recent onset (ineffective if cords); collagenase injections though no long-term studies; surgery or percutaneous needle aponeurotomy for advanced disease if functional impairment but high recurrence rate

Carpal Tunnel Syndrome

Painful tingling, hypoesthesia, or both, in one or both hands in distribution innervated by median nerve. Causes include:

- Repetitive activities
- DM
- Thyroid disease
- Amyloidosis
- RA
- Space-occupying lesions (eg, lymphoma)
- Trauma (eg, Colles fracture)

Physical exam demonstrates decreased sensation in palm, thumb, index finger, middle finger, and thumb side of ring finger, weak handgrip, and tapping over median nerve at wrist causes pain to shoot from wrist to hand (Tinel sign). Acute flexion of wrist for 60 sec (Phalen test) should also cause pain.

Lab studies should include fasting glucose, TSH, nerve conduction velocity testing (confirms diagnosis and should be done before surgery).

Management: (combined modalities may be effective if single modalities fail)

Nonpharmacologic Interventions

Modify work or leisure activities to avoid repetitive movement, carpal tunnel mobilization (moving bones in wrist through PT or OT), and yoga may provide symptom relief. Splinting in neutral position, especially at night; surgery (more effective than splinting) is indicated for prolonged (>6 mo) moderate to severe symptoms (pain, numbness, diminished hand function, thenar eminence atrophy) after confirming median nerve injury by electrodiagnostic testing. Nerve and tendon gliding maneuvers are not effective.

Pharmacotherapy

Injectable corticosteroids (eg, methylprednisolone 15 mg into proximal or distal tunnel; distal is more painful) are more effective than night resting splinting or oral corticosteroids[BC] (eg, prednisone 20 mg/d po for 1 wk followed by 10 mg/d for a second wk). Perineural dextrose (D5%) injections may help.

OSTEOARTHRITIS (see also specific sites [pp 216–220])

Classification

- Noninflammatory: pain and disability are typically the only complaints; also tenderness, bony prominence, crepitus
- Inflammatory: may also have morning stiffness lasting >30 min and night pain; findings may include joint effusion on exam or radiograph, warmth, and synovitis on arthroscopy (pp 216-220).

Management of Osteoarthritis and General Musculoskeletal Disorders

- Consider needs and preferences of the patient. Begin with nonpharmacologic interventions.

Nonpharmacologic Interventions **(Table 85)**

- Superficial heat: hot packs, heating pads, paraffin, or hot water bottles (moist heat is better): 20 min on, 20 min off
- Deep heat: microwave, shortwave diathermy, or ultrasound
- Superficial cooling using ice packs or fluoromethane spray (eg, *Gebauer's Spray and Stretch*)
- Biofeedback and TENS
- Exercises:
    - All programs should include isometric strengthening, stretching, and range of motion.
    - Those who can tolerate basics can progress to isotonic strengthening and aerobic exercises.
    - Swimming, bicycling, walking, and tai chi have low joint-loading and may protect the knee. Splints may also help protect the joints.
    - Closed-chain (the limbs are stationary while the body moves) avoid joint torsion.
    - Supervised settings have better adherence than unsupervised home-based exercise.
- Weight loss: especially for low-back, hip, and knee OA
- Splinting and orthotics: Avoid splinting for long periods (eg, >6 wk) because periarticular muscle weakness and wasting may occur.
- Assistive devices: Cane should be used in the hand contralateral to the affected knee or hip. Cane length should be to the level of the wrist crease. Use walker if moderate or severe balance impairment, bilateral weakness, or unilateral weakness requiring support of >15–20% of body weight.
- Acupuncture as an adjunct to NSAIDs or analgesics for knee OA or chronic low-back pain
- Dry needling performed by PT may provide short-term pain improvement for up to 12 wk.
- Trigger-point injections with anesthetic agents may be valuable for myofascial pain.
- Chiropractic tx as an adjunct to medical tx for back pain
- Surgical intervention (eg, debridement, meniscal repair, prosthetic joint replacement)

Table 85. ACR Recommendations for Physical, Psychosocial, and Mind-Body Approaches for the Management of Osteoarthritis of the Hand, Knee, and Hip

Intervention	Joint		
	Hand	Knee	Hip
Exercise	++	++	++
Balance training		+	+
Weight loss		++	++
Self-efficacy and self-management programs	++	++	++
Tai chi		++	++
Yoga		+	
CBT	+	+	+
Cane		++	++
Tibiofemoral knee braces		++	
Patellofemoral braces		+	
Kinesiotaping	+[1]	+	

(cont.)

Table 85. ACR Recommendations for Physical, Psychosocial, and Mind-Body Approaches for the Management of Osteoarthritis of the Hand, Knee, and Hip (cont.)			
	Joint		
Intervention	Hand	Knee	Hip
Hand orthosis	++[1]		
Hand orthosis (other joints)	+		
Acupuncture	+	+	+
Thermal interventions	+	+	+
Paraffin	+		
Radiofrequency ablation		+	

++ strongly recommended; + conditionally recommended; empty cell = no recommendation.

[1] first carpometacarpal

Modified from Kolasinski SL et al. *Arthritis Rheum.* 2020;72(2):220–233.

Pharmacotherapy Overview

- If mild to moderate pain, 3-day trial of scheduled APAP. For most patients, ineffective as monotx.
- If unsuccessful, moderate to severe, or inflammatory, topical (if 1 or few joints) or oral NSAIDs, with appropriate cautions, at the lowest dose for as short as possible; can add capsaicin if incomplete control of symptoms.
- If inadequately relieved and only one or a few joints, glucocorticoid or hyaluronate (if knee) joint injections.
- Duloxetine may be helpful, especially in knee OA.
- Tramadol may have modest long-term effects.
- Avoid opioids.[CW]
- If pain is still uncontrolled, consider surgery.

Table 86. Recommendations for the Pharmacotherapy of Osteoarthritis of the Hand, Knee, and Hip			
	Joint		
Intervention	Hand	Knee	Hip
Topical NSAIDs	+	++	
Topical capsaicin	–	+	
Oral NSAIDs	++	++	++
Intra-articular glucocorticoid injection	+	++	++
Ultrasound-guided intra-articular glucocorticoid injection			++
Intra-articular glucocorticoid injection compared to other injections	+	+	+
APAP	+	+	+
Duloxetine	+	+	+
Tramadol	+	+	+
Chondroitin sulfate	+	– –	– –

++ strongly recommended; + conditionally recommended; – conditionally recommended against; – – strongly recommended against; empty cell = no recommendation.

Modified from Kolasinski SL at al. *Arthritis Rheum.* 2020;72(2):220–233.

Topical Analgesics **(Table 87):** Liniments containing methyl salicylates (**Table 101**), capsaicin crm (p 223), menthol counterirritants, lidocaine (all OTC lidocaine preparations are 4%; lidocaine 5% pch *[Lidoderm]* is not OTC).

Intra-articular, Bursal, and Trigger-point Injections:

- Corticosteroids (eg, methylprednisolone acetate, triamcinolone acetonide, triamcinolone hexacetonide [longest acting]) may be particularly effective if monoarticular symptoms. May provide moderate short-term improvement of pain and small improvement of function. Ultrasound-guided corticosteroid and local anesthetic of the hip with advice and guidance reduced pain and improved function more at 6 mo than advice and education alone. Typical doses for all these drugs:
  - 40 mg for large joints (eg, knee, ankle, shoulder, hip with fluoroscopy or ultrasound guidance)
  - 30 mg for wrists, ankles, and elbows
  - 10 mg for small joints of hands and feet

Often mixed with lidocaine 1% or its equivalent (some recommend giving equal volume with corticosteroids, whereas others give 3–5× the corticosteroid volume depending on size of joint) for immediate relief. Effect lasts 1–2 mo. Typically given ≤3×/y.

- Chemonucleolysis (enzymatic) injections of disc may have limited benefit.
- Etanercept, botulinum toxin, and methylene blue are not beneficial.
- Blocks and radiofrequency ablation of medial branch of the primary dorsal ramus show limited effectiveness.
- Prolotherapy (repeated injection of irritants to increase inflammation and strengthen surrounding ligaments) has little evidence of effectiveness.
- Hyaluronate preparations *(Euflexxa, Hyalgan, Orthovisc, Synvisc, Supartz)* 3–5 injections 1 wk apart for knee OA. *Synvisc-One* requires only one injection. Benefit is similar to NSAIDs, but may last ≥6 mo.

Nutraceuticals: Some evidence of short-term (≤3 mo) benefit from collagen hydrolysate, passion fruit peel extract, Curcuma longa extract, Boswellia serrata extract, curcumin, pycnogenol, and L-carnitine. ACR recommends against chondroitin sulfate (400 mg q8h) for hip and knee OA, but it may have modest effects on hand OA.

APAP (acetaminophen): APAP is ineffective in managing acute low-back pain and has minimal short-term benefit in knee and hip OA.

NSAIDs: Topicals are preferred over orals in persons aged >75 with knee or hand OA. Diclofenac gel (1%) or pch and ketoprofen (5%, 10%, 20%) have comparable improvement and fewer AEs than oral NSAIDs and relieve pain. Oral NSAIDs have higher rates of AEs than APAP (**Table 87**). Not recommended for long-term use. If one NSAID is not effective at the maximum dose, switch to a different NSAID. Combining with APAP is slightly more effective but may increase risk of bleeding. PPIs (**Table 64**), H_2 blockers (**Table 64**), or misoprostol 100–200 mg q6h with food may be valuable prophylaxis against NSAID-induced ulcers in high-risk patients. Salsalate and celecoxib, a selective COX-2 inhibitor, are less likely to cause gastroduodenal ulcers than nonselective NSAIDs and do not inhibit platelets. Except for ASA, NSAID-induced platelet effects reverse when the NSAID is cleared. All can have renal effects and may increase INR in patients taking warfarin. Avoid in persons with HTN, HF, or CKD of all causes, including DM.[CW]

Other:

- Colchicine (0.6 mg q12h) may be of benefit in inflammatory OA with recurrent symptoms.
- Duloxetine[BC], begin at 30 mg/d po and increase to 60 mg/d po after 1 wk, may benefit chronic low-back pain and OA, particularly knee.

Table 87. APAP and NSAIDs	
Class, Drug (Formulation)	**Geriatric Dosage for Arthritis (Excretion)**
✓**APAP** (T, C, S)	No anti-inflammatory properties and less effective than NSAIDs; hepatotoxic above 4 g/d po; at high dosages (≥2 g/d po) may increase INR in patients receiving warfarin; reduce dosage 50–75% if liver or kidney disease or if harmful or hazardous alcohol intake
	650 mg po q4–6h (q8h if CrCl <10) (L, K)
ER	1300 mg po q8h
ASA	650 mg po q4–6h (K)
ER	1300 mg po q8h or 1600–3200 mg po q12h
Enteric-coated[OTC,1]	1000 mg po q6h
Liquid-filled C *(Vazalore)*	325–650 mg po daily
Nonacetylated Salicylates	Do not inhibit platelet aggregation; fewer GI and renal AEs; no reaction in ASA-sensitive patients; monitor salicylate concentrations
✓Choline magnesium salicylate (S)	3 g/d po in 1, 2, or 3 doses (K)
Choline, magnesium, trisalicylate (T, S)	1 tab or tbsp po q8–12h
✓Magnesium salicylate[OTC,1] (T) *(Doan's)*	2 tabs q6–8h, max 4800 mg po q24h; avoid in kidney failure
✓Salsalate (T)	1500 mg to 4 g/d po in 2 or 3 doses (K)
Nonselective NSAIDs	Avoid chronic oral use without GI protection; avoid in HF.[BC]
Diclofenac (T)	50–150 mg/d po in 2 or 3 doses (L)
(Voltaren-XR) (T)	100 mg/d po (L)
(Zipsor) (C)	25 mg po up to q6h (L)
(Zorvolex) (C)	18–25 mg po q8h (L)
(Pennsaid) (sol) 1.5%	apply 40 gtt (10 gtt at a time) per knee q6h (L)
(pump) 2%	2 pump activations, q 12 h (L)
✓Enteric-coated	
(Arthrotec 50) (T)	1 tab po q8–12h (L)
(Arthrotec 75) (T)	1 tab po q12h (L)
✓Gel[OTC] 1%	2 g (upper extremity)–4 g (lower extremity) q6h (L)
✓Patch *(Flector)*	1 q12h (L)
Diflunisal (T)	500–1000 mg/d po in 2 doses (K)
✓Etodolac (T)	200–400 mg po q6–8h; fewer GI AEs (L)
(Lodine XL) (C)	400–1000 mg/d po (L)
Fenoprofen (C, T)	200–600 mg po q6–8h; higher risk of GI AEs (L)
Flurbiprofen (T)	200–300 mg/d po in 2, 3, or 4 doses; higher risk of GI AEs (L)

(cont.)

Table 87. APAP and NSAIDs (cont.)	
Class, Drug (Formulation)	**Geriatric Dosage for Arthritis (Excretion)**
✓Ibuprofen (T, ChT, S)	1200–3200 mg/d po in 3 or 4 doses; fewer GI AEs (L)
with famotidine *(Duexis)* (T)	1 tab po q8h
Injectable *(Caldolor)*	400–800 mg IV q6h (max 3200 mg/d)
✓Ketoprofen (T, C)	50–75 mg po q8h (L)
SR *(Oruvail* [Canadian brand]) (C)	200 mg/d po (L)
gel[OTC]	2–4 g 2–4×/d (max 15 g) topically
(Active-Ketoprofen, Sound Frotek, Ketophene RapidPaq)	1 g 3×/d topically
Ketorolac (T, Inj)	10 mg po q4–6h, 15 mg IM or IV q6h; duration of use should be limited to 5 d (K)
Meclofenamate sodium (C)	200–400 po mg/d in 3 or 4 doses; high incidence of diarrhea; some COX-2 selectivity (L)
Mefenamic acid (C)	250 mg po q6h (L)
✓Meloxicam (T, S)	7.5–15 mg/d po; some COX-2 selectivity; fewer GI AEs (L)
✓Nabumetone (T)	500–1000 mg po q12h; fewer GI AEs (L)
✓Naproxen (T, S)	220–500 mg po q12h (L)
Delayed-release *(EC-Naprosyn)* (T)	375–500 mg po q12h (L)
ER *(Naprelan)* (T)	750–1000 mg/d po (L)
Naproxen sodium (T)	275 mg or 550 mg po q12h (L)
✓Oxaprozin (C)	1200 mg/d po (L)
Piroxicam (C)	10 mg/d po; can cause delirium (L)
Sulindac (T, C)	150–200 mg po q12h; may have higher rate of renal impairment (L)
Tolmetin (T, C)	600–1800 mg/d po in 3 or 4 doses (L)
Trolamine salicylate[OTC] *(Aspercreme* and others) (crm)	3–4×/d topically
Selective COX-2 Inhibitor	Avoid in HF.[BC]
✓Celecoxib (C)	100–200 mg po q12h; less GI ulceration; does not inhibit platelets; may increase INR if taking warfarin; avoid if moderate or severe hepatic insufficiency; may induce renal impairment; contraindicated if allergic to sulfonamides (L)

✓= preferred for treating older adults; CrCl unit = mg/mL

[1] Also OTC in a lower tab strength

RHEUMATOID ARTHRITIS

Evaluation and Diagnosis

Evaluation: RF; anticitrullinated peptide antibodies (ACPAs), which has similar sensitivity but more specificity than RF; antinuclear antibody (ANA); CBC; ESR; CRP; LFTs; BUN; Cr; eye exam (if starting hydroxychloroquine); hepatitis B screen; hepatitis C screen (if at increased risk); TB test (if starting biologic); x-ray hands, wrists, and feet

Diagnosis: inflammatory arthritis involving ≥3 joints; positive RF, ACPA, or both; disease duration ≥6 wk; and elevated CRP or ESR, but without evidence of diseases with similar clinical features. Also confirmed if seronegative RA, clinically quiescent disease, and recent onset RA with findings or clinical features consistent with those that meet the ACR/EULAR classification criteria for RA.

Table 88. 2010 American College of Rheumatology/European League Against Rheumatism (ACR/EULAR) Criteria for Diagnosis of Rheumatoid Arthritis[1]

A. Joint involvement (any swollen or tender joint excluding first carpometacarpal, metatarsophalangeal, and distal and proximal interphalangeal joints)	
1 large joint (shoulders, elbows, hips, knees, ankles)	0
2 to 10 large joints	1
1 to 3 small joints (with or without involvement of large joints)	2
4 to 10 small joints (with or without involvement of large joints)	3
>10 joints (at least 1 small joint)	5
B. Serology (at least 1 test result is needed for classification)	
Negative RF and negative ACPA	0
Low-positive (<3 × upper limit of normal) RF or low-positive ACPA	2
High-positive (>3 × upper limit of normal) RF or high-positive ACPA	3
C. Acute-phase reactants (at least one test result is needed for classification)	
Normal CRP and normal ESR	0
Abnormal CRP or abnormal ESR	1
D. Duration of symptoms (by patient self-report)	
<6 wk	0
≥6 wk	1

Scoring: Add score of categories A–D; a score of ≥6/10 is needed for classification of a patient as having definite RA.

[1] Aimed at classifying newly presenting patients; patients with erosive disease or long-standing disease with a hx of presenting features consistent with these criteria should be classified as having RA.

Adapted from Aletaha D et al. *Arthritis Rheum* 2010;62(9):2569–2581. Reproduced with permission of John Wiley & Sons, Inc.

Staging

- Duration: early <6 mo, intermediate 6–24 mo, late >24 mo
- Activity: low, moderate, high by any of 11 instruments, 5 of which are recommended (onlinelibrary.wiley.com/doi/epdf/10.1002/acr.24042)
- Poor prognostic factors: functional limitation, extra-articular disease, RF positivity ± ACPA, or bony erosions by radiography

Management

- See 2021 ACR guidelines (rheumatology.org/Practice-Quality/Clinical-Support/Clinical-Practice-Guidelines). *Note:* modifications in the guideline for comorbid disease (ie, CHF, hepatitis, malignancy, serious infections); comanagement with rheumatology
- All patients with established disease should be offered DMARDs as soon as possible; goal is to induce remission and then lower dosages to maintain remission. Tight control of disease activity is associated with better radiographic and functional outcomes.
- Monitor q1–3 mo if active disease (tight control of tx); if no improvement by 3 mo or target not reached by 6 mo, adjust tx.

Nonpharmacologic Interventions

- Patient education
- Exercise
- PT and OT
- Atherosclerosis risk factor modification
- Splints and orthotics
- Surgery for severe functional abnormalities due to synovitis or joint destruction
- Bone protection (see Osteoporosis, p 246)

Pharmacotherapy

- Analgesics (**Table 87** and Pain, p 252): Opioids typically used only in severe or end-stage disease or in flares. Associated with increased risk for serious infection.
- NSAIDs (**Table 87**): Often used as bridging tx until DMARDs are effective.
- Conventional synthetic DMARDs: hydroxychloroquine, sulfasalazine, methotrexate, leflunomide
- Biologic DMARDs (bDMARDs): TNF inhibitors (etanercept, adalimumab, infliximab, golimumab, certolizumab pegol), T-cell costimulatory inhibitor (abatacept), IL-6 receptor inhibitors (tocilizumab, sarilumab), anti-CD20 antibody (rituximab)
- Targeted synthetic DMARDs: JAK inhibitors (tofacitinib, baricitinib, upadacitinib)

Principles of Treatment

- Initial tx is based on disease activity.
- For specific populations (eg, pulmonary disease, HF, previous severe infection), order of preference differs.
- Treat-to-target includes frequent monitoring of disease activity using validated instruments and modification of tx to reach a predefined target (low disease activity or remission).
- Patients should be at target ≥6 mo before tapering.
- For DMARD-naive patients with low disease activity, order of preference is hydroxychloroquine, sulfasalazine, methotrexate, leflunomide.
- For DMARD-naive patients with moderate-to-high disease activity, methotrexate is recommended over hydroxychloroquine, sulfasalazine, leflunomide, or biologic or targeted synthetic DMARDs. Begin with monotx. Check for hepatitis B and C. Monitor CBC, LFTs q8wk.
- Dual and triple nonbiologic DMARD combinations with hydroxychloroquine, sulfasalazine, or leflunomide are also used with methotrexate as one component. Monitor CBC, LFTs q8wk.
- Glucocorticoids (eg, prednisone ≤15 mg/d po or equivalent) with osteoporosis prevention measures (Osteoporosis, p 246). Often used as bridging tx until DMARDs are effective. Avoid in delirium.[BC] Low-dose prednisone (10 mg/d) po has benefit as an adjunct to methotrexate. Limit use to lowest effective dose for the shortest time.
- Flares can be treated with increased dose of oral or pulse IV glucocorticoids (eg, 3 infusions of up to 1000 mg methylprednisolone per wk).

- Frequent or severe flares should prompt consideration of escalation of dose or modification of regimen.
- Biologic DMARDs Use only after failure of nonbiologic DMARDs.[CW] If a first biological has failed, treat with a different biological.
- Don't perform MRI of the peripheral joints to routinely monitor inflammatory arthritis.[CW]

GOUT

Definition

Urate crystal disease that may be expressed as acute gouty arthritis, typically in a single joint of foot, ankle, knee, or olecranon bursa; intercritical (between flairs), or chronic arthritis and tophaceous gout.

Precipitating Factors

- Alcohol, heavy ingestion
- Allopurinol, stopping or starting
- Binge eating
- Dehydration
- Diuretics (except potassium-sparing)
- Fasting
- Infection
- Serum uric acid concentration, any change up or down
- Surgery

Evaluation of Acute Gouty Arthritis

- Joint aspiration to remove crystals and microscopic exam to establish diagnosis; serum urate (can be normal during flare)
- Ultrasound, including bedside, may show hyperechoic linear density overlying joint cartilage surface or tophaceous deposits in joints or tendons.
- Dual-energy CT can identify urate deposits and differentiate urate from calcium deposition.

Management

Pharmacotherapy of Acute Gouty Flare: Any of the following are appropriate first-line options (ACR):

- Intra-articular injections (p 224) if only 1 or 2 joints involved
- NSAIDs (**Table 87**) for 5–7 d; avoid ASA, indomethacin[BC]
- Prednisone 30–40 mg po daily or in 2 divided doses until flare resolves, then taper over 7–10 d. If npo, can give IV or IM. If tx is prolonged, consider osteoporosis tx (see Osteoporosis).
- Colchicine 1.2 mg po (2 tabs) for the first dose, followed 1 h later by 0.6 mg po (total dose 1.8 mg) unless patient has received this regimen within the last 14 d. Then begin 0.6 mg po 1×/d or q12h.
- If polyarticular or multiple large joint involvement or severe pain, consider combination tx of colchicine, NSAIDs, and methylprednisolone 0.5–2 mg/kg po q12h or 20 mg IV 2×/d with taper or ACTH 25–40 IU SC; may repeat daily for 3 d.
- IL-1 inhibitors (canakinumab *[Ilaris]* (highest pain reduction among different agents at day 2) and anakinra *[Kineret]*) (not superior to triamcinolone injection) may be useful if cannot tolerate other options.

Pharmacologic anti-inflammatory prophylaxis: Colchicine 0.6 mg/d po or 2×/d for 2–4 wk before and for 3–6 mo after beginning any tx in **Table 89**, if no tophi. Naproxen 250 mg po 2×/d may also be effective. If tophi, 6 mo after resolution or indefinitely if tophi persist.

- If neither of the above are tolerated, or if either are contraindicated or ineffective, low-dose prednisone or prednisolone (<10 mg/d po)

Table 89. Medications Useful in Managing Chronic Gout		
Medication	**Geriatric Dosage**	**Comments (Metabolism, Excretion)**
Xanthine oxidase inhibitors		
✓Allopurinol	100–900 mg/d po in divided doses if >300 mg/d	Consider if nephrolithiasis, tophi, Cr ≥2 mg/dL, 24-h urinary uric acid >800 mg. Starting dosage should not exceed 100 mg/d and 50 mg/d in ≥Stage 4 CKD. Do not initiate during flare; reduce dosage in renal or hepatic impairment; increase dose by 100 mg q2–5wk to normalize serum urate level; monitor CBC; rash is common; if Han Chinese, Thai, Korean, or Black, screen for HLA-B*5801 before initiating (K)
Febuxostat *(Uloric)*	40–80 mg/d po	Begin 40 mg/d; increase to 80 mg/d if uric acid >6 mg/dL at 2 wk; not recommended if CrCl <30; increased risk of cardiovascular and all-cause mortality (K, L)
Uricosurics		Avoid if urolithiasis and if increase risk of urate nephropathy; less effective in urate overproducers
Probenecid[OTC]	500–1500 mg po in 2–3 divided doses	Contraindicated as first-line if hx of urolithiasis. Measure urinary uric acid before initiating and if >800 mg/24 h, contraindicated. Adjust dose to normalize serum urate level or increase urine urate excretion; inhibits platelet function; may not be effective if renal impairment[BC] (CrCl <50) (K, L)
Lesinurad *(Zurampic)*	200 mg/d po	Must be taken with allopurinol or febuxostat; should not be started if CrCl <45 (L, K)
Uricase		
Pegloticase *(Krystexxa)*	8 mg IV q2wk	Effective in reducing flares in patients with high uric acid levels intolerant of or refractory to allopurinol; may cause anaphylaxis, gout flares, and infusion reactions; contraindicated if G6PD deficiency (K)
Rasburicase *(Elitek)*	0.2 mg/kg IV 1×/mo	Hypersensitivity reactions; do not administer if G6PD deficiency
Other agents		
Colchicine[1] *(Colcrys)*[2]	0.5–0.6 mg/d (po, IV)	Lower dose and monitor AEs if CrCl <30.[BC] May also be effective in prevention of recurrent pseudogout; monitor CBC (L)
Losartan *(Cozaar)*	12.5–100 mg po q12–24h	Modest uricosuric effect that plateaus at 50 mg/d; may be useful in patients with HTN or HF

✓ = preferred for treating older adults; CrCl unit = mL/min. G6PD, glucose-6-phosphate-dehydrogenase.

[1] Probenecid (500 mg) and colchicine (0.5 mg) combinations are available as generic.

[2] No longer available as generic.

Management of Chronic Gout

Nonpharmacologic Interventions

Lifestyle modification (weight loss if overweight, decrease saturated fats, substitute low-fat dairy products for red meat or fish, limit alcohol use, avoid organ meats [eg, sweetbread, liver, kidney]; avoid high fructose corn syrup–sweetened sodas). D/C nonessential medications that induce hyperuricemia (eg, thiazides, loop diuretics, niacin).

Pharmacotherapy

Strong recommendations for pharmacotherapy (ACR). Established diagnosis of gouty arthritis and:

- Tophus or tophi, clinical
- Frequent attacks (≥2/y)
- CKD with CrCl <60

Monitor uric acid q12mo if stable, q6mo if ongoing symptoms or tophi.

ACR strongly recommends treating to target <6 mg/dL (**Table 89**). First-line is allopurinol. If Stage ≥3 CKD, allopurinol or febuxostat beginning with low doses, is strongly recommended over probenecid. Initiate concomitant anti-inflammatory prophylaxis (eg, colchicine, NSAIDs, corticosteroids) for 3–6 mo. Pegloticase is reserved for patients in whom tx fails to reach target and who have frequent flares (≥2/y) or nonresolving tophi.

PSEUDOGOUT

Definition

Crystal-induced arthritis (especially in knees and wrists) associated with calcium pyrophosphate that may be asymptomatic or present with acute or chronic crystal inflammatory arthritis (pseudo-RA), severe joint degeneration, or spinal involvement.

Risk Factors

- Advanced OA
- DM
- Gout
- Hemochromatosis
- Hypercalcemia
- Hyperparathyroidism
- Hypomagnesemia
- Hypophosphatemia
- Hypothyroidism
- Neuropathic joints
- Older age

Precipitating Factors

- Acute illness
- Dehydration
- Minor trauma
- Surgery

Evaluation of Acute Pseudogout

Joint aspiration and microscopic exam to establish diagnosis; radiograph indicating chondrocalcinosis (best seen in wrists, knees, shoulder, symphysis pubis). Ultrasound, including bedside, may show pseudo–double contour sign when calcium pyrophosphate crystals deposit in the hyaline cartilage. Some recommend screening for associated conditions with calcium, phosphorus, PTH, magnesium, alkaline phosphatase, iron, and transferrin.

Management of Acute Flare

If 1 or 2 joints, aspiration and intra-articular glucocorticoid may be effective. If multiple joints, see Gout, Management (p 229). NSAIDs (eg, naproxen 500 mg po 2×/d) or prednisone (30–50 mg/d po with taper over 7–10 d after flare resolves) are often used first, because colchicine is less effective in pseudogout. Anakinra or tocilizumab may be effective if refractory.

Most flares resolve within 7–14 d.

Prevention of Recurrence and Chronic Inflammatory Arthritis

If >3 attacks/y, consider colchicine 0.6 mg po q12h.

If chronic calcium pyrophosphate crystal inflammatory arthritis (ie, pseudo-RA), NSAIDs +/– colchicines and, if needed, followed by hydroxychloroquine or magnesium carbonate. Methotrexate and anakinra may also help.

POLYMYALGIA RHEUMATICA, GIANT CELL (TEMPORAL) ARTERITIS

Polymyalgia Rheumatica

Proximal limb and girdle stiffness typically lasting ≥30 min without tenderness but with constitutional symptoms (eg, fatigue, malaise, weight loss) for ≥1 mo and sedimentation rate elevated to >50 mm/h (7–22% will have normal sedimentation rate), and CRP (virtually always abnormal); consider ultrasound to demonstrate effusions within shoulder bursae or MRI to demonstrate tenosynovitis or subacromial and subdeltoid bursitis if diagnosis is uncertain.

Provisional ACR/EULAR classification criteria include:

- required criteria: age >50, bilateral shoulder aching, abnormal CRP or ESR
- morning stiffness >45 min (2 points)
- hip pain or limited range of motion (1 point)
- absence of RF, ACPA, or both (2 points)
- absence of peripheral joint pain (1 point)

Scores ≥4 had 68% sensitivity and 78% specificity. Specificity is higher (88%) for discriminating shoulder conditions from polymyalgia rheumatica and lower (65%) for discriminating RA from polymyalgia rheumatica. A single-site study showed better test characteristics in an unselected population with early inflammatory articular disease. The clinical usefulness of these criteria has yet to be determined.

Other recommended tests include RF, CBC, comprehensive metabolic panel, and dipstick UA.

Giant Cell (Temporal) Arteritis

Medium to large vessel vasculitis that presents with (likelihood ratios for disease) limb claudication (6.0), jaw claudication (4.9), temporal artery thickening (4.7) or loss of pulse (3.3), scalp tenderness (3.1), elevated sedimentation rate (3.1 if >100 mm/h), or CRP (1.7 if >2.5 mg/d), symptoms of polymyalgia rheumatica (1.3), headache (1.3), unexplained fever (1.2), or anemia (1.2), or visual disturbances (1.2). Synovitis suggests an alternate diagnosis. Color Doppler ultrasound and MRI may help. Giant cell arteritis is confirmed by temporal artery biopsy, which can be performed after starting tx; may need contralateral biopsy if first is negative and suspicion is high.

Management

Polymyalgia Rheumatica

- Low-dosage (eg, 15 mg/d po) prednisone[BC] or its equivalent; increase dosage if symptoms are not controlled within 1 wk. If symptoms are not controlled by 20 mg/d, consider alternate diagnosis (eg, giant cell arteritis, paraneoplastic syndrome).
  - Begin tapering 2–4 wk after aching and stiffness have resolved by 2.5 mg/d q2–4wk to oral dose of 10 mg/d. Dosage is 10 mg 1×/d, taper in 1-mg/4-wk decrements. Monitor symptoms and CRP or sedimentation rate (minor fluctuations in labs alone do not need dose increases). If relapse, increase to pre-relapse dose and decrease gradually within 4–8 wk. Minimum duration of tx is 1 y.
- Methylprednisolone[BC] 120 mg IM q3–4 wk is an alternative with reduction to 100 mg at wk 12 and reduce by 20 mg q12 wk until wk 48, then by 20 mg q16 wk.
- Consider adding methotrexate, tocilizumab *(Actemra)*, or rituximab if patient has comorbidities that increase steroid complications, has multiple relapses, and if tx fails.
- Consider osteoporosis prevention medication (p 248).

Giant Cell (Temporal) Arteritis

- Tx should not be delayed while waiting for pathologic diagnosis from temporal artery biopsy. Begin prednisone 40–60 mg/d po (if no vision loss) or methylprednisolone

500–1000 mg IV/d for 3 d (if vision loss) while biopsy and pathology are pending. Consider GI bleed prophylaxis with PPI.[BC] Pneumocystis prophylaxis only if also using methotrexate.

- If symptoms respond, begin taper by 10 mg prednisone/d after 2 wk and another 10 mg/d at 4 wk, then taper by 10% or 5 mg q1–2 wk over 9–12 mo. Once-daily dose is 10 mg, taper 1-mg/mo. Monitor Hb, ESR, CRP before dose changes, but treat based on symptoms, not lab tests. Treat relapses with increased glucocorticoids.
- Glucocorticoid-sparing agents. Use if high risk of developing AEs due to prednisone or relapsing course.
  - Methotrexate 7.5–15 mg/wk po and folate 5–7.5 mg/d po
  - Tocilizumab *(Actemra)* 162 mg SC qwk or every other week or abatacept *(Orencia)* 10 mg/kg SC on days 14, 21, 29, and wk 8
- For relapsing or refractory cases, adding IL-6 receptor inhibitor tocilizumab *(Actemra)* or cyclophosphamide, mean dose 100 mg/d po may help.
- Use low-dosage ASA (81–100 mg/d po) to reduce risk of visual loss, TIA, or stroke. Combine with PPI or misoprostol.
- Be aware of higher rates of systemic infection during first 6 mo of tx and higher rates of CVD.
- Monitor symptoms and CRP or sedimentation rate.
- Maintain tx for 1 y to prevent relapse; 35% relapse within 21 mo.
- Consider osteoporosis prevention medication (p 248).
- Monitoring for development of thoracic aortic aneurysm, especially ascending, with CT is on a case-by-case basis.

NEUROLOGIC DISORDERS

TREMORS

Table 90. Classification of Tremors

Tremor Type	Hz (cycles/sec)	Associated Conditions	Features	Treatment
Cerebellar	3–5	Cerebellar disease	Present only during movement; ↑ with intention; ↑ amplitude as target is approached	Symptomatic management
Essential	4–12	Familial in 50% of cases	Varying amplitude; common in upper extremities, head, neck; ↑ with antigravity movements, intention, stress, medications	Long-acting propranolol (**Table 21**); or primidone *(Mysoline)* 100 mg qhs start, titrate to 250–750 mg/d po in 3–4 divided doses; or gabapentin[BC] (**Table 96**)
Parkinson	4–7	Parkinson disease, parkinsonism	"Pill rolling;" present at rest; ↑ with emotional stress or when examiner calls attention to it; commonly asymmetric	See Parkinson disease (p 238)
Physiologic	4–12	Normal	Low amplitude; ↑ with stress, anxiety, emotional upset, lack of sleep, fatigue, toxins, medications	Tx of exacerbating factor

[BC] Avoid if CrCl <60 mL/min.

DIZZINESS

- Medications commonly associated with orthostatic hypotension include:
  - Cardiac: α blockers, β blockers, ACEIs, diuretics, nitrates, clonidine, hydralazine, methyldopa, reserpine, dipyridamole
  - CNS: antipsychotics, opioids, medications for Parkinson disease, skeletal muscle relaxants, TCAs
  - Urologic: antimuscarinic agents for UI, PDE5 inhibitors
- Caffeine, alcohol, nicotine, and head trauma can also cause or contribute to dizziness.

Table 91. Classification of Dizziness

Primary Symptom	Duration	Diagnosis	Management
Dizziness			
Lightheadedness 1–30 min after standing	Seconds to minutes (E)	Orthostatic hypotension	p 75
Wobbly/off balance gait; impairment in >1 of the following: vision, vestibular function, spinal proprioception, cerebellum, lower-extremity peripheral nerves	Occurs with ambulation (C)	Multiple sensory impairments including peripheral neuropathy; Parkinson disease	Correct or maximize sensory deficits; PT for balance and strength training; walking aid

(cont.)

Table 91. Classification of Dizziness (cont.)			
Primary Symptom	**Duration**	**Diagnosis**	**Management**
Unsteady gait with short steps; ↑ reflexes and/or tone	Occurs with ambulation (C)	Ischemic cerebral disease	ASA; modification of vascular risk factors; PT
Provoked by head or neck movement; reduced neck range of motion	Seconds to minutes (E)	Cervical spondylosis	Behavior modification; reduce cervical spasm and inflammation
Drop attacks			
Provoked by head or neck movement, reduced vertebral artery flow seen on Doppler or angiography	Seconds to minutes (E)	Postural impingement of vertebral artery	Behavior modification
Vertigo			
Brought on by position change, positive Dix-Hallpike test	Seconds to minutes (E)	Benign paroxysmal positional vertigo	Epley or Semont maneuver to reposition crystalline debris[1]
Acute onset, nonpositional	Days	Labyrinthitis/ vestibular neuronitis	Methylprednisolone, 100 mg/d po × 3 d with subsequent gradual taper over 3 wk to improve vestibular function recovery; meclizine[BC] (**Table 67**) for acute symptom relief
Low-frequency sensorineural hearing loss (usually begins unilaterally) and tinnitus, ear pain, sense of fullness in ear	Minutes to hours (E)	Ménière disease	Meclizine[BC] (**Table 67**) for acute symptom relief; diuretics and/or salt restriction for prophylaxis
Vascular disease risk factors, cranial nerve abnormalities	10 min to several hours (E)	TIAs	ASA; modification of vascular risk factors

C, chronic; E, episodic.

[1] youtube.com/watch?v=nX1HU-CCg2Y or youtube.com/watch?v=hiP7ifVxb0Q

MANAGEMENT OF ACUTE STROKE

Examination

- Cardiac (murmurs, arrhythmias, enlargement)
- Neurologic (serial examinations)
- Optic fundi
- Vascular (carotids and other peripheral pulses)

Diagnostic Testing

- Emergent noncontrast brain MRI or noncontrast CT
  - TIA: transient neurologic deficits without infarction on imaging
  - Stroke: neurologic deficits with infarction on imaging
- The NIH Stroke Scale (NIHSS; stroke.nih.gov/documents/NIH_Stroke_Scale.pdf) can quantify stroke severity and prognosis. NIHSS score >15 signifies major or severe stroke with high risk of death or significant permanent neurologic disability; NIHSS score <8 has a good prognosis for neurologic recovery.
- Bloodwork: BUN, CBC with platelet count, Cr, electrolytes, glucose, cardiac troponins, INR, PT, PTT, oxygen saturation

- ECG
- Other tests as indicated by clinical presentation:
  - ABG if hypoxia is suspected
  - Thrombin time and/or ecarin clotting time if patient is taking direct thrombin inhibitor or factor Xa inhibitor
  - Intracranial angiography by MRA, CT angiography, or Doppler ultrasound if intraarterial fibrinolysis or mechanical thrombectomy is being contemplated
  - Echocardiography (transesophageal preferred over transthoracic) for detection of cardiogenic emboli
  - Carotid duplex and transcranial Doppler studies for detection of carotid and vertebrobasilar embolic sources, respectively

Stroke Center Referral and Supportive Care

- If available, presenting stroke patients should be immediately referred to either a certified Comprehensive Stroke Center (preferred), which has 24/7 access to endovascular procedures, or a certified Primary Stroke Center.
- While waiting for transport to the stroke center, or if managing stroke when a certified stroke center is not available, provide supportive care as follows:
  - Maintain O_2 saturation >94%.
  - Correct metabolic and hydration imbalances.
  - Detect and treat coronary ischemia, HF, arrhythmias.
  - In patients with ischemic stroke and restricted mobility, implement DVT/PE prophylaxis with UFH, LMWH, or fondaparinux[BC] (Avoid if CrCl <30 mL/min) (**Table 17**).
  - Monitor and treat hyperthermia, using antipyretics (eg, APAP) for temperature >100.4°F.
  - Monitor for depression.
  - Refer to rehabilitation when medically stable.
  - Discharge on statin drug (**Table 19** and **Table 20**).

Thrombolytic Therapy for Ischemic Stroke (adapted from 2018 AHA/American Stroke Association Guidelines)

- Consider IV thrombolysis if patient presents within 180 min of symptom onset and emergently transport patient to a Comprehensive Stroke Center, if available.
- IV thrombolysis can be considered up to 9 h after symptom onset; additional relative exclusion criteria include age >80 or NIHSS >25.
- There are numerous contraindications to thrombolytic tx; see www.ncbi.nlm.nih.gov/pmc/articles/PMC4530420/

Antiplatelet Therapy for Ischemic Stroke

- Antiplatelet tx should be initiated within 24 h for patients with TIA or nondisabling stroke (ie, deficits that do not impair ADLs) and patients not receiving thrombolytic tx. Assess risk status of TIA using ABCD2 score: 1 point each for age ≥60, BP ≥140/90, speech disturbance without weakness, symptom duration 10–59 min, and hx of DM; 2 points for unilateral weakness and symptom duration ≥60 min.
  - For TIA with ABCD2 score <4, use ASA 162–325 mg/d po (initial dose 325 mg). If patient has had prior TIA or stroke, use single antiplatelet tx: ASA 50–325 mg/d po or clopidogrel 75 mg/d po or combination form of ASA and long-acting dipyridamole *(Aggrenox)* 1 tab po q12h.
  - For TIA with ABCD2 score ≥4 or nondisabling stroke, use dual antiplatelet tx ASA 325 mg po and clopidogrel 300–600 mg po on day 1, followed by ASA 50–325 mg/d po and clopidogrel 75 mg/d po on days 2–21, with single antiplatelet tx after day 21.

- Chronic tx for patients after thrombolysis or EVT: single antiplatelet tx with ASA 50–325 mg/d po or clopidogrel 75 mg/d po or combination form of ASA and long-acting dipyridamole *(Aggrenox)* 1 tab po q12h
- In the absence of AF, warfarin tx is no more effective and is associated with more bleeding than ASA in preventing strokes in patients with prior TIA or stroke.
- Anticoagulants are not recommended except in DVT/PE prophylactic dosages for medical patients with restricted mobility (**Table 17**).

Endovascular Thrombectomy (EVT)

- EVT should be considered in patients with large vessel occlusion presenting within 24 h of symptoms, ideally within 6 h of symptom onset.
- EVT is more likely to be beneficial in larger strokes with more significant deficits (NIHSS ≥6). Compared to medical tx alone, EVT produces significantly better functional outcomes with no added risks.

Management of Acute Hypertension in Ischemic Stroke

- If patient is otherwise eligible for IV thrombolysis (see contraindications, p 236), attempt to lower BP to ≤185/110 mm Hg so that patient may undergo reperfusion tx. Options for lowering BP are:
  - Labetalol 10–20 mg IV over 1–2 min, may repeat once; ***or***
  - Nicardipine 5 mg/h IV, increasing by 2.5 mg/h q5–15 min to max of 15 mg/h
- If patient is ineligible or not being considered for thrombolytic tx, do not lower BP if SBP ≤220 mm Hg or if DBP ≤120 mm Hg; higher BP may be lowered gently, with goal of 15% reduction over first 24 h. Choice of BP-lowering agent should reflect patient's comorbidities (**Table 21**).

Management of Hypertension in Acute Intracranial Hemorrhage

- Do **not** lower BP if SBP is between 150 and 220 mm Hg.
- If SBP >220 mm Hg, consider lowering BP gently with IV agents and continuous BP monitoring.

STROKE PREVENTION

Risk Factor Modification

- Smoking cessation.
- HTN tx (see Hypertension, p 54):
  - Goal BP <130/80 mm Hg if prior TIA or stroke; adjust goal according to comorbidities, function, and patient preference.
  - If previously treated, restart oral antihypertensive medication a few days after TIA or stroke.
  - If hypertensive but not previously treated, initiate oral antihypertensive medication a few days after TIA or stroke.
- Dyslipidemia tx (**Table 19** and **Table 20**).
- Antiplatelet tx if prior ischemic stroke (p 236)
- Anticoagulation (**Table 17**) or antiplatelet (**Table 16**) tx for AF.
- Low-sodium (≤2.4 g/d), Mediterranean-type diet
- Exercise (≥30 min of moderate-intensity activity daily)
- Weight reduction
- Screen for DM if prior TIA or stroke

- Consider the addition of agents that have shown some evidence of further lowering of stroke risk when added to standard antiplatelet, antihypertensive, and lipid-lowering tx: ezetimibe, PCSK9 inhibitors, eicosapentaenoic acid enhancers, pioglitazone, GLP-1 receptor agonists, and folic acid.
- Treat carotid stenosis (**Table 92**).

Table 92. Treatment Options for Carotid Stenosis in Older Adults

Presentation	% Stenosis	Treatment Options	Comments
Prior TIA or stroke	≥70	CA/CE or MM	CE superior to medical tx only if patient is reasonable surgical risk and facility has track record of low complication rate for CE (<6%)
Prior TIA or stroke	50–69	CE or MM	Serial carotid Doppler testing may identify rapidly developing plaques
Prior TIA or stroke	<50	MM	CE of no proven benefit in this situation
Asymptomatic	≥70	CA/CE[CW] or MM	Don't recommend CE for asymptomatic carotid stenosis unless the complication rate is low (<3%).[CW]
Asymptomatic	<70	MM	CE of no proven benefit in this situation

CA, carotid angioplasty with stent placement in patients with multiple comorbidities and/or at high surgical risk; CE, carotid endarterectomy; MM, medical management.

PARKINSON DISEASE

Diagnosis Requires

- Bradykinesia, eg:
  - Slowness of initiation of voluntary movements (eg, glue-footedness when starting to walk)
  - Reduced speed and amplitude of repetitive movements (eg, tapping index finger and thumb together)
  - Difficulty switching from one motor program to another (eg, multiple steps to turn during gait testing)
- ***and*** one or more of the following:
  - Muscular rigidity (eg, cogwheeling)
  - 4–7 Hz resting tremor
  - Impaired righting reflex (eg, retropulsed during sternal push or shoulder pull test)
- Other clinical features of Parkinson disease:
  - Postural instability and falls
  - Hyposmia
  - Hypophonia
  - Micrographia
  - REM sleep behavior disorder
  - Constipation
  - Masked facies
  - Infrequent blinking
  - Drooling
  - Seborrhea of face and scalp
  - Festinating gait
- Neuropsychiatric conditions are also common usually later in the clinical course: anxiety, depression, dementia, visual hallucinations, dysthymia, psychosis, delirium

Table 93. Distinguishing Early Parkinson Disease From Other Parkinsonian Syndromes					
Condition	**Tremor**	**Asymmetric Involvement**	**Early Falls**	**Early Dementia**	**Postural Hypotension**
Parkinson disease	+	+	–	–	–
Drug-induced parkinsonism	+/–	–	–	–	–
Vascular parkinsonism	–	+/–	+/–	+/–	–
LBD	+/–	+/–	+/–	+	+/–
Progressive supranuclear palsy	–	–	+	+/–	–
Corticobasal ganglionic degeneration	–	+	+	–	+
Multiple-system atrophy	–	+/–	+/–	–	+

+ = usually or always present; +/– = sometimes present; – = absent.

Source: Adapted from Christine CW et al. *Am J Med* 2004;117:412–419.

Nonpharmacologic Interventions

- Patient education is essential, and support groups are often helpful.
- Monitor for orthostatic hypotension (p 75).
- PT/Exercise programs to improve physical functioning, stability, and constipation:
  - Regular aerobic exercise (eg, treadmill training)
  - Balance and flexibility exercises (eg, tai chi)
  - Resistance training
- OT to maximize fine-motor functioning with adaptive equipment (eg, specialized eating utensils) and to perform home safety evaluations
- Speech-language tx to improve dysarthria and hypophonia
- Diet with increased fiber and hydration to minimize constipation; adequate vitamin D and calcium as osteopenia is common

Surgical Treatment—Deep Brain Stimulation (DBS)

- DBS of the globus pallidus or subthalamic nucleus is used for tx of motor complications of Parkinson disease.
- DBS is best suited for patients who have fluctuating motor problems (tremor and other dyskinesias) despite medical tx and who have few comorbidities, especially no dementia.
- Compared with medical tx in selected patients, DBS can significantly increase motor function (several more hours per day of "on" time) and decrease troubling dyskinesias.
- Early (0–3 mo) complications include surgical site infection (~10%), symptomatic intracranial hemorrhage (~2%), death (~1%), cognitive and speech problems (10–15%), and an increased risk of falls.

Pharmacotherapy (Tables 94 and **95**)

- Begin tx when symptoms interfere with function.
- First-line tx is dopamine or dopamine agonist.
- Start at low dose and titrate upward gradually.
- Monitor orthostatic BP during titration of medications.
- Tailor tx to symptoms.

Table 94. Symptom-Directed Treatment of Parkinson Disease

Category	Symptoms	Treatment Options
Motor	Tremor, bradykinesia, rigidity	Use dopamine, dopamine agonists
	Persistent tremor despite dopamine/dopamine-agonist tx	Add β blocker or clozapine; consider DBS
	Bradykinesia, motor fluctuations, increased "off time" despite dopamine tx	Increase dopamine dose; add inhaled L-DOPA or dopamine agonist or COMT inhibitor or MAO B inhibitor (**Table 95**); consider DBS for refractory motor fluctuations
	Postural instability or gait impairment despite dopamine tx	Add amantadine or cholinesterase inhibitor
Nonmotor	Depression	Try SSRI or SNRI; consider careful trial of TCA[BC]; consider trial of pramipexole
	Cognitive impairment/ Parkinson disease/ Dementia	Consider trial of cholinesterase inhibitor (rivastigmine as preferred choice, donepezil, galantamine), monitoring carefully for exacerbation of tremor or GI side effects
	Orthostatic hypotension	See Orthostatic (Postural) Hypotension (p 75)
	REM sleep behavior disorder	Try high-dose melatonin 3–15 mg hs (**Table 131** and p 350); if not effective, consider careful trial of clonazepam 0.25–1 mg po hs only in healthier patients without dementia or sleep apnea at low risk of falls
Drug-Induced	Dyskinesias	Carefully reduce dopamine dose (if motor symptoms worsen, try adding low dose of dopamine agonist); add amantadine; consider clozapine
	Nausea	Slowly titrate dopamine dose; consider domperidone; avoid metoclopramide, prochlorperazine, and promethazine[BC]
	Impulse-control disorders	Reduce or D/C dopamine agonists; consider trial of amantadine
	Hallucinations/psychosis	Exclude systemic illness; carefully reduce antiparkinsonian drugs; try pimavanserin *(Nuplazid)* 34 mg po 1×/d, which can take up to 3 wk to be effective; alternatives are quetiapine or clozapine (avoid all other antipsychotics[BC])

Table 95. Medications for Parkinson Disease

Class, Medication	Comments (Metabolism, Excretion)
Dopamine	
Carbidopa-levodopa	Mainstay of Parkinson disease tx; initiate with 1/2 tab of 25/100 mg po q8–12h; increase dose by 1/2–1 tab q1–2wk to achieve minimal target dose of 1 tab q8h, then titrate upward gradually prn; watch for GI AEs, orthostatic hypotension, confusion; long-term tx associated with motor fluctuations and dyskinesias (addition of dopamine agonist may attenuate these effects) (L)
Enteral suspension *(Duopa)*	For use in patients with enteral feeding

(cont.)

Class, Medication	Comments (Metabolism, Excretion)
SR carbidopa-levodopa *(RYTARY)*	Useful at daily dopamine requirement ≥300 mg; slower absorption than carbidopa-levodopa; can improve motor fluctuations (L)
Inhaled levodopa *(Inbrija)*	Indicated as an option to treat "off" episodes in patients already on carbidopa-levodopa
Dopamine Agonists	More CNS AEs than dopamine
Apomorphine	For acute, intermittent tx of "off" episodes
(Apokyn)	Increase gradually to max 0.6 mL (6 mg)
(Kynmobi)	Increase gradually to max 30 mg
Pramipexole	Initial dose 0.125 mg/d po; increase gradually to effective dosage (0.5–1.5 mg q8h) (K)
ER pramipexole	Increase gradually to effective dosage (1.5–4.5 mg 1×/d) (K)
Ropinirole	Initial dose 0.25 mg/d po; increase gradually to effective dosage (up to 1–8 mg q8h) (L)
ER ropinirole	Increase gradually to effective dosage (up to 6–24 mg 1×/d) (L)
Rotigotine *(Neupro)*	Increase weekly to effective dosage (max 6 mg/24 h for early stage disease, 8 mg/24 h for advanced disease) (K)
Catechol *O*-Methyl-transferase (COMT) Inhibitors	Adjunctive tx with L-DOPA
Tolcapone *(Tasmar)*	Monitor LFTs q6mo (L, K)
Entacapone *(Comtan)*	Watch for nausea, orthostatic hypotension (K)
Opicapone *(Ongentys)*	Avoid food within 1 h before and at least 1 h post dose (L, K)
Anticholinergics	
Benztropine	Can cause confusion and delirium; helpful for drooling. Avoid.[BC] (L, K)
Trihexyphenidyl	Same as above. Avoid.[BC] (L, K)
Dopamine Reuptake Inhibitor	
Amantadine	Useful in early and late Parkinson disease; watch closely for CNS AEs; do not D/C abruptly (K)
ER Amantadine *(Gocovri)* *(Osmolex ER)*	Can be used for tx of dyskinesia in patients on dopamine tx; many behavioral AEs (K)
Monoamine Oxidase B (MAO B) Inhibitors	
Rasagiline *(Azilect)*	Interactions with numerous drugs and tyramine-rich foods; expensive (L, K)
Safinamide *(Xadago)*	Use as adjunctive tx with dopamine to treat "off" episodes; many AEs and drug interactions (K)
Selegiline	Use as adjunctive tx with dopamine; do not exceed a total dosage of 10 mg/d; metabolized to amphetamine derivatives (L, K)
Combination Medication	
Carbidopa-levodopa + entacapone *(Stalevo)*	Should be used only after individual dosages of carbidopa, L-DOPA, and entacapone have been established (L, K)

MULTIPLE-SYSTEM ATROPHY (MSA)

Diagnosis (see also **Table 93**)

- Diagnosis is made on hx and physical findings.
- May have early nonmotor phase characterized by urinary and/or sexual dysfunction, orthostatic hypotension, REM sleep behavior disorder.
- Clinical hallmarks are (in varying combinations):
  - Progressive autonomic failure—erectile dysfunction, genital hyposensitivity in women, urinary dysfunction, orthostatic hypotension.
  - Parkinsonism—bradykinesia, rigidity, falls; resting pill-rolling tremor is not usually seen but may have postural action tremor.
  - Cerebellar dysfunction—wide-based gait ataxia, uncoordinated limb movements.
- Other common features include:
  - Inspiratory stridor
  - Pronounced neck flexion (antecollis)
  - Depression and/or anxiety
  - Absence of dementia and hallucinations
  - Frontal lobe executive dysfunction and attention deficits

Clinical Course

- Rapid progression of motor symptoms once they appear (about half of patients will require a walking aid within 3 y after onset of motor manifestations)
- Progressive course over approximately 6–10 y, culminating in death
- Late stage characterized by frequent falls, profound bradykinesia, unintelligible speech, recurrent aspiration pneumonia

Management

- Tx is for symptom management of above conditions; there are no known disease-altering tx.
- Up to 40% of patients will respond transiently to L-DOPA tx, which should be continued if there are no side effects.
- Neurorehabilitation programs can be helpful for maximizing mobility, preventing falls, increasing communication ability, and preventing choking episodes.

SEIZURES

Classification

- Generalized: All areas of brain affected with alteration in consciousness
- Partial: Focal brain area affected, not necessarily with alteration in consciousness; can progress to generalized type

Initial Evaluation, Assessment

- History: neurologic disorders, trauma, drug and alcohol use
- Physical exam: general, with careful neurologic
- Routine tests: BUN, calcium, CBC, Cr, ECG, EEG, electrolytes, glucose, head CT, LFTs, magnesium
- Tests as indicated: head MRI, lumbar puncture, oxygen saturation, urine toxicity or drug screen

Common Causes

- Advanced dementia
- CNS infection
- Drug or alcohol withdrawal
- Idiopathic causes
- Metabolic disorders
- Prior stroke (most common)
- Toxins
- Trauma
- Tumor

Management

- Treat underlying causes.
- Institute anticonvulsant tx (**Table 96**). Virtually all anticonvulsant medications can cause sedation and ataxia.
- Avoid the following drugs, which can lower seizure threshold: bupropion, chlorpromazine, clozapine, maprotiline, olanzapine, thioridazine, thiothixene, and tramadol.[BC]
- Consider discontinuing anticonvulsant tx if seizure-free for 2 y; recurrence can occur in 30–50% of patients. If discontinuing carbamazepine or oxcarbazepine, should be tapered over 6 mo.

Table 96. **Anticonvulsant Medications**

Medication	Comments (Metabolism, Excretion)
◆Carbamazepine	Many drug interactions; mood stabilizer; may cause SIADH[BC], thrombocytopenia, leukopenia (L, K)
◆Gabapentin	Used as adjunct to other agents; watch for peripheral edema; reduce dosage if CrCl <60[BC] (K)
Lacosamide *(VIMPAT)*	Used as adjunct to other agents for partial-onset seizures; not studied in older adults (L, K)
Lamotrigine	Prolongs PR interval; risk of severe rash; when used with valproic acid, begin at 25 mg q48h, titrate to 25–100 mg q12h (L, K)
ER lamotrigine	Dose is dependent on presence of other anticonvulsants in drug regimen, especially valproic acid (L, K)
Levetiracetam	Reduce dosage in renal impairment[BC]: CrCl 30–50: 250–750 q12h CrCl 10–29: 250–500 q12h CrCl <10: 500–1000 q24h (K)
Oxcarbazepine *(Trileptal)*	Can cause hyponatremia[BC], leukopenia (L)
Phenobarbital	Many drug interactions; not recommended for use in older adults (L)
Phenytoin	Many drug interactions; exhibits nonlinear pharmacokinetics (L)
◆Pregabalin	Indicated as adjunct tx for partial-onset seizures only; watch for peripheral edema; adjust dosage on basis of CrCl[BC] (K)
Tiagabine	AE profile in older adults less well described (L)
Topiramate ER topiramate	May affect cognitive functioning at high dosages (L, K)
Valproic acid ER	Can cause weight gain, tremor, hair loss; several drug interactions; mood stabilizer; monitor LFTs and platelets (L)
Zonisamide	Anorexia; contraindicated in patients with sulfonamide allergy (K)

◆ = also has primary indication for neuropathic pain. CrCl unit = mL/min.

APHASIA

Table 97. Aphasias in Which Repetition Is Impaired

Type	Fluency	Auditory Comprehension	Associated Neurologic Deficits	Comments
Broca	–	+	Right hemiparesis	Patient aware of deficit; high rate of associated depression; message board helpful for communication
Wernicke	+	–	Often none	Patient frequently unaware of deficit; speech content usually unintelligible; tx often focuses on visually based communication
Conduction	+	+	Occasional right facial weakness	Patient usually aware of deficit; speech content usually intelligible
Global	–	–	Right hemiplegia with right field cut	Most commonly due to left middle cerebral artery thrombosis, which has a poor prognosis for meaningful speech recovery

+ = present; – = absent.

PERIPHERAL NEUROPATHY

History and Physical Exam

- Time course: acute (<4 wk), subacute (1–3 mo), chronic (>3 mo)
- Family hx: Charcot-Marie-Tooth disease is most common hereditary neuropathy
- Drug and toxin exposure hx: alcohol, amiodarone, antibiotics (eg, metronidazole, dapsone), chemotherapeutic agents, phenytoin, statins, solvents, heavy metals, insecticides
- Distribution (focal, multifocal, symmetric/asymmetric) and type (sensory, motor, and/or autonomic) of deficit

Diagnosis

- Most neuropathies can be diagnosed clinically (**Table 98**)

Table 98. Diagnostic Features of Selected Neuropathies

Distribution	Type of Deficit	Common Causes
Lower extremities symmetric polyneuropathy	Sensory predominant (burning, tingling, numbness)	DM (~30% of all neuropathies), idiopathic, B_{12} deficiency, MGUS, CKD, alcohol, chemotherapy
Upper and lower extremities symmetric polyneuropathy	Sensory +/- motor +/- autonomic	Idiopathic, Guillain-Barré, CIDP, Lyme disease, HIV
Mononeuropathy or radiculopathy	Sensory +/- motor	Carpal tunnel, ulnar neuropathy, Bell palsy, radiculopathy
Asymmetric polyneuropathy	Sensory +/- motor +/- autonomic	Vasculitis, DM, ALS

CIDP, chronic inflammatory demyelinating polyneuropathy; MGUS, monoclonal gammopathy of undetermined significance.

- Reasonable blood screening tests would include CBC, glucose, Cr, BUN, TSH, LFTs, vitamin B_{12} level, ESR, SPEP
- Nerve conduction studies can help distinguish the more common axonal pathologies (DM, medication effects, alcohol, kidney failure, malignancy) from demyelinating ones (including Guillain-Barré syndrome and chronic inflammatory demyelinating polyneuropathy [CIDP])

- About 30% of cases are idiopathic.

Management

Prevention of Complications

- Protect distal extremities from trauma—appropriate shoe size, daily foot inspections, good skin care, avoidance of barefoot walking.
- Prevent falls (p 138)—balance and strength training; assess for other fall risk factors
- Maintain appropriate glycemic control in diabetic neuropathy.

Medications for Painful Neuropathy

- Expected to achieve a 30–50% reduction in pain in roughly 1/3 of patients
- Help only pain, not other neurologic symptoms
- Should be started at low dosage and increased as needed and tolerated
- In older adults, anticonvulsants are reasonable as first-line oral agents:
  - Gabapentin can begin 100–200 mg po qhs but may need up to 100–600 mg po q8h. If CrCl ≤15 mL/min, dose at 100–300 mg/d. If CrCl 16–29 mL/min, dose at 200–600 mg/d over 1–2 doses. If CrCl 30–49 mL/min, dose at 300–900 mg/d over 2–3 doses. Reduce dose if CrCl <60 mL/min.[BC]
  - Pregabalin 75–300 mg po q12h, extended-release *(Lyrica CR)* 165–660 mg po q24h; lower dosage according to CrCl if CrCl <60 mL/min[BC]; primary indication is for management of postherpetic neuralgia, diabetic peripheral neuropathy, or fibromyalgia.
  - Carbamazepine 200–400 mg po q8h; (carbamazepine ER) 200 mg po q12h
- Other oral agents that may be effective include:
  - TCAs[BC] (eg, nortriptyline 10–100 mg po qhs or desipramine 10–75 mg po qam); benefits often outweighed by side effects in older adults
  - Duloxetine[BC] 20–60 mg/d po; avoid if CrCl <30 mL/min
  - SSRIs[BC] have not been shown to be as effective as TCAs (**Table 42**)
  - Lamotrigine (**Table 96**) 400–600 mg/d po
  - Opioids[BC]: watch for AEs of itching, mood changes, weakness, confusion
  - Tramadol[BC] 100–300 mg/d po; reduce dose for IR[BC] or avoid for ER[BC] if CrCl <30 mL/min
- Topical agents that may be effective include:
  - Capsaicin applied q6–8h, starting at low dose and titrating upward as needed (available in crm, gel, S, lot, or pch, range 0.025–0.15%); see **Table 101** for further information.
  - Capsaicin 8% cutaneous pch *(Qutenza)* applied by health professional, using a local anesthetic, to the most painful skin areas (max of 4 pch). Apply for 30 min to feet, 60 min for other locations. Risk of significant rise in BP after placement; monitor patient for at least 1 h.
  - TENS
  - Lidocaine 5% pch *(Lidoderm)* 1–3 patches covering the affected area up to 24 h/d; lidocaine 4% patches are available OTC; see **Table 101** for further information.
  - Other topical lidocaine preparations 2–4×/d

OSTEOPOROSIS

COMMONLY USED DEFINITIONS

- Osteoporosis: a skeletal disorder characterized by compromised bone strength (bone density and bone quality) predisposing to an increased risk of fracture
- Established osteoporosis: prior fragility fracture defined as those occurring from a fall from a standing height or less, or due to minor trauma (eg, not a car or sports accident). Fragility fractures occur particularly at the spine, hip, wrist, humerus, rib, and pelvis. Certain skeletal locations, including the face, skull, cervical spine, fingers, and toes are not considered fragility sites.
- Clinical Osteoporosis:
  - BMD 2.5 SD or more below that of young normal individuals (T score) (WHO). Scores between 1 and 2.5 SD below young normals are termed osteopenia. For each SD decrement in BMD, hip fracture risk increases about 2 fold; for each SD increment in BMD, hip fracture risk is about halved.
  - Elevated risk of fracture (eg, based on Fracture Risk Assessment Tool [FRAX]: sheffield.ac.uk/FRAX/tool.aspx?country=9) estimated 10-y probability of hip fracture ≥3% or 10-y risk of all major osteoporotic fracture ≥20%) regardless of BMD or prior fragility fracture

RISK FACTORS FOR OSTEOPOROTIC FRACTURE

- Increasing age[1]
- Female sex[1]
- BMI (both low and high)[1]
- Previous low-trauma fracture as adult[1]
- Parent fractured hip[1]
- Current smoking[1]
- Oral glucocorticoids (ever used ≥3 mo at a dose of prednisolone of 5 mg daily or equivalent)[1]
- RA[1]
- Secondary osteoporosis (type I DM, osteogenesis imperfecta in adults, untreated long-standing hyperthyroidism, hypogonadism or premature menopause (<45 y), chronic malnutrition, or malabsorption and chronic liver disease; if BMD entered into FRAX, no need to enter these variables[1]
- Alcohol (>3 drinks/d)[1]
- Lower BMD[1]
- Lower trabecular bone score
- Frailty
- Dementia
- Depression
- Impaired vision
- Low physical activity
- Recurrent falls
- Nocturia
- CKD (GFR <45 mL/min) BSA
- DM2

[1]indicates risk factors included in FRAX

TOXINS AND MEDICATIONS THAT CAN CAUSE OR AGGRAVATE OSTEOPOROSIS

- Alcohol
- ADT
- Anticonvulsants
- Antipsychotics
- Corticosteroids
- Heparin
- Lithium
- Nicotine (ie, smoking)
- Phenytoin
- PPIs (if ≥1 y; Controversial: observational studies with mixed results)
- SSRIs (Controversial: observational studies with mixed results)
- Thyroxine (if over-replaced or in suppressive dosage)

EVALUATION

- BMD (hip and spine preferred) at least once in all women after age 65; insufficient evidence to support screening in men (USPSTF) but Bone Health and Osteoporosis Foundation (BHOF) recommends BMD in all men after age 70, and in men with prior clinical fracture after age 65 (**Table 107**); reimbursement for BMD in men is difficult. Do not use BMD screening in women aged <65 or men aged <70 with no risk factors.[CW] Uncertain how often to repeat. Some suggest in 3 y for patients with osteopenia and in 5–15 y for those with normal BMD. Do not routinely repeat more than every 2 y.[CW]
  - A measure of bone strength, Trabecular Bone Score, can be generated with software add-ons to some BMD systems and can be entered into FRAX (see below).
  - BHOF recommends screening with vertebral imaging (dual-energy x-ray absorptiometry or x-ray) for women aged ≥65 with ≤-1.0 at femoral neck and women aged ≥70 and men aged ≥80 (70–79) with T score ≤1.0 (1.5) at lumbar spine, total hip, or femoral neck. However, this is controversial and is not covered by Medicare.
- FRAX (sheffield.ac.uk/FRAX/tool.aspx?country=9)—Practitioners in some countries use FRAX first and perform BMD only if tx decision is equivocal.
  - FRAX does not include fracture risk factors such as falls, cognitive impairment, UI, and most medications, nor does it address persons with <10 y of anticipated survival. However, the benefits of osteoporosis drugs may occur within 6–12 mo.
  - Some recommend assessing FRAX score every 5 y and obtain BMD if score is close to tx threshold (eg, 10-y risk of major osteoporotic fracture >15%).
- There is insufficient evidence about screening for serum 25(OH)D deficiency (USPSTF) and it is not recommended.[CW] BHOF recommends monitoring levels and maintaining between >30 ng/mL and <50 ng/mL if bone disease.
- BHOF recommends excluding secondary causes (serum PTH, TSH, calcium, phosphorus, albumin, alkaline phosphatase, bioavailable testosterone in men, kidney function tests, LFTs, CBC, UA, electrolytes, SPEP). Less consensus on 24-h urinary calcium excretion (consider if GI disorders or after gastrectomy or bariatric surgery), cortisol, and antibodies associated with gluten enteropathy. Bone turnover markers are not routinely used.

MANAGEMENT

Universal Recommendations

- Elemental calcium, 1200 mg/d (diet plus supplement) for women aged >50 and men aged >70, 1000 mg/d for men aged <70. The amount of elemental calcium in supplements is listed on the product label under "Supplement Facts." Doses ≤600 mg, 2×/d are better absorbed but may result in worse adherence. For most patients, calcium carbonate (40% elemental calcium) is sufficient and least expensive.
- For patients on H2RA or PPIs (**Table 101**) or who have achlorhydria, calcium citrate (20% elemental calcium) should be used.
  - For patients who have difficulty swallowing calcium citrate tabs, smaller tabs of 125 mg *(Freeda Mini Cal-citrate)* and granules, 1 tsp = 760 mg *(Freeda Calcium Citrate Fine Granular)*, are available.
  - Dietary sources of calcium include:
    - Milk (per 8 oz): whole 276 mg; reduced fat 293 mg; low fat 305 mg; nonfat 316 mg
    - Yogurt (per 6 oz): whole 209 mg; low fat 311 mg
    - Cheese: American (per slice) 293 mg; cheddar (per 1 oz) 201 mg; Swiss (per 1 oz) 252 mg
    - Cottage cheese (per cup): 174–187 mg
    - Ice cream (per cup): 144–168 mg
    - Calcium supplementation probably does not increase risk of CVD. Data on the risk of dementia and stroke-related dementia are inconclusive. Risk of kidney stones is

increased. Some experts recommend getting as much calcium through dietary sources as possible.

- Vitamin D 800–1000 IU (Institute of Medicine); Each 8-oz glass of milk or fortified orange juice has approximately 100 IU. D_3 (cholecalciferol) is the preferred form of supplementation. Taken without calcium, vitamin D may not reduce fracture risk, but taken with calcium it may reduce any fractures by 6% and hip fractures by 16%. In unselected men (age ≥50) and women (age ≥55), supplementation with 2000 IU does not reduce fractures.
- OTC calcium plus vitamin D preparations vary considerably in amounts of each, so ask patients to read labels (look for elemental calcium) to ensure they are getting adequate amounts.
- Avoid tobacco.
- Fall prevention, including exercise for muscle strengthening and balance training (**Table 61**)
- No more than moderate alcohol use (≤1 drink/d in women, ≤2 drink/d in men)
- If hyperparathyroid, in a cohort study, parathyroidectomy reduced risk of hip and any fracture.

Pharmacotherapeutic Prevention and Management

Indications for Pharmacotherapy

- Established osteoporosis (prior fragility fracture)
  - Oral pharmacotherapy can begin in hospital if hip or vertebral fracture. Do not wait for BMD.
  - IV and SC tx can begin 2 wk after surgery; if severely vitamin D deficient, replete first. Contraindicated if hypocalcemia.
- Clinical osteoporosis
  - No prior fracture but osteoporosis by BMD (−2.5 or less)
  - High risk based on FRAX estimated 10-y probability of hip fracture ≥3% or 10-y risk of all major osteoporotic fracture ≥20%.
- Osteopenia (BMD −1 to −2.5)
  - No consensus on tx
  - 4 infusions of zoledronic acid at 18-mo intervals reduced fragility fractures (vertebral or nonvertebral) by 37% in women.

Treatment Principles (**Table 99** for specific drugs)

- Vitamin D levels should be normal (25[OH]D ≥30 ng/mL) before initiating pharmacotherapy because bisphosphonates and denosumab can precipitate symptomatic hypocalcemia if vitamin D levels are low.
- When initiating tx with bisphosphonates or denosumab, discuss the risk factors for developing osteonecrosis of the jaw (ONJ) (eg, IV administration, cancer and cancer tx, glucocorticoid tx, smoking, DM, and preexisting dental disease) and review the symptoms of ONJ. A routine dental visit before starting tx is not necessary; if the patient has any active and unevaluated dental problems, a preinitiation dental visit is advisable. If an invasive dental procedure (eg, dental implant or extraction) is planned, many experts delay bisphosphonate tx until healing of the jaw is complete.
- Monitoring BMD in patients already receiving tx is controversial. Some recommend repeating BMD 1 y after tx initiation or change.
- If discontinuing denosumab, teriparatide, abaloparatide, or romosozumab, initiate bisphosphate tx if kidney function permits.

Bisphosphonates

- First-line tx but are contraindicated in renal failure. If CrCl <35 mL/min, denosumab is an alternative.
  - Time to benefit is 12.4 mo to prevent 1 nonvertebral fracture, 20.3 mo to prevent 1 hip fracture, and 12.1 mo to prevent 1 clinical vertebral fracture per 100 postmenopausal women.
- IV bisphosphonates if GI contraindications (eg, esophageal disorders), intolerant of oral bisphosphonates, or are unable to sit up after oral dosing.
- Some experts recommend using oral bisphosphonates (alendronate or risedronate) that have demonstrated efficacy in reducing hip fractures.
- PPIs reduce the effectiveness of oral bisphosphonates; some experts recommend holding the PPI the day before bisphosphonate administration and not giving the PPI until >60 min after the bisphosphonate has been taken.
- Bisphosphonates are more effective in preventing hip fracture when adherence is >80% (compared with adherence <50%). Adherence is highest with monthly compared to weekly regimens, which is higher than daily regimens.
- Bisphosphonates increase the risk of atypical femoral fractures, with more risk with longer duration of tx, especially beyond 8 y. Risk-benefit varies by race/ethnic group and is most pronounced for Whites (eg, at 3 y, 2 atypical fractures would occur and 139 hip and 541 clinical fractures would be prevented). After discontinuing bisphosphonates, the risk of atypical fractures decreases rapidly.
- The optimal duration of bisphosphonate tx is uncertain. The risk of subtrochanteric or femoral shaft fractures increases with tx beyond 3 y. An FDA analysis concluded neither clear benefit nor harm for overall osteoporotic fracture risk by continuing bisphosphonates beyond 5 y. Some recommend discontinuing, at least temporarily, after 5 y of oral tx or 3 y of IV tx for those at modest risk; BMD should be monitored q2–3y. After bisphosphonates have been discontinued, there are no data on whether or when to resume tx. Others recommend that those with highest risk (ie, T score <-2.5, recent fracture, or both) continue for up 10 y for oral drugs or 6 y for zoledronic acid.

Denosumab

- An alternative for those who are intolerant of bisphosphonates or have CKD. The efficacy of denosumab in Stage 4 and 5 CKD is unknown, and CKD increases risk of hypocalcemia with denosumab tx.
- Compared to bisphosphonates, risk of atypical fracture is at least as high and risk of osteonecrosis of the jaw is higher.
- Discontinuation of denosumab results in bone loss to pretreatment levels within 2 y and vertebral fractures within a short period (8–16 mo). If denosumab is discontinued, start a bisphosphonate if CrCl ≥30 mL/min.

Parathyroid Hormone (PTH) and Parathyroid Hormone–related Protein Analog Therapy

- Consider teriparatide (PTH) or abaloparatide (PTH-related protein analog):
  - For patients who are intolerant of bisphosphonates or denosumab
  - For patients at very high risk of fracture, including those with:
    - osteoporosis-range BMD and patient has had a spine or hip fracture
    - continued fracture after 1 y of bisphosphonate tx
    - multiple spine fractures regardless of BMD
    - T score <-3.0
    - FRAX 10-y risk of major osteoporotic fracture >30% or hip fracture >4.5%
- Some experts use teriparatide for prolonged fracture-related pain or nonhealing but evidence is conflicting and use is not standard practice.

- Maximum duration of use is 2 y (teriparatide) or 1.5 y (abaloparatide) and usually a bisphosphonate or denosumab is started after stopping PTH-based tx. If severe risk, some experts recommend a second course after intercurrent use of bisphosphonates.
- Teriparatide is more effective than risedronate at preventing vertebral and clinical (nonvertebral and symptomatic vertebral) but not nonvertebral fractures. Some recommend teriparatide as initial tx if severe spinal osteoporosis (≥2 moderate or 1 severe vertebral fracture by radiography).

Romosozumab-aqqg

- Monoclonal antibody that blocks the effects of the protein sclerostin and works mainly by increasing new bone formation. Used for persons at very high risk of fracture.
- More effective than teriparatide on BMD and more effective than placebo or alendronate alone if followed by alendronate after 12 mo of tx on fracture outcomes.
- Bone-forming effect wanes after 12 mo and patients should be switched to bisphosphonates or denosumab.
- Increased risk of heart attack and stroke (do not use if these occurred in previous year) and cardiovascular death

Other treatments

- Raloxifene can be used in women who cannot tolerate other medications or are at high risk for breast cancer.
- Calcitonin is less often used because it is less effective and has higher risk of AEs.
- Conjugated estrogens/bazedoxifene is not well studied for osteoporosis.

Osteoporosis in Men

- For men, nonpharmacologic tx, indications for pharmacotherapy, and choices of drugs, other than estrogen, are the same as for women. Bisphosphonate tx has been evaluated less in men. Zoledronic acid reduces the risk of morphometric vertebral fractures.
  - If symptomatic hypogonadism or a medical reason for hypogonadism, add testosterone replacement. (p 326)

Table 99. Pharmacotherapeutic Prevention and Management of Osteoporosis[1]

Medication	Administration/Comments
Bisphosphonates	All contraindicated in CKD (CrCl <30–35). Orals must be taken fasting with water, patient must remain upright and npo for 30–60 min after taking. All IV can cause acute phase reaction (flu-like symptoms), particularly after first dose. *Class effect:* Esophagitis; bone, joint, or muscle pain; osteonecrosis of jaw (estimated 1–28 cases/100,000 patient-years with oral tx)[2]; occipital inflammation; possibly AF); association with atypical femoral fractures rare.
Alendronate	Prevention: 5 mg/d po or 35 mg/wk po, Tx: 10 mg/d po or 70 mg/wk po
Effervescent *(Binosto)* with cholecalciferol	Same as above
Ibandronate	Tx and prevention: 150 mg/mo po or 2.5 mg/d po; 3 mg IV q3mo
Risedronate	Tx and prevention: 35 mg/wk po, 5 mg/d po, or 150 mg/mo po

(cont.)

Table 99. Pharmacotherapeutic Prevention and Management of Osteoporosis[1] (cont.)	
Medication	**Administration/Comments**
Delayed-release *(Atelvia)*	35 mg/wk po
Zoledronic acid	Prevention: 5 mg IV given over >15 min q2y ; Tx: 5 mg IV given over >15 min every y. May cause acute renal failure in patients using diuretics.
Parathyroid Hormone and Parathyroid Hormone–related Protein Analogs	Avoid in patients with Paget disease, prior skeletal radiation tx, hx of skeletal malignancies, hypercalcemic disorders, or metabolic bone disease other than osteoporosis; can cause hypercalcemia.
Abaloparatide *(Tymlos)*	Tx for no more than 2 y; may cause orthostatic hypotension (K)
Teriparatide *(Forteo)*	Tx for 1 y followed by 1 y of bisphosphonates or raloxifene can maintain 1-y gains in BMD (L, K)
Others	
Denosumab *(Prolia)*	Skin infections, dermatitis, osteonecrosis of jaw, hypocalcemia especially if CrCl <30, hypoparathyroidism, malabsorption, or uncorrected calcium. Risk of atypical fracture is expected to be similar to bisphosphonates. Rapid bone loss when drug is discontinued.
Romosozumab-aqqg *(Evenity)*	Tx is limited to 12 mo. D/C if MI or stroke during tx. Hypocalcemia, especially if eGFR 15–29 or on dialysis, osteonecrosis of jaw, atypical fractures, arthralgia

CrCl unit = mL/min; eGFR unit = mL/min

[1] Unless specified, medication can be used for prevention or tx.

[2] Risk factors include IV tx (little data on osteoporosis doses); cancer; dental extractions, implants, and poor-fitting dentures; glucocorticoids; smoking; and preexisting dental disease. Some experts recommend that bisphosphonates be stopped for several months before and after elective complex oral procedures, or, if procedures are emergent, that bisphosphonates be held for several months after.

PAIN

DEFINITION

An unpleasant sensory and emotional experience associated with actual or potential tissue damage (International Association for Study of Pain taxonomy)

Acute Pain

Distinct onset, usually evident pathology, short duration; self-limiting; common causes: trauma, postsurgical pain

Persistent or Chronic Pain

Pain that does not remit in the expected amount of time; due to ongoing nociceptive, neuropathic, or mixed pathophysiologic processes, often associated with functional and psychologic impairment; may occur in absence of any past injury or evident body damage; can fluctuate in character and intensity over time (**Table 100**). Chronic pain occurs on at least half of the days for 6 mo or more (National Pain Strategy 2016, iprcc.nih.gov/national-pain-strategy-overview/national-pain-strategy-report), referred to as persistent pain hereafter.

Table 100. Types of Pain, Examples, and Management

Type of Pain and Examples	Typical Description	Nonpharmacologic Interventions and Effective Drug Classes
Peripheral		
Nociceptive: somatic (eg, tissue injury of bones, soft tissue, joints, muscles)		
Arthritis, low-back pain, myofascial pain, bursitis, tendonitis, burn, muscle spasms, contractures	Well localized, constant; aching, stabbing, gnawing, throbbing	Motor-control exercises (yoga, tai chi), PT and manipulation, CBT, acupuncture/acupressure, massage, TENS, other nondrug tx, APAP, topical anesthetics/NSAIDs, intraarticular corticosteroid, salsalate, NSAIDs, duloxetine, opioids
Acute postoperative, fracture, bone metastases	Well localized, constant; aching, stabbing, gnawing, throbbing	APAP, topical anesthetics/NSAIDs, nondrug tx (eg, massage, music), NSAIDs, opioids
Nociceptive: visceral (eg, tissue injury of visceral organs including heart, lungs, testes, and biliary system)		
Renal colic, gastritis, peptic ulcer, cholecystitis, bowel obstruction, peritonitis, constipation	Diffuse, poorly localized, referred to other sites, intermittent, paroxysmal; dull, colicky, squeezing, deep, cramping; often accompanied by nausea, vomiting, diaphoresis	Tx of underlying cause, APAP, IV NSAID, opioids (not for constipation) with nondrug tx

(cont.)

Table 100. Types of Pain, Examples, and Management (cont.)		
Type of Pain and Examples	**Typical Description**	**Nonpharmacologic Interventions and Effective Drug Classes**
Neuropathic: peripheral nervous system (eg, injury to nervous system—nerves and spinal cord)		
Cervical or lumbar radiculopathy, postherpetic neuralgia, trigeminal neuralgia, diabetic neuropathy, phantom limb pain, herniated intervertebral disk, spinal cord injury, drug toxicities	Prolonged, usually constant, but can have paroxysms; sharp, burning, pricking, tingling, pins-and-needles, shooting electric-shock–like; associated with other sensory disturbances (eg, paresthesias, dysesthesias); allodynia, hyperalgesia, impaired motor function, atrophy, or abnormal deep tendon reflexes	Nondrug tx, topical anesthetics, TCAs, SNRIs, anticonvulsants, opioids
Nociplastic or Mixed (eg, pain from altered nociception despite no clear evidence of actual or threatened tissue damage; neurologic dysfunction or combined and uncertain causes)		
Myofascial pain syndrome, somatoform pain disorders, fibromyalgia; poststroke; TMJ dysfunction, tension headache	No identifiable pathologic processes or symptoms out of proportion to identifiable organic pathology; widespread musculoskeletal pain, stiffness, and weakness; fatigue, sleep disturbance; taut bands of muscles and trigger points; sensitivity to sensory stimuli	Exercise, PT, and CBT, other nondrug psychologic tx, antidepressants, antianxiety agents

Note: Cancer pain may present with any of the types described above.

OVERVIEW

Comprehensive evaluation of pain is important in establishing an individualized tx plan that incorporates unique risks and characteristics. **Figure 9** provides overview of approaches described in more detail to follow.

EVALUATION

Key Points, Approach

- Perform comprehensive evaluation for underlying cause of pain, pain characteristics, and impact on physical and psychosocial function and quality of life. Identify multiple factors (eg, anxiety, depression, beliefs, insomnia, fear avoidance, biomechanical issues) that when combined with pain can cause impairment or dysfunction.
- Geriatricpain.org for provider and caregiver tools and resources for pain assessment
- Use interprofessional assessment and tx (eg, pharmacists, physical therapists, psychologists) when possible, particularly for persistent pain.
- Patient's report is the most reliable evidence of pain intensity and impact on function.
- Assess for pain on each presentation (older adults may be reluctant to report pain).
- Use synonyms for pain (eg, burning, aching, soreness, discomfort).
- Use a standard pain scale (eg, Numeric Rating Scale, Verbal Descriptor Scale, or Faces Pain Scale); adapt for sensory impairments (eg, large print, written vs spoken).
- Reassess regularly for improvement, deterioration, and complications/AEs, and document.

- Be aware of own implicit biases related to pain perception and tolerance in historically marginalized groups, especially Black people, that impact pain tx choices.

History and Physical Exam

- Evaluate underlying diseases that are known to be painful in older persons (**Table 100**); note hx of chronic pain. Most common sites of pain include back, neck, hip, knee, foot, and hand.
- Consider potential drug toxicities due to neuropathies (eg, amiodarone, bortezomib, leflunomide, ixabepilone, chemotherapeutic agent neuropathy, antibiotic-induced neuropathies). Note if neuropathy is acute after starting medication, or if there is an increase in existing neuropathy after adding a new medication.
- Focus on a complete examination of pain source and on musculoskeletal, peripheral vascular, and neurologic systems, as well as any body part that might be the source of referred pain.
- Physical exam essential to identify physical pain contributions (eg, leg length discrepancy, hip OA, myofascial pain, sacroiliac joint syndrome).
- Distinguish new illness from chronic condition.
- Analgesic and other tx hx: effectiveness, AEs, current and previous prescription and OTC drugs, "natural" remedies.
- Lab and diagnostic tests to establish etiologic diagnosis. More than half of patients who report being pain-free have radiographic evidence of degenerative joint disease, thus not useful as evidence of pain etiology.
  - Avoid imaging studies (MRI, CT, or x-rays) for acute low-back pain without specific indications.[CW] *Note:* Comparative plain film x-ray may be highly important in identifying new vertebral compression fractures in symptomatic patient.
  - Don't recommend advanced imaging (eg, MRI) of the spine within the first 6 wk in patients with nonspecific acute low-back pain in the absence of red flags (eg, trauma hx, unintentional weight loss, immunosuppression, cancer hx, IV drug use, steroid use, osteoporosis, age >50, focal neurologic deficit, and progression of symptoms).[CW]
  - Do not use electromyography and nerve conduction studies to determine cause of axial lumbar, thoracic, or cervical spine pain.[CW]

Characteristics of Pain Complaint

Provocative (aggravating) and **P**alliative (relieving) factors—what makes better or worse?
Quality (eg, burning, stabbing, dull, throbbing)—to establish type of pain to guide tx
Region (eg, pain map)—anticipate multiple pain locations and conditions
Severity (eg, scale of 0 for no pain to 10 for worst pain possible)—ask how tolerable pain is
Timing (eg, when pain occurs, frequency and duration)—to guide tx plan

Psychosocial Assessment

- Depression, anxiety, mental status (p 2 for screen). Impact on family or significant other. Enabling behaviors by others (eg, over-solicitousness, codependency, reinforcing debility).
- Evaluate pain coping, fear avoidance, and pain self-efficacy that impact tx success.

Functional Assessment

- ADLs, impact on activities, and quality of life
- Evaluate sleep pattern and perception of quality sleep.

Figure 9. Assessment and Treatment Approaches for Pain Management in Older Adults.

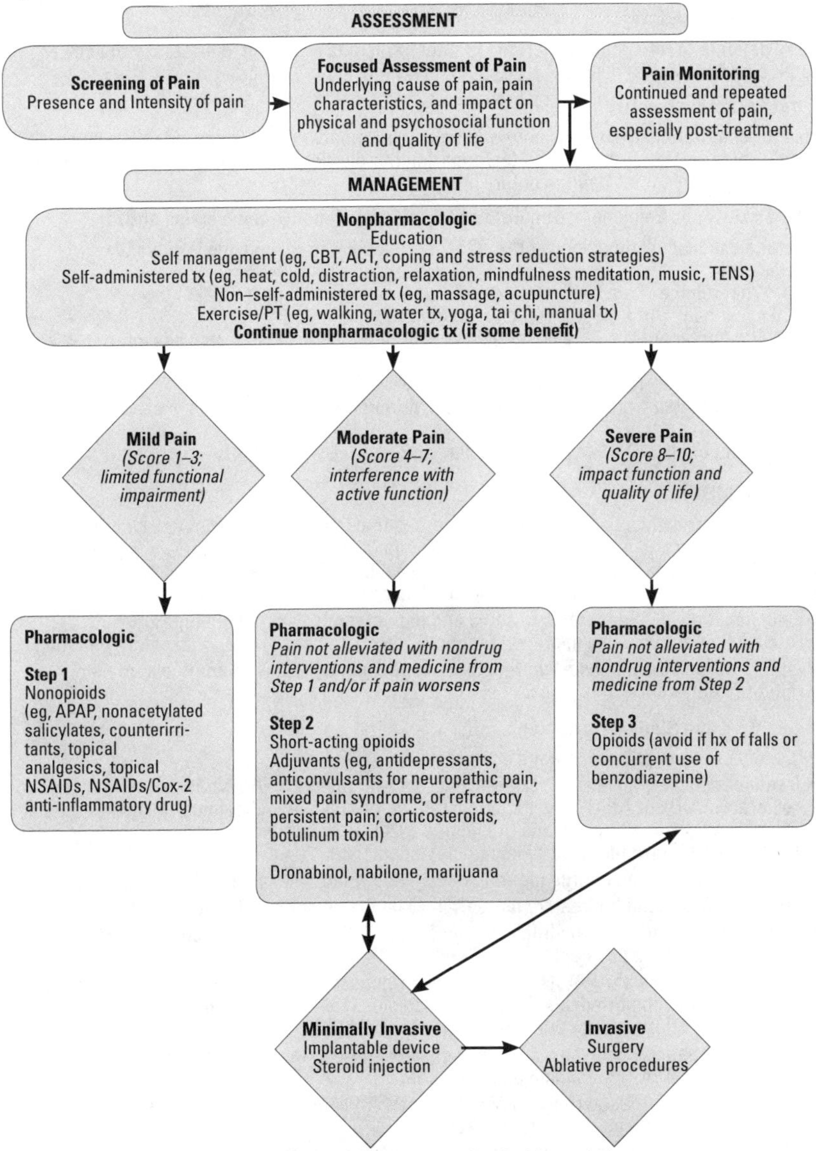

Source: K Herr, University of Iowa, College of Nursing, 2020. Used with permission.

Assessing Pain and Impact on Function

Functional Pain Scale

Asks patients to rate pain as tolerable or intolerable and how pain interferes with activity (active and passive activities)

Brief Pain Inventory (BPI)

Use for comprehensive assessment of pain and its impact (https://www.mdanderson.org/research/departments-labs-institutes/departments-divisions/symptom-research/symptom-assessment-tools/brief-pain-inventory.html).

PEG Scale (Pain, Enjoyment, General Activity; VA-developed 3-item version of BPI)

Average 3 individual question scores. 30% improvement from baseline is clinically meaningful.

Q1: What number from 0–10 best describes your pain in the past week?
  0 = "no pain", 10 = "worst you can imagine"

Q2: What number from 0–10 describes how, during the past week, pain has interfered with your enjoyment of life?
  0 = "not at all", 10 = "complete interference"

Q3: What number from 0–10 describes how, during the past week, pain has interfered with your general activity?
  0 = "not at all", 10 = "complete interference"

MANAGEMENT

Goal: To find optimal balance in pain relief, functional improvement, and AEs. Nondrug (complementary and alternative tx) can be beneficial and considered early in tx plan, particularly in managing persistent pain problems. Combination of drug and nondrug approaches may lower dosing of analgesics and reduce ADRs.

- Establish realistic measurable tx goals and expectations with patient (eg, 30% pain reduction or significantly improved function), social and family supports, before initiating tx.
- Involve caregivers and seek out resources (eg, community-based programs) to help reinforce adherence to tx plans.

Acute Pain and Short-term Management

- Identify cause of pain and treat if possible.
- Treat acute pain from musculoskeletal injuries with topical NSAIDs with or without menthol gel, oral NSAIDs or APAP, specific acupressure, or TENS. Avoid opioids, including tramadol (American College of Physicians Guidelines 2020). Tx that reduces inflammatory processes may actually contribute to chronic pain development.
- Teach patient to use nondrug techniques (eg, heat/cold, relaxation, TENS).
  - Do not recommend bedrest for more than 48 h when managing low-back pain.[CW]
- Refer to PT for selected nondrug strategies (eg, TENS, joint mobilization, stabilizing exercises, assistive devices).
- Use fixed schedule of APAP, NSAIDs (consider nonselective vs celecoxib depending on risk factors and comorbidities, **Figure 9**), or opioids (**Table 101**). Combination of APAP and NSAIDs may offer superior analgesia than either alone.
  - Do not exceed 3000 mg maximum daily dose of APAP in those with normal liver function and no other APAP-containing pain medications.
  - Local anesthetic-based regional anesthesia techniques; continuous nerve block provides postoperative analgesia with fewer AEs.
  - Topical local anesthetic agents reduce discomfort of procedural pain, including lidocaine topical 5%, vapocoolant anesthetic sprays, and lidocaine gel.

- NSAIDs shortest possible time postoperatively, D/C or lower dose after 24–48 h.
- Older adult postop pain management often includes combination of APAP, celecoxib, and gabapentin.
- When opioids required, use should taper with healing of injury.
  - Prescribe lowest dose of IR opioids and no greater quantity than needed for expected duration of pain severe enough to require opioids.
  - Do not prescribe ER or LA opioids for acute pain.
  - When increasing doses of ≥50 morphine milligram equivalent dose (MME)/d, reassess risk-benefit ratio.
  - Buprenorphine HCl (*Buprenex*OTC) 0.15 mg inj q6h slow IV has favorable safety profile with reduced risk for respiratory depression; better tolerated but nausea common during titration. Consider before Schedule II (eg, fentanyl, oxycodone) or Schedule IV (eg, tramadol) options based on patient's underlying conditions.

Persistent Pain

- Identify and treat local causes of pain with local tx (eg, manipulation, massage, heat, PT, TENS), topical anesthetics (eg, lidocaine oint/pch or diclofenac gel/pch/gtt), minor interventions (eg, steroid joint injection), or surgery.
- Educate patient and promote self-management and coping. Include caregiver when possible.
  - Use positive messaging and establish realistic expectations and goals for pain relief. Complete absence of pain may not be possible, but reduction in severity to maximize function and quality of life is priority.
  - Identify and address attitudes, beliefs, and barriers that interfere with tx success (eg, concerns about pain, beliefs that impact willingness to try a pain tx, concerns about tx considered).
  - Promote healthy behaviors including physical activity, weight control, and sleep.
  - Refer to Pain Self-Management program and resources (healthinaging.org/a-z-topic/pain-management).
  - Refer to Arthritis Foundation or community resources such as senior centers (arthritis.org)
  - Geriatricpain.org for provider and caregiver tools and resources for pain management
  - Consider age, gender, education, income/insurance impact on use. Younger, female with higher education more likely to use complementary and psychological interventions. Older, female, insured, and highly educated more likely to use PT, OT, and rehabilitative tx.
- Emphasize self-administered tx (eg, heat, cold, massage, liniments, topical agents, distraction, relaxation, music, virtual reality) and self-management approaches (eg, CBT). Prescribe exercise for analgesic effects (p 295).
- Establish exercise or movement-based program and consider barriers to adherence (eg, lack of time, fear of exacerbating pain, lack of perceived need, lack of motivation). Ask about exercise habits at each visit.
  - Strength training, aerobic conditioning, and flexibility exercises optimal
    - Intensities up to 80% of 1 repetition maximum (RM) for resistance training and 60% maximum HR or maximum oxygen update are safe for patients with OAs.
  - Progressive exercise key component
    - Isometric exercises progressed gradually from 30–75% muscle maximum voluntary contraction
    - Isometric resistance training increased by 5–10% weekly
    - Aerobic intensity increased by 2.5% weekly

  - Individual measures of intensity frequency and duration should be specified and gradually increased.
- In those overweight with mild to moderate pain, start with weight loss (eg, MOVE!® Weight Management program, cardiovascular or resistance land-based exercises, aquatic program).
- Exercise, rest, heat/cold application, massage, distraction, relaxation, and support groups are useful in long-term care settings.
- Add tx taught or conducted by professionals (eg, coping skills, biofeedback, imagery, hypnosis) as needed.
- To target interventions, the common problem of chronic low-back pain benefits from careful evaluation of potential etiologies (eg, hip OA, lumbar spinal stenosis, myofascial pain, fibromyalgia, depression, leg length inequality, sacroiliac joint pain, iliotibial [IT] band pain, insomnia).
  - Trigger-point tx (including dry and wet needling, stretching, and strengthening exercises) by manual PT, chiropractic, or acupuncture can be useful for neck, shoulder, and lower torso muscular pain.
  - See Musculoskeletal chapter for nondrug tx for hand, knee, and hip (**Table 85**).
- Combine pharmacotherapy and nonpharmacologic strategies as needed.
- Treat comorbid psychiatric conditions associated with persistent pain, including anxiety, depression, and PTSD.
  - Options include psychotherapy, biofeedback, mindfulness training, counseling (relationship, social, financial, substance abuse)
- Consider therapeutic injections (eg, steroid injections, nerve blocks) to treat acute and persistent pain syndromes (see Musculoskeletal chapter for specific indications).
  - Injections are rarely sole tx.
  - Diagnostic value can be determined by response to an injected local anesthetic.
  - Spinal cord stimulation may be useful for failed back syndrome (ie, postlaminectomy), complex regional pain syndrome, and neuropathic pain.
  - Intrathecal infusions may be indicated for both cancer and noncancer pain.
- When appropriate, refer for:
  - Consult PT and OT for mechanical devices to minimize pain and facilitate activity (eg, splints, assistive devices for joint unloading), TENS, range-of-motion and ADL programs.
  - Pain clinic with interdisciplinary team approach for complex pain syndromes with poor response to first-line tx.
  - Psychiatric pain management consult for somatization or severe mood or personality disorder.
  - Anesthesia pain management consult for possible interventional tx (eg, neuraxial analgesia, injection tx, neuromodulation, radiofrequency denervation) when more conservative approaches are ineffective.
  - Pain or chemical dependency specialist referral for management of at-risk patients and those with substance misuse or substance use disorder.

Pharmacotherapy

Approach

- Base initial choice of analgesic on the severity and type of pain and impact on function; consider cost, availability, patient preference, comorbidity, impairments, safety, and adverse outcomes (**Figure 9** and **Table 101**).
- For ongoing tx, careful risk-benefit analysis should be completed when determining appropriate drug and use.

- Standing analgesic orders used consistently at specified intervals should minimize need for prn doses.
  - Write order for type of pain and level of pain with guidance on how and when to select a prn medication from options as ordered in **Table 101**.
  - Dosage range should be provided with fixed time interval (appropriate to drug pharmacokinetics) and adequate to permit appropriate and safe titration based on patient's status and need (typically limited to 2–3× lower dose).
  - Avoid therapeutic duplication of prn opioid analgesics. Clarify criteria for route if >1 route ordered.

Table 101. Principles of Analgesic Management for Persistent Pain in Older Adults

Drug Class and Dosing	Practical Considerations
Step 1: Treatment of Mild Pain (Score of 1–3 and limited functional impairment)	
Acetaminophen (APAP) (**Table 87**)	Mixed evidence in management of chronic low-back pain and OA, but first line due to safety profile. Continue evaluating risk vs benefit for prescribing APAP due to recent evidence of uncertain analgesic benefit and increased safety concerns. Advise against alcohol use; schedule around-the-clock. Ask about all OTC with APAP.
Nonacetylated salicylates (eg, salsalate) (**Table 87**)	Consider if inflammatory pain.
Aspirin (ASA) *(Vazalore)*	Liquid-filled gel C preparation with faster absorption in GI and reduced GI erosions and ulcers associated with IR ASA; not OTC
Counterirritants	Use in localized musculoskeletal pain. May be effective for arthritic pain, but effect limited when pain affects multiple joints. Apply to affected area and monitor for skin injury, especially if used with heat or occlusive dressing. Ideal for minor pains due to minimal side effects. Avoid applying to wounds or damaged skin. Many available OTC with limited evidence to support use.
✓Camphor-menthol-phenol^{OTC}	lot: camphor 5%, menthol 5%, phenol 5% prn; max q6h
✓Camphor and phenol^{OTC}	S: camphor 5%, phenol 4.7% prn; max q8h
✓Methyl salicylate and menthol	Monitor for salicylate toxicity if used over several areas.
(eg, *BenGay* oint^{OTC}, *Icy Hot* crm^{OTC})	methyl salicylate 18.3%, menthol 16% q6–8h
(eg, *BenGay* extra strength crm ^{OTC})	methyl salicylate 30%, menthol 10% q6–8h
✓Trolamine salicylate (*Aspercreme* rub^{OTC})	trolamine salicylate 10% q6h or more frequently
OTC counterirritants	Use 1 pch at a time.
Icy Hot pch 5% menthol^{OTC}	May moderately reduce musculoskeletal or neuropathic pain
Icy Hot Advanced^{OTC} pch 7.5% menthol	Burning is common, but decreases with time. Do not leave patch on for >1 h (max 2 pch/24 h)
BenGay Pain Relieving^{OTC} pch 5% menthol	Patches may have advantage if nongreasy

(cont.)

Table 101. Principles of Analgesic Management for Persistent Pain in Older Adults (cont.)

Drug Class and Dosing	Practical Considerations
Salonpas Pain Relief OTC pch 3% menthol/10% methyl salicylate *Salonpas Pain Relieving Patch* OTC 3.1% camphor/6% menthol/10% methyl salicylate *Salonpas Original* OTC 1.2% camphor/5.7% menthol/6.3% methyl salicylate	Caution applying near eyes, genitals Use no more than 2 pch/d and for no more than 3 d in a row.
Topical Analgesics (Musculoskeletal Disorders p 213; Neurologic Disorders p 234)	Temporary tx of minor pain associated with muscles and joints due to backache, strains, sprains, cramps, arthritis; pain associated with diabetic neuropathy OTC compounded topical analgesics available, although no evidence to support use Never apply over broken or compromised skin. Wash hands after applying or use glove. Do not use heating pad.
✓Capsaicin (eg, *Capsin, Capzasin-HP, No Pain-HP, R-Gel, Zostrix, Qutenza*)	Evidence for localized peripheral neuropathic pain, particularly postherpetic neuralgia and HIV neuropathy. Only use in dermal neuropathic pain. Renders skin and joints insensitive by depleting and preventing reaccumulation of substance P in peripheral sensory neurons; may cause burning sensation (which is intolerable to some) up to 2 wk; instruct patient to wash hands after application to prevent eye contact; do not apply to open or broken skin. Pch should be applied by health professional, using a local anesthetic, to the most painful skin areas (max of 4 pch). Apply for 30 min to feet, 60 min to other locations. Repeat no more often than every 3 mo. Risk of significant rise in BP after placement; monitor patient for at least 1 h. Crm effective in OA.
Salonpas Hot OTC pch 0.025% capsaicin	
✓Lidocaine *(Lidoderm)*	*Lidoderm* safe, effective for localized peripheral neuropathic pain, approved for postherpetic neuralgia. Limited evidence for other painful conditions (low-back pain, OA). Monitor for rash or skin irritation; potential for systemic absorption; dosing limit of 3 pch applied up to 24 h/d
OTC lidocaine <5% available	OTC products: no comparative studies. Apply up to 12 h.
Topical NSAIDs (Table 87) Diclofenac OTC	As effective as oral NSAIDs with fewer systemic and GI AE for chronic localized musculoskeletal pain, particularly hand and knee OA. Lack of clear efficacy data in acute or chronic low-back pain, neuropathic pain. Don't combine topical plus oral NSAIDs. Evaluate serum Cr as some systemic absorption. *Note:* Some topical tx are expensive and insurer may not cover.

(cont.)

Table 101. Principles of Analgesic Management for Persistent Pain in Older Adults (cont.)	
Drug Class and Dosing	**Practical Considerations**
NSAIDs/Cox-2 anti-inflammatory drug (Musculoskeletal Disorders p 213, **Table 87**)	Avoid nonselective NSAIDs for chronic use (>6 wk) and in patients with hx of gastric or duodenal ulcers, unless other alternatives are not effective and patient can take gastroprotective agent.[BC] Use NSAIDs with caution in highly selected patients (eg, acute-on-chronic pain flare or new acute pain problem [eg, gout] in existing persistent pain disorder [eg, chronic low-back pain]) for short-term use (<2 wk) with nonacetylated salicylate, or ibuprofen or celecoxib. Avoid scheduled use of PPI for >8 wk unless for high-risk patients (eg, chronic NSAID use).[BC] See **Table 7** Periodically assess for GI and renal toxicity, HTN, HF, and drug-drug and drug-disease interactions
Step 2: Treatment of Moderate Pain (Score 4–7 and interference with active function [eg, exercise, mobility-related], pain not alleviated with medicine from Step 1, and/or if pain worsens)	
Adjuvants (**Table 102**)	Consider adjuvant analgesics, including antidepressants and anticonvulsants, for patients with neuropathic pain or mixed pain syndromes, or refractory persistent pain. Tailor to pain characteristics/etiology and risk factors. Effects may be enhanced when used in combination with other analgesics and/or nondrug strategies. Select agents with lowest AE profiles. Begin low and titrate slowly; allow adequate therapeutic trial (eg, 2–3 wk for onset of efficacy).
Short-Acting Opioids	See section on Opioid Use (p 264). MME[1] provided below to use in converting from one opioid to another due to differences in opioid potency.

Drug/Formulations	**MME[1]**	**Starting Dosage for Opioid-Naive**	**Comments**
Hydrocodone + APAP (formerly *Vicodin*)	30 mg po	2.5–5 mg q4–6h	*Caution:* Total APAP dosage should not exceed 3 g/d
Hydrocodone + ibuprofen	30 mg po	7.5/200 mg	Monitor renal function and use gastric protection ER T without abuse-deterrent formulation
Oxycodone	20 mg po	2.5–5 mg q4–6h	Limited information on dosing in renal failure; use caution despite weak active metabolites and avoid if CrCl <30 ER abuse-deterrent products available
Oxycodone + APAP	20 mg po	2.5–5 mg oxycodone q6h including 325 mg APAP	
(Magnacet)	20 mg po	2.5–5 mg oxycodone q6h including 400 mg APAP	

(cont.)

Table 101. Principles of Analgesic Management for Persistent Pain in Older Adults (cont.)

Drug Class and Dosing		Practical Considerations	
Drug/Formulations	**MME[1]**	**Starting Dosage for Opioid-Naive**	**Comments**
Oxycodone + ASA	20 mg po	2.25–4.5 mg oxycodone q6h	Monitor renal function and use gastric protection
Oxycodone + ibuprofen	20 mg po	1 tab po q6h; do not exceed 4 tabs in 24 h	Monitor renal function and use gastric protection. Tx not to exceed 7 d.
Tramadol[BC]	150–300 mg po	25 mg q4–6h; increase 25–50 mg in divided doses over 3–7 d to max dose of 100 mg 4×/d; not >300 mg for those aged >75 Oral sol available 5 mg/1 mL for flexibility in titrating dosing and for patients with swallowing difficulties	Not first-line tx; consider before starting pure opioids. Avoid in seizure disorders.[BC] Risk of seizures (↑ risk with higher doses and combination with SSRI/TCA) and orthostatic hypotension; withdrawal symptoms can occur. Higher risk of hip fracture on initiation than codeine and commonly used NSAIDs. Higher mortality in older adults with OA over 1 y follow-up compared to NSAIDs, not codeine. Higher all-cause mortality, cardiovascular AEs, and fractures compared to codeine. When CrCl <30, reduce dose for IR; Avoid ER.[BC]
Tramadol[BC] + APAP	150–300 mg po	2 tabs q4–6h; max 8 tabs/d	*Caution:* total APAP dosage should not exceed 3 g/d.

Drug Class and Dosing	Practical Considerations
Marijuana (Substance-Related and Addictive Disorders, p 352)	*Chronic pain:* Limited evidence but effective in controlling noncancer persistent pain
Cannabidiol (CBD)	Mixed results on efficacy of CBD products in relieving pain in older adults; inconsistent labeling of OTC CBD products impacting safety and quality control; CBD legalization varies by state. Avoid CNS depressants and alcohol while on CBD tx. Avoid activities requiring mental acuity.
Dronabinol *(Marinol)* Nabilone *(Cesamet)*	Starting dose 2.5 mg po 2×/d, 1 h before lunch and dinner. If unable to tolerate, initiate 1×/d 1 h before dinner or at bedtime to reduce risk of CNS symptoms.
Step 3: Treatment of Moderate to Severe Pain (Score 6–10), pain not alleviated with nondrug interventions and medicine from Step 2, and severe enough to impact function and quality of life	
Opioids	Avoid if hx falls or concurrent benzodiazepine use.[BC] See section on Opioid Use (p 264).

(cont.)

Table 101. Principles of Analgesic Management for Persistent Pain in Older Adults (cont.)

Drug Class and Dosing	Practical Considerations		
Drug/Formulations	**MME[1]**	**Starting Dosage for Opioid-Naive**	**Comments**
Morphine *(MSIR, Astramorph PF, Duramorph, Infumorph, Roxanol, OMS Concentrate, MS/L, RMS, MS/S)*	30 mg po 10 mg IV, IM, SC	5 mg po q4h; 1–2 mg IV q3–4h; 2.5–5 mg IM, SC q4h; 5–10 mg Sp q3–4h	Not recommended in renal failure; metabolites accumulate
Hydromorphone	7.5 mg po 1.5 mg IV, IM, SC 6 mg rectal	1–2 mg po q3–6h; 0.1–0.3 mg IV q2–3h; 0.4–0.5 mg IM, SC q4–6h; 3 mg Sp q4–8h	Considered safer in renal insufficiency
Oxymorphone *(Opana, Opana injectable)*	10 mg po 1 mg IV, IM, SC	5 mg po q4–6h; 0.5 mg IM, IV, SC q4–6h 5 mg Sp q4–6h	Use carefully in renal failure and liver impairment ER option with abuse-deterrent properties

Drug Class and Dosing	Practical Considerations
Extended-Release and Long-Acting Opioids Transdermal buprenorphine ER Hydrocodone bitartrate *(Zohydro ER)* ER Hydromorphone *(Exalgo)* ER Morphine ER Oxycodone Oxycodone/acetaminophen ER *(Xartemis XR)* Tramadol ER[BC] *(Ultram ER, ConZip)* Tapentadol ER *(Nucynta ER)* Transdermal fentanyl	When opioids are indicated, ER products reduce dosing frequency and may be useful in adherence and in those with cognitive impairment. Not for use with opioid-naive patients and avoid in frail older adults with cachexia. Given that the long-term use of opioids is not recommended unless clearly warranted, ER and LA opioids are less often used. FDA label indication for ER opioids for management of pain severe enough to require daily, around-the-clock, long-term opioid tx and for which alternative tx options are inadequate. Tapentadol decreased pain with limited psychophysical or cognitive change in older patients. Transdermal fentanyl and buprenorphine are options when need for long-acting opioid and patient unable to take oral or enteral medications. See product information for starting dose for ER products.
Methadone	Due to variability of pharmacokinetics and pharmacodynamics of methadone, referral to and consult with an expert in methadone dosing should occur before attempting to change to or from methadone. Risk of dose accumulation; associated with prolonged QTc interval. Acceptable in renal insufficiency. Consult palliative care or pain service. For details on methadone prescribing and monitoring, see https://www.samhsa.gov/medication-assisted-treatment/medications-counseling-related-conditions/methadone
Rapid-acting opioids Fentanyl *(Actiq, Abstral, Fentora, Lazanda, Subsys, Onsolis)*	Do not use in opioid-naive patients. Use is for breakthrough pain in those on opioid tx. May be used in oncology and palliative care. Consult package information and consult with palliative care or pain specialist.

NA, not applicable; CrCl unit = mL/min.

[1] Morphine milligram equivalent dose (MME), dose of opioid equivalent to 10 mg of parenteral morphine or 30 mg of oral morphine with chronic dosing.

Opioid Use in Persistent Pain

Considerations in Opioid Use

- Nonpharmacologic interventions and nonopioid tx are preferred for persistent pain. If not effective, consider opioids if moderate to severe pain impacts function and quality of life and expected benefits for both pain and function are anticipated to outweigh risks to the patient. Careful risk-benefit analysis is essential.
  - Establish potential benefits of opioid use in improved function and quality of life. Situations in which opioids may be beneficial include high-intensity cancer-related pain, daily or almost daily frequent or continuous severe pain related to serious underlying conditions, and high-intensity neuropathic pain due to partially or totally uncorrectable underlying cause (eg, spinal nerve-root compression).
  - Assess for medical risks (eg, respiratory, sleep apnea), potential for misuse or abuse of opioid medication, and potential adverse effects of opioids.
  - Before starting opioids for chronic pain, establish tx goals for pain and function and consider how opioid tx will be discontinued if benefits do not outweigh risks. See below for creating an opioid plan and abuse-prevention approaches.
  - Before starting opioid tx, discuss with patients known risks and realistic benefits of opioid tx as well as patient and clinician responsibilities for managing tx.
  - Increased risk of falls, fall injuries, and fractures during first 2 wk of use. Educate older adults and family on preventive actions, including slow rising with time to stabilize before walking, removal of throw rugs, use of walker or cane or other supports until dizziness or unsteadiness resolves.
  - Establish standard expectations for use to reduce risks and protect others from unintentional or intentional diversion in practice setting. Communicate to patients verbally and in simple written materials.
  - Screen for risks of opioid misuse with thorough hx, medical record review, prescription drug monitoring program (PDMP) review, and standard opioid risk tool (eg, ORT-OUD, SOAPP-R). (See digital text for more information on PDMPs.)
  - Risks of opioid abuse/misuse behaviors and overdose deaths are lower in older adults.
- Select patients who may benefit from low-dose opioid tx in combination with other tx (eg, specific somatic, peripheral, or neuropathic pain).
  - Avoid opioids in chronic central or visceral pain syndromes such as fibromyalgia, headaches, or abdominal pain.
- Evaluate benefits and harms within 1–4 wk of initiating opioid tx for persistent pain or of dose escalation. Evaluate continued tx q90d or more frequently.
  - Continue opioid tx only if there is clinically meaningful improvement in pain and function that outweighs risks to patient safety.
  - If benefits do not outweigh harms, optimize other tx and work to taper opioids to lower dosages or to taper and D/C opioids.
  - Discuss availability of naloxone with patients and caregivers when beginning and renewing opioid prescriptions (FDA labeling recommendation).

Changing

- Use long-acting or SR analgesics for continuous pain after stabilizing dose with short-acting opioid. Administer around-the-clock for continuous pain.
- Use MMEs as a common denominator for all dose conversions to avoid errors, and titrate to effectiveness. See hopweb.org/index.cfm?cfid=101993669.
- When changing opioids, decrease equivalent analgesic dose by 25–50% because of incomplete cross-tolerance.

Tapering

- Unless person exhibits life-threatening issues or warning signs of impending overdose (eg, confusion, sedation, slurred speech), opioid tx should not be discontinued abruptly, and clinicians should not rapidly reduce opioid dosages from higher dosages.
- Decision to taper down or off opioids should be based on individualized assessment of benefits and risks considering diagnosis, circumstances, and unique needs. See *HHS Guide for Clinicians on the Appropriate Dosage Reduction or Discontinuation of Long-term Opioid Analgesic* (hhs.gov/opioids/sites/default/files/2019-10/Dosage_Reduction_Discontinuation.pdf).

Management of Opioid Adverse Events

- Older adults more sensitive to AEs and may present atypically. Higher risk for falls and fractures; lower risk for opioid misuse and overdose.
- Monitor for dry mouth, constipation, sedation, nausea, delirium, urinary retention, and respiratory depression. Growing evidence supports concerns related to cognitive impairment, sleep, endocrine dysfunction (hypogonadism), immunosuppression, and hyperalgesia.
- Tolerance can develop to most adverse effects of opioids, except constipation. Reduce dosage or consider adding medication to counter ADRs, if troublesome, until tolerance develops.
- Warn about risk of APAP toxicity when using combination products and the importance of including all OTC products with APAP in daily APAP total (not to exceed 4 g/d po in healthy and 3 g/d po in frail older adults).
- Sedation: Warn patient about the risk of sedation with opioids that gradually resolves within 1 wk.
- Delirium or agitation: Opioid-induced urinary retention can present as delirium or agitation.
- Constipation
  - Anticipate, prevent, and vigorously treat. Begin prophylactic, osmotic, or stimulant laxative when initiating opioid tx **(Table 66).** Titrate laxative dose up with opioid dose. Docusate is not recommended because it has shown limited efficacy.
- OIC can result. If prophylactic and first-line interventions (dietary changes, OTC tx, exercise) are not effective, evaluate for OIC using Bowel Function Index focused on 3 items rated on 0–100 scale: in the past 7 d, (1) ease of defecation, (2) feeling of incomplete bowel evacuation, and (3) personal judgment of constipation. Score of 30 or higher merits the consideration of prescription OIC medication.
- Opioid antagonists are approved to treat OIC. Careful titration and observation are necessary because some patients may experience partial analgesia reversal (also **Table 66**, p 151). See Palliative Care, Pain.

Prevention of Opioid Harm, Misuse, Abuse, and Withdrawal

Opioids should be initiated as a trial, to be continued if progress is documented toward functional goals, and if there is no evidence of complications, including misuse or diversion. An ongoing tx plan for all patients receiving opioid tx that includes the following is good practice:

- Evaluate for risk of harm. Known risk factors include:
  - Illegal drug use; prescription drug use for nonmedical reasons
  - Hx of substance use disorder or overdose
  - Mental health conditions (eg, depression, anxiety)
  - Sleep-disordered breathing
  - Concurrent benzodiazepine use

- Assess for risk of opioid misuse or abuse (eg, ORT-OUD or SOAPP-R); Substance-Related and Addictive Disorders, p 352, https://nida.nih.gov/sites/default/files/opioidrisktool.pdf.
  - A score of 3 or higher on the ORT-OUD is considered high risk for opioid use disorder. Prescribe opioids only after all other tx modalities exhausted, under close supervision—ideally in consultation with a pain or addiction specialist.
  - In at-risk patients requiring opioid management, abuse-deterrent agents may be useful (eg, *Embeda, Targiniq ER*).
- Consult CDC for resources and tools to support safe opioid prescribing, monitoring, and education of patients (https://www.cdc.gov/opioids/healthcare-professionals/prescribing/index.html)

Adjuvant Medication Use

- Medications not typically used for pain may be helpful for its management, depending on the etiology (eg, antidepressants, antiseizure medications).
- Use alone or in combination with nonpharmacotherapy and other analgesics (**Table 102**).

Table 102. Adjuvant Medications for Pain Relief in Older Adults[1]

Class, Medication	Indications/Comments
Anticonvulsants (also **Table 96** and p 231)	Indicated for neuropathic pain, fibromyalgia If one does not work, try another. Numerous drug interactions (fewer for gabapentin and pregabalin); adverse effects include sedation, dizziness, peripheral edema Increased risk of falls due to dizziness and somnolence. Avoid if hx of falls or fractures.[BC] See **Table 7.**
Carbamazepine	Many drug interactions; mood stabilizer; used for trigeminal or glossopharyngeal neuralgia; may cause SIADH[BC], thrombocytopenia, leukopenia
Gabapentin[BC] (p 243)	Recommended as first line or as co-analgesic in postherpetic neuralgia and/or dermatosis papulosa nigra. Mixed evidence for neuropathic pain. Slow titration based on analgesic response increasing every 3–7 d (may take several mo). If CrCl >15–29, dose at 200–700 mg/d po; if CrCl >30–59, dose at 200–700 mg/d po q12h; if CrCl ≤15, dose at 100–300 mg/d po; reduce dose if CrCl <60.[BC]
Pregabalin *(Lyrica)*[BC] (p 243)	Primary indication is for management of postherpetic neuralgia, diabetic peripheral neuropathy, and fibromyalgia; fewer AEs and titration to analgesic effect more rapid. Start 100 mg/d po in divided doses increasing to 300 mg/d po over several wk. Effect in 3–4 wk. Reduce dose if CrCl <60.[BC]
Antidepressants (Table 42)	Indicated for neuropathic pain, fibromyalgia, chronic musculoskeletal pain, including OA and chronic low-back pain, depression. TCAs often helpful for migraine or tension headaches and arthritic conditions. Avoid tertiary amines due to increased AEs.[BC] Of TCAs, low-dose desipramine or nortriptyline best side-effect profile, however avoid due to anticholinergic, sedating, and orthostatic hypotension.[BC] Older adults more sensitive to anticholinergic effects, use cautiously with comorbid disease. SNRIs lower anticholinergic properties. Data on SSRIs for pain management lacking, but may increase bleeding risk if combined with ASA or NSAIDs; taper dose before discontinuing. Avoid if hx of falls or fractures.[BC]

(cont.)

Table 102. **Adjuvant Medications for Pain Relief in Older Adults[1] (cont.)**	
Class, Medication	**Indications/Comments**
Duloxetine	Preferred SNRI for older adults, typically well tolerated with reduced side effects Significant drug-drug interactions. Monitor for serotonin syndrome. Slow taper when discontinuing, may require 10 mg po for days (open capsule and put half in applesauce).
Venlafaxine *(Effexor XR)*	Analgesic effect is dose dependent and often requires higher dosing than for antidepressant effect.
Milnacipran *(Savella)*	Dual reuptake inhibitor; used to treat pain of fibromyalgia; contraindicated with MAOI or within 2 wk of MAOI discontinuation
Corticosteroids (Table 52)	Low-dose medical management may be helpful in inflammatory pain conditions. Intraarticular injection first-line tx for hip OA; taper dose if discontinuing
Skeletal Muscle Relaxants[BC]	Limited evidence of effectiveness, predominantly sedating with limited analgesic effect. High risk for older adults due to anticholinergic ADRs, excessive sedation, and weakness. Recommended for short-term use to relieve acute pain associated with true spasticity (baclofen and tizanidine may be useful). Avoid or use with caution in older adults due to limited efficacy and adverse effects.[BC] Monitor for muscle weakness, urinary function, cognitive effects, sedation, orthostasis; potential for many drug-drug interactions. Avoid abrupt discontinuation because of CNS irritability.
Neuromuscular Blocking Agent	Injected into muscles to treat myofascial pain syndrome resulting from skeletal muscle spasm and migraines when source is neck or facial muscles
Onabotulinum toxin A *(Botox)*	Dosing individualized based on muscle affected, severity of muscle activity, and prior experience; not to exceed 360 U IM q12–16wk

CrCl unit = mL/min

[BC]Avoid.

[1] Useful for moderate and/or severe pain depending on pain etiology.

Medical Marijuana Use for Chronic Pain

- Medical marijuana is legal in most US states and provides an alternative to opioids for moderate to severe pain.
- No cannabinoid is currently FDA approved as analgesic, although there is evidence of efficacy. Little information on optimal dosing.
- Monitor for signs of excessive use or abuse; neurologic or psychiatric AEs (eg, dysphoria, euphoria, somnolence, vertigo).
- Oral, synthetic cannabis products with high THC:CBD ratios (>98% THC) and sl extracted cannabis products with comparable THC:CBD ratios may be associated with short-term improvements in chronic pain but increased risk of dizziness and sedation.
- For patients who tell you that they are already or will be starting to use CBD or THC, provide guidance:
  - THC products: typically 1:1 THC:CBD is preferred to minimize THC psychoactive effects. Starting dose of THC 0.5 mg to 3 mg (initially at night) and increase to a maximum of 30–40 mg.

- For persistent pain, suggest edibles or capsules: start 1/4 to 1/2 of a single serving; standard serving is 10 mg.
  - Beware of lag time to effect (1–2 h). If patients are expecting a psychoactive effect and do not feel it quickly, they might take more doses and have more AEs.
- For breakthrough pain, suggest solutions and tinctures: starting dose 1–2 mg po 3×/d.
- Avoid inhaled or vaporized, unless the patient insists. If so, recommend vaporized cannabis flower; avoid high-THC strains. Most vaporized products provide approximately 2 mg for a 3-sec inhalation. Always check the product guide. Might be better for patients with short-lasting symptoms or to avoid prolonged psychoactive effects.
- Caution patients:
  - On the additive effects with their CNS active medications; drug interactions with warfarin, anticholinergics, alcohol, other highly protein-bound medications (glipizide, loop diuretics, statins)
  - No driving for 6 h after inhalation; for 8–9 h after edible ingestion of a high-THC product
  - Beware of withdrawal symptoms (eg, when hospitalized), including anxiety, headache, and hypersomnia
- Caution patients that products labeled as CBD frequently also contain THC above state limits for CBD-only products and the amount of CBD in products might not be reliable. Monitor LFTs at 1, 3, and 6 mo.

◦ CBD-alone products have very limited data on analgesia but are a reasonable starting place for cannabis-naive patients.
- Good safety profile with respect to nonsedating, no misuse potential, minimal AEs
- Starting dose should not be more than 5–10 mg; may increase to 40–50 mg.
- Little data on topicals, but feasible that, if carrier has lipid solubility, agent could be useful for musculoskeletal pain.

PAIN IN THE COGNITIVELY IMPAIRED OLDER ADULT

Assessment and Management

- Pain is highly prevalent in all subtypes of dementia. Use simple pain tools (eg, scale with none, mild, moderate, or severe pain; yes/no questions) to solicit self-report of pain in persons with moderate cognitive impairment.
- Assess pain in persons with severe cognitive impairment or inability to communicate pain using the Pain Assessment algorithm (**Figure 10**), including medical hx and physical exam to identify potential pain etiologies.
- Use nonverbal pain behavior tool, such as Pain Assessment in Advanced Dementia (PAINAD) or Pain Assessment Checklist for Seniors with Limited Ability to Communicate (PACSLAC-II), to identify potential pain problems. PAINAD is useful with cognitively impaired Black patients.
- Attempt nondrug interventions relevant to etiology of pain and most useful in persons with dementia, including distraction, massage, heat, exercise or activity, music, and relaxation or rest.
- In cognitively impaired persons with behavioral disturbances or agitation suspected of an underlying pain etiology for which other causes have been ruled out and with behaviors not responding to nondrug interventions, try an analgesic trial for diagnostic purposes to evaluate pain etiology. The following is a guide to be adjusted based on individual comorbidities and contraindications:
  - Try APAP first (if no hepatic dysfunction). Order scheduled rather than prn. APAP is often effective in improving behaviors, function, or both.

    - If no response to APAP after 24–48 h and if localized inflammatory pain is suspected, try topical NSAIDs, lidocaine, or both.
    - If no response after 24 h, try morphine sulfate sol (5–10 mg po q4–6h) or oxycodone 5–10 mg po q6–8h. Consider buprenorphine transdermal pch (5 mcg/h to max 10 mcg/h for 7 d) if unable to take oral analgesic. *Caution:* monitor for changes in neuropsychiatric status in frail older adults, particularly in combination with antidepressants.
  - If no response to APAP after 24–48 h and if neuropathic pain is suspected, try pregabalin 50 mg po 3×/d (Reduce dose if CrCl <60 mL/min[BC]). If pain diagnosis is supported by a response to pregabalin, consider a tx plan that includes pregabalin or gabapentin.
- Carefully monitor response to analgesics with each change as agent and dose are titrated to achieve pain relief yet avoid undesirable AEs.
- If behavior improves with pain tx, establish pain tx plan considering risks, benefits, and costs of tx options.
- For analgesic consideration:
  - Limited evidence is available on the safety and efficacy of analgesics or adjuvants for persons with dementia.
  - APAP appears to be generally safe and well tolerated.
  - NSAIDs use appears to be associated with increased risk of GI and cardiovascular AEs; short-term NSAID use has not been investigated.
  - Opioid AEs—limited data about safety for persons with dementia.

Figure 10. Pain Assessment in Older Adults with Severe Cognitive Impairment

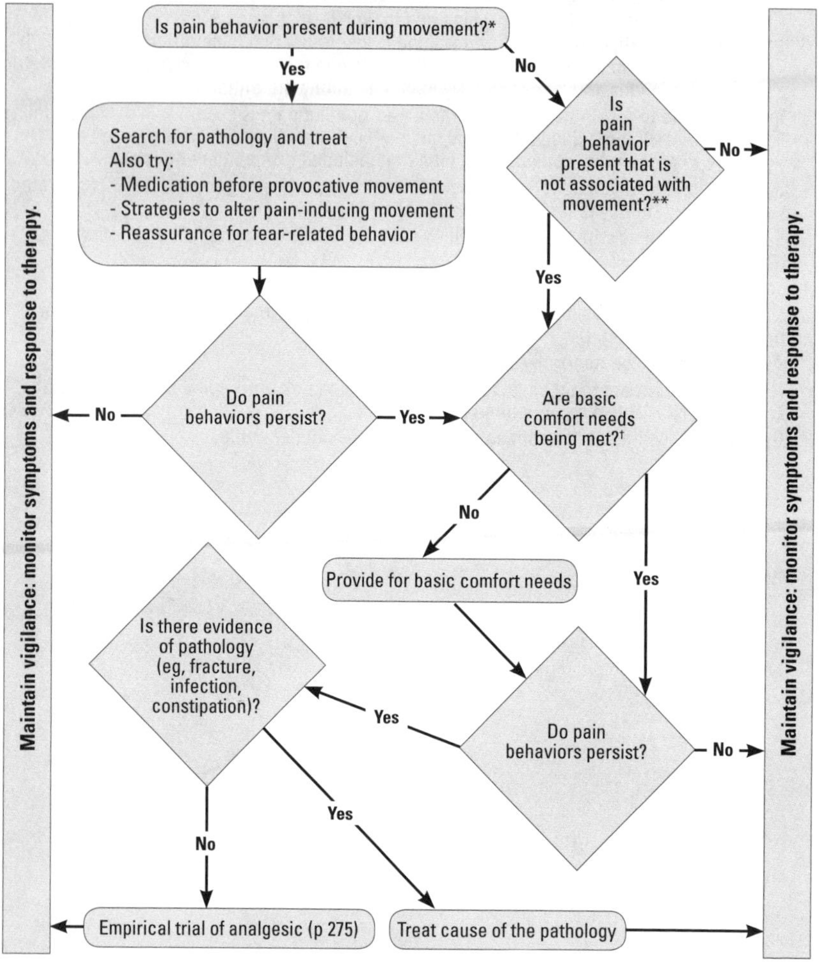

*Examples: facial expressions (eg, grimacing, frowning, expressive eyes, raised upper lip, mouth opening); body movements (eg, guarding, rigid/stiff, rubbing, resisting care, restlessness); vocalizations (eg, pain-related words, sighing, complaining, shouting, groaning)

**Examples: agitation, fidgeting, sleep disturbance, diminished appetite, irritability, reclusiveness, disruptive behavior

†Examples: toileting, thirst, hunger, visual or hearing impairment

Sources: American Geriatrics Society. *J Amer Geriatr Soc* 2002; 50(6 Suppl):S205–S240; Kunz et al. *Euro J Pain* 2019; 24(1): 192-208; Ersek et al (2019). *Pain Medicine* 2019; 20(6): 1093–1104.

PALLIATIVE CARE AND HOSPICE

DEFINITION

Palliative care is a patient- and family-centered approach that optimizes quality of life by anticipating, preventing, and treating suffering associated with serious life-threatening or terminal illness. Palliative care is not setting specific and occurs throughout the course of serious illness addressing physical, psychosocial, and spiritual needs to facilitate patient autonomy, access to information, and choice. Hospice care is palliative care provided by an interprofessional team for patients who are no longer seeking curative tx and who have a prognosis of ≤6 mo if the disease follows its normal trajectory. Hospice care is neither intended to shorten nor extend life expectancy, but evidence suggests that hospice could prolong life for some patients with certain conditions (eg, advanced lung cancer, advanced HF).

APPROACH

- Initiate palliative care at the time of diagnosis of serious or life-threatening disease.
  - Key predictors of survival include dependency of ADLs, presence of comorbidities, poor nutritional status and weight loss, abnormal vital signs and lab values.
  - Disease-specific predictors of survival include dementia, COPD, cancer, Parkinson disease, and HF.
- Enlist a comprehensive, interprofessional team (physicians, nurses, social workers, chaplain, pharmacist, PTs, OTs, dietitian, family and caregivers, volunteers) as appropriate and available to develop culturally sensitive palliative care plans to anticipate, prevent, and treat physical, psychological, social, and spiritual needs.
- Advance care planning (ACP) should occur early to enable patients to:
  - define goals and preferences for medical tx and care
  - discuss these with family and healthcare providers
  - record, review, and update these preferences, as needed
- High-quality ACP or goals of care conversations can occur over video.
  - Consider partially filled out forms based on discussion and send to patient to complete; in some states, a witnessed digital or phone consent may be acceptable for orders for life-sustaining care (eg, POLST).
- Educate, plan, and document advance directives; final wishes; healthcare and financial proxy; family awareness of decisions (see Assessment and Approach, p 8).
- Facilitate early access to hospice care when possible.
  - Refer to a Medicare-certified hospice program. The Medicare Hospice Benefit is comprehensive and may relieve the family of considerable financial burden. Interview local hospice programs to determine scope of clinical services, especially complex pain management (ie, interventional approaches) and access to inpatient hospice care, if needed.
- Support, educate, and treat both patient and family.
  - Communicate, listen, and support decision-making
  - Focus on attainable goals
  - Teach stress management skills, coping
  - Encourage conflict resolution
  - Help complete unfinished business
  - Urge focus on non–illness-related affairs and one day at a time

- Address physical, psychologic, social, and spiritual needs.
  - Promote physical and psychological comfort
  - Encourage spiritual practices
  - Anticipate grief, losses, and completion of unfinished business
  - Refer to PT
- Coordinate care among providers. Help integrate potentially curative, disease-modifying, and palliative tx.
- Focus on the continuum of needs, from symptom management, comfort, meeting goals, completing "life business," healing relationships, and bereavement.
- Offer bereavement support.

PAYMENT

- Except for hospice, all palliative-care services are reimbursed though public or private payers using the same mechanism used for physician payment, or have a variety of funding from grants and healthcare system subsidy.
  - Medicare-certified hospices are funded primarily through the Medicare Hospice Benefit (that is also observed by most private insurers).

DECISIONS ABOUT PALLIATIVE CARE

Palliative care is a low-risk intervention that improves many patient-facing outcomes. Recommend without reservation.

Follow principles of informed decision-making (**Figure 1**) to determine decisional capacity of the patient (p 8).

Goals of Care Discussions and Planning

Patients need to be alerted to the expected trajectory of their serious or life-threatening disease, and advanced care planning should be initiated at the time of first diagnosis. Updates on the progression of the patient's disease along the trajectory of the illness should be communicated with the patient and their family at least annually or more frequently depending on the needs of the patient. Focus on living as well as you can for as long as you can.

Goals of care discussions can occur at diagnosis of a serious illness, progression of disease, functional decline, poor quality of life, limited prognosis, and transitions in care settings. These are opportunities to review patient progress and then establish or revisit patient goals and preferences.

Table 103. Examples of Illness Trajectory of Functional Decline Before Dying

Trajectory	Condition	End-of-Life Needs and Prognosis
Short period of functional decline before death	Cancer	Predictable decline over weeks or months Plan palliation and eventually hospice care
Chronic illness with exacerbations and sudden dying	CHF, COPD, end-stage liver disease, AIDS	Periods of acute exacerbations; variability day to day and week to week; may stabilize for periods; aggressive symptom relief. Discuss hospice home care if frequent unscheduled emergent medical visits or hospitalizations.

(cont.)

Trajectory	Condition	End-of-Life Needs and Prognosis
Progressive deterioration	Dementia, Parkinson disease, advanced MS	Prolonged course; gradual physical and cognitive decline with increase fatigue, weight loss, and oral intake; multiple comorbidities; challenge for caregivers; infectious complications are late and often terminal events; address benefits and burdens of artificial nutrition and hydration. Follow course of disease using Palliative Performance Scale (PPS) or FAST to help guide hospice discussion and referral.
Sudden, severe neurologic injury	Stroke, traumatic brain injury	Death in acute stage or from complications or after tx withheld; uncertainty of neurologic outcomes and physical and cognitive ability and chance for improvement. Best option for home-based care if desired during last days-to-weeks via hospice.

Table 103. Examples of Illness Trajectory of Functional Decline Before Dying (cont.)

Source: Periyakoil V et al. *Primer of Palliative Care*. 7th Ed. Chicago IL: American Academy of Hospice and Palliative Care; 2019.

Communicating Bad News (SPIKES)

S=Setting: Prepare for discussion by ensuring all information, facts, and data are available. Deliver in person in a private area without interruptions or physical barriers. Determine individuals who patient may want involved.

P=Establish patients' perception of their illness (knowledge and understanding) by asking open-ended questions. Use vocabulary patient uses when breaking bad news.

I=Secure invitation to impart medical information. Determine what and how much the patient wants to know.

K=Deliver knowledge and information in a sensitive, straightforward manner; avoid technical language and euphemisms. Check for understanding after small chunks of information and clarify concepts and terms.

E=Use empathetic and exploratory responses; use active listening, encourage expression of emotions, acknowledge patient's feelings.

S=Strategize and summarize and organize an immediate tx plan that addresses patient's concerns and agenda. Provide opportunities to raise important issues. Reassess understanding of condition and tx plan and determine the need for further education and follow-up with patient and family.

Communicating Prognosis

- Estimating prognosis is challenging and evolves with patient location in disease trajectory, response to tx, complications, and other factors.
- Communicating prognosis is to prepare patients and families for what is to come and support informed decision-making.
- Sources of data to estimate prognosis include patient physiological status, functional status scales (eg, Karnofsky Performance Scale, PPS, FAST), disease-based prediction rules, web-based programs, and hospice eligibility criteria.
  - PPS scores of 10–60% and ≥70% provide distinct survival curves.
  - *Prognostat Tool* estimates chances of survival in palliative-care patients based on sex, age, diagnosis, and initial PPS score.
  - The *ePrognosis* calculator is an interactive prognostic tool for older adults with mortality estimates derived from geriatric prognostic indices (eprognosis.org).

- Most—but not all—patients and families want to know prognosis. Establish the desire and expectations for communicating prognosis.
- Frame delivery with uncertainty using ranges and exceptions. Be honest, but provide hope for meaningful remaining life.

Advance Directives

- Any written or verbal statement that provides guidance of what tx the patient might desire. Living wills document tx patient might refuse in a life-threatening situation and typically require the patient's witnessed signature.
- Designed to respect patient's autonomy and determine their wishes about future life-sustaining medical tx if unable to indicate wishes (p 8).
- Written by the patient and documented, although not accepted by emergency medical services as legally valid forms; vary from state to state.
- Spoken conversations with relatives, friends, and clinicians should be thoroughly documented in the medical record for later reference; these documented conversations carry the same ethical and legal weight as those recorded, if properly verified.
- The role of the team in assisting with advance directives and ACP is to ensure that the patient's wishes are met, wherever they may lie on the spectrum of care.
- Discussions related to advance directives are billable (see Assessment and Approach, p 8).

Durable Power of Attorney (POA) for Healthcare or Healthcare Proxy

- A written document that enables a capable person to appoint someone else to make future medical tx choices for them in the event of decisional incapacity (**Figure 1**).

Instructional Advance Directives (DNR Orders, Living Wills, MOLST, POLST, POST)

- Do-Not-Resuscitate (DNR) orders written by the physician based on the wishes previously expressed by the individual in their advanced directive or living will.
- Physician Orders for Life-Sustaining Treatment (POLST), Physician Orders for Scope of Treatment (POST) or Medical Orders for Life-Sustaining Treatment (MOLST) include written instructions about starting, continuing, withholding, or withdrawing particular forms of life-sustaining medical tx.
- POLST documents differ from state to state, but are designed to be recognizable (eg, bright pink; posted on refrigerator), used by first responders, and transferred across settings.
- Clinicians who comply with such directives are provided legal immunity for such actions.
- POLST form can be very useful in formalizing patient preferences (polst.org). May be revoked or altered at any time by the patient.
- Key elements of POLST Plan of Care address cardiopulmonary resuscitation, level of medical intervention desired in the event of an emergency (comfort only, limited tx, or full tx), and use of artificial nutrition and hydration. Some states include use of antibiotics, hospitalization, and mechanical ventilation.
- To determine whether POLST should be completed, ask "Would I be surprised if this person died in the next year?" If no, the POLST is appropriate.

Key Interventions, Treatment Decisions to Include in Advance Directives

- Resuscitation procedures
- Mechanical respiration
- Chemotherapy, radiation tx
- Dialysis
- Simple diagnostic tests
- Pain control
- Blood products, transfusions
- Intentional deep sedation
- ICD and pacemakers

Withholding or Withdrawing Therapy

- Any person can refuse tx at any time. Withholding tx (not starting) has same legal and ethical standing as withdrawing tx (stopping it after it has been started), although withdrawal is clinically and emotionally more challenging.
- Beginning a tx does not preclude stopping it later; a time-limited trial may be appropriate.
- Palliative care should not be limited, even if life-sustaining tx are withdrawn or withheld.
- Decisions on artificial feeding should be based on the same criteria applied to the use of ventilators and other medical tx.
- Initiate discussion about pacemaker deactivation only if potential patient benefit; consider the potential negative effects of deactivation before disabling the pacemaker. *Note*: Pacemaker is not a resuscitative device and typically does not keep palliative-care patients alive.
- Reanalyze risk-to-benefit ratio of ICD tx in patients with terminal illness. Life-prolonging tx may no longer be desired.

Death Certificate Completion (see Assessment and Approach, p 13)

- Certification of death at the end of life may be completed by the hospice medical director or primary provider and provides personal information about the decedent and about circumstances and cause of death.
- Information is important for settlement of estate and provides family members closure, peace of mind, and documentation of the cause of death.

HOSPICE

Hospice is comprehensive and coordinated bio-psycho-social-spiritual approach to interdisciplinary care at the end of life that also incorporates grief and bereavement services.

Referral and Eligibility

- Patients, families, or other healthcare providers can make a referral to hospice; eligibility for service is confirmed by a certification of terminal illness (CTI) from the primary care provider or the hospice medical director (**Table 104**).
  - CTI must state the objective reasons for established prognosis, which often includes the diagnosis, its rate of change, the patient's functional status, and various biometric markers of decline.
  - **Table 104** provides guidelines for disease-specific prognosis, but multiple comorbidities and unique circumstances necessitate a carefully documented statement of the best rationale for admission. A patient may not be referred simply because "they need more help." Some states may have expanded eligibility criteria or concurrent care demonstration projects, though most follow the recommendations in **Table 104.**
  - Patients are evaluated for eligibility upon admission and every 60–90 d thereafter.
- Referral is appropriate when curative tx is no longer indicated (ie, ineffective, AEs too burdensome) and life is limited to months. A simple tool to help with decision-making is to ask "Would I be surprised if this patient died within 6 months"? If "no," cite and document specific reasons to support this conclusion.

Approach

- Hospice is designed for people who have a prognosis of <6 mo, but there is no limit on how long a person may spend enrolled in hospice as long as their illness continues to cause decline.
- Patients may rescind hospice if their illness improves, and then return to hospice without penalty at a later point.

- Hospice must be accepted by the patient or family, or both, and can be rescinded at any time.
- Hospice provides palliative medications, medical supplies, durable medical equipment, team member visits as needed and desired by patient and family (physician, nurse, home health aide, social worker, chaplain), and volunteer services. Refer to Medicare Conditions of Participation that define requirements (eg, interdisciplinary team composition [physicians, nurses, social workers, bereavement counselors], levels of care, visits, team meetings, plan of care, documentation).
- Optimal hospice care requires adequate time in the program; waiting to refer until death is imminent does not take full advantage of hospice care.
- Hospice care is typically delivered in patient's home, but can occur in a nursing home or residential care facility (long-term care, assisted living) or in an inpatient setting (hospice-specific or contracted facility) if acuity or social circumstances warrant.
- Coverage of hospice services varies (eg, inpatient availability, amount of home care, sites for care), so determine and discuss with patient and family.

Table 104. Typical Trajectory and Hospice Eligibility for Selected Diseases

Disease	Typical Determinants for Hospice Eligibility[1]
Cancer	Clinical findings of malignancy with widespread, aggressive, or progressive disease evidenced by increasing symptoms, worsening lab values, and/or evidence of metastatic disease Impaired performance status with a PPS value of ≤70% Refuses further curative tx or continues to decline in spite of definitive tx
End-stage heart disease	Optimally treated for heart disease or either not candidates for surgical procedures or who decline those procedures (optimally treated: not on vasodilators have a medical reason for refusing [eg, hypotension or renal disease]) ***and*** Significant symptoms of recurrent HF at rest and classified as NYHA Class IV (ie, unable to carry on any physical activity without symptoms, symptoms present at rest, symptoms increase if any physical activity is undertaken) Documentation of the following supports eligibility but are not required: • tx-resistant symptomatic supraventricular or ventricular arrhythmia • hx of cardiac arrest or resuscitation or unexplained syncope • brain embolism of cardiac origin • concomitant HIV disease • documented EF of ≤20%
Dementia	FAST Scale Stage 7 (p 84) ***and*** Have had 1 of the following in the past 12 mo: • aspiration pneumonia • pyelonephritis or other upper UTI • decubitus ulcer (multiple, Stage 3–4) • fever (recurrent after antibiotics) • inability to maintain sufficient fluid and calorie intake with 10% weight loss during previous 6 mo, or serum albumin <2.5 g/dL • septicemia

(cont.)

Table 104. Typical Trajectory and Hospice Eligibility for Selected Diseases (cont.)	
Disease	**Typical Determinants for Hospice Eligibility[1]**
End-stage pulmonary disease	Disabling dyspnea at rest, poorly or unresponsive to bronchodilators, resulting in decreased functional capacity, eg, bed to chair existence, fatigue, and cough (documentation of FEV_1, after bronchodilator, <30% of predicted is objective evidence for disabling dyspnea, but is not necessary to obtain) ***and*** Progression of end-stage pulmonary disease, as evidenced by *prior* increased visits to emergency department or *prior* hospitalization for pulmonary infections and/or respiratory failure or increasing physician home visits before initial certification (documentation of serial decrease of FEV_1 >40 mL/y is objective evidence for disease progression, but is not necessary to obtain) ***and*** Hypoxemia at rest on room air, as evidenced by pO_2 ≤55 mm Hg or O_2 sat ≤88% or hypercapnia, as evidenced by $PaCO_2$ ≥50 mm Hg. Values may be obtained from EMR within 3 mo. Documentation of the following will support eligibility, but not required: • right HF secondary to pulmonary disease (cor pulmonale) • unintentional progressive weight loss of >10% of body weight over preceding 6 mo • resting tachycardia >100 bpm
End-stage liver disease	PT >5 sec over control or INR >1.5 and Serum albumin <2.5 g/dL and one or more of the following: ascites refractory to tx or patient noncompliant, spontaneous bacterial peritonitis, hepatorenal syndrome (elevated Cr and BUN; oliguria [<400 mL/d], urine Na <10 mEq/L, cirrhosis, and ascites), hepatic encephalopathy refractory to tx or patient noncompliant, recurrent variceal bleeding despite intensive tx Documentation of the following will support eligibility: • progressive malnutrition • muscle wasting with reduced strength and endurance • continued active alcoholism (>80 g ethanol/d) • hepatocellular carcinoma • HBsAg (hepatitis B) positivity
Chronic renal failure	Not seeking dialysis or renal transplant or discontinuing dialysis ***and*** CrCl <10 mL/min (<15 mL/min for DM) ***or*** Serum Cr >8 mg/dL (>6 mg/dL for DM) (<15 mL/min with comorbid CHF; <20 mL/min for people with DM) Documentation of the following signs and symptoms of renal failure support eligibility: • uremia • intractable hyperkalemia (>7) not responsive to tx • hepatorenal syndrome • oliguria (<400 mL/d) • uremic pericarditis • intractable fluid overload not responsive to tx
Failure to thrive[2]	BMI <22 kg/m^2 and either declining enteral/parenteral nutritional support or not responding to such support, despite adequate caloric intake ***and*** Karnofsky score ≤40 or PPS value ≤40% ***and*** Must have chronic disease diagnosis (eg, HF, COPD)

[1] May vary depending on fiscal intermediary; additional supportive indications available for most diagnoses. Source: Adapted from montgomeryhospice.org/health-professionals/end-stage-indicators (extracted from CMS documentation LCD for Hospice-Determining Terminal Status [L13653]).

[2] Adult failure to thrive can be used to determine hospice eligibility, but should not be listed as principal diagnosis.

MANAGEMENT OF COMMON END-OF-LIFE SYMPTOMS

Pain

Primary goal: to alleviate suffering and improve quality of life at end of life as defined by the patient and family

- See Pain chapter (p 252) for assessment and interventions.
- The most distressing symptom for patients and caregivers
- Placement of Foley catheters, limited repositioning to prevent increased pain are acceptable for comfort measures at the end of life.
- Alternate (nonoral) routes may be needed (eg, transdermal, transmucosal, rectal, vaginal, topical, SC or IV catheter, epidural, intrathecal) for analgesics and all medications.
- Organ system insufficiencies (eg, hepatic, renal) necessitate reduced dosing and increased intervals.
  - Methadone and fentanyl are not dialyzable
  - Monitor carefully for sedation and respiratory depression
- Provide orders for breakthrough IR pain medications when using long-acting opioids (ie, 10% total daily opioid dose)
- A white paper outlines appropriate methadone use in palliative care (McPherson ML et al. *J Pain Symptom Manage* 2019; 57[3]:635–645).
- Recommend expert pain management consult if pain not adequately relieved with standard analgesic guidelines and interventions.
- Additional tx may include:
  - radionuclides and bisphosphonates (for metastatic bone pain)
  - radiation tx or chemotherapy directed at source of pain
  - cannabinoids have analgesic properties, reduce nausea, and improve appetite and sleep
    - knowledge of prior use can guide informed care
  - nerve blocks effective for deep visceral pain and local plexopathy-related pain
    - consult with interventional pain specialist
- Pain crisis: Palliative sedation for intractable pain and suffering is an important option to discuss with patients. While evaluating cause, bolus of 10% opioid total daily dose can be administered. If no relief in 10–15 min, can administer higher dose. Subsequent doses q15min until relief obtained. Establish new equianalgesic dose. Other options include:
  - Ketamine 0.1 mg/kg IV bolus. Repeat prn q5min. Follow with infusion of 0.015 mg/kg/min IV (if IV access not available, SC at 0.3–0.5 mg/kg). Decrease opioid dosage by 50%.
  - Benzodiazepines may be used to induce sleep state in the event of excruciating pain unrelieved by other options. Observe for problems with increased secretions and treat (p 282).

Altered Mental Status, Delirium (Delirium, p 77)

- In inpatient palliative care, delirium prevalence increases to 88% in the last weeks and hours of life. The most common causes are medications (eg, opioids, anticholinergics, benzodiazepines), metabolic insufficiency from progressive organ failure, and infection. Other often overlooked causes include substance abuse, constipation, UTI, pain, skin infections, medications, and environmental overstimulation.
- Causes comorbidities (eg, falls, fracture impairment, psychological distress for family) and increased mortality
- Regular screening with validated tool (CAM, *DSM-5*, ICD-10)
- Collateral hx from caregiver with Single Question in Delirium (SQiD): Do you feel that (person's name) has been more confused lately?

- Optimize nondrug approaches: orientation, therapeutic activities, optimized sleep-wake pattern, mobilize, sensory aids use; hydration and nutrition monitoring, bladder and bowel function, supportive care, education.
- Investigate and manage reversible factors (if consistent with agreed-upon goals of care), including deprescribing opioid rotation, treating infection, fluid replacement, addressing environmental and other factors.
- Consider pharmacotherapy if needed for distress and safety. Haloperidol preferred: 1 mg po or 0.5 mg IV or SC (parenteral 2× as potent as oral) hourly prn until calm, then q6–12h in divided doses to maintain.
- Using benzodiazepines remains controversial. Cautious use as a trial in patients with agitation in whom haloperidol or nonpharmacologic tx failed.
- Although commonly used to manage delirium in palliative care, recent evidence suggests that antipsychotics are associated with both increased delirium symptoms and reduced patient survival.
- Lorazepam (3 mg) IV and haloperidol (2 mg) IV are reserved for severe cases or when seizures or alcohol withdrawal are suspected.
- Provide communication, education, and emotional support to patients, family, and healthcare team.

Anorexia, Cachexia, Dehydration

See also Malnutrition (p 204) and volume depletion (p 197). Universal symptom of patients with serious and life-threatening illness.

Note: Percutaneous feeding tubes are not recommended in patients with dementia; instead offer oral assisted feeding.[CW]

Reassure patient and caregivers that appetite abates with age and dehydration is not uncomfortable.

Nonpharmacologic Interventions

- Educate patient and family on effects of disease progression that result in lack of appetite and weight loss.
- Promote interest, enjoyment in meals (eg, alcoholic beverage if desired, involve patient in meal planning, small frequent feedings, cold or semifrozen nutritional drinks).
- Good oral care is important.
- Alleviate dry mouth with ice chips, popsicles, moist compresses, or artificial saliva.

Pharmacotherapy

- Corticosteroids: dexamethasone 1–2 mg po q8h; methylprednisolone 1–2 mg po q12h; prednisone 5 mg po q8h. Proven beneficial for palliative-care patients with cancer, but no evidence for patients with end-stage nonmalignant disease. Insufficient evidence for any particular corticosteroid or dosing regimen.

Note: Avoid prescription appetite stimulants or high-calorie supplements for tx of anorexia or cachexia in older adults; instead, optimize social supports, provide feeding assistance, and clarify patient goals and expectations.[CW]

Anxiety, Depression

- Provide opportunity to discuss feelings, fears, existential concerns. Short-term counseling.
- Referral to appropriate team members (spiritual, nursing)
- Medicate (Anxiety, p 47, and Depression, p 92)
- Psychostimulants (methylphenidate and modafinil) may be useful in terminally ill because of rapid onset and immediate energizing effects.
- Methylphenidate or ketamine can be used for depression in palliative care.

- Virtual reality can improve mental health through cognitive stimulation, improved mood, and reduced agitation and anxiety in palliative care and hospice setting.
- Most patients with cancer and concomitant anxiety and depression show substantial sustained improvements with experimental psychedelic use, (eg, peyote, psilocybin, synthetic LSD, ketamine) using guided sessions, monitoring, and counseling
  - Patients with terminal conditions can use state or federal "right to try" laws to gain access to psychedelic-assisted tx.
  - Unprescribed and unsupervised use is concerning and asking patient about alternative tx is wise.

Bowel Obstruction

Indications for Radiographic Evaluation

- To differentiate between constipation and mechanical obstruction
- To confirm the obstruction, determine site and nature if surgery is being considered

Nonpharmacologic Interventions

- Nasogastric intubation: only if surgery is being considered, for high-level obstructions, and poor response to pharmacotherapy
- Percutaneous venting gastrostomy: for high-level obstructions and profuse vomiting not responsive to antiemetics
- Palliative surgery
- Hydration: IV or hypodermoclysis

Pharmacotherapy (aimed at specific symptoms)

- Nausea and vomiting: haloperidol 0.5–5 mg (≤10 mg) po, IM q4–8h prn; ondansetron 4 mg IV (over 2–5 min) q12h, 8 mg po q12h (**Table 67**).
- Spasm, pain, and vomiting: scopolamine 0.3–0.65 mg IM, IV, SC q4–6h prn; 0.4–0.8 mg po q4–8h prn; transdermal 2.5 cm^2 pch applied behind the ear q3d ***or*** hyoscyamine 0.125–0.25 mg sl q6–8h.
- Diarrhea and excessive secretions: loperamide (**Table 68**); octreotide 0.15–0.3 mg SC q12h, expensive.
- Pain: **Table 102**.
- Inflammation due to malignant obstruction: dexamethasone 4 mg po q6h × 5–7 d.

Constipation (p 150)

- Most common cause: opioid AEs, medications with anticholinergic AEs, low intake food, fluid, and fiber, impaired mobility. Use stimulant or osmotic laxative (**Table 66**). Consider enema if no bowel movement for 4 d. Evaluate for bowel obstruction or fecal impaction. Treat OIC not responsive to laxative tx.
- Instances of severe OIC may respond to naloxone 0.8–2 mg po q12h, titrated to a max of 12 mg/d po given in water or juice, along with routine bowel regimen.
  - Methylnaltrexone bromide *(Relistor)* approved for OIC in adults with chronic, noncancer pain and those with advanced illness receiving palliative care 8 mg SC (38–62 kg) to 12 mg SC (62–114 kg) and 0.15 mg/kg for other weights with one dose q48h or 450 mg po 1×/d.
  - Naloxegol *(Movantik)* 25 mg po 1×/d is indicated for OIC in adult patients with chronic noncancer pain. D/C all maintenance laxative tx before initiating naloxegol. Use laxatives prn if no response to naloxegol after 3 d.

Cough (p 307)

Dysphagia (also p 144)

Nonpharmacologic Interventions

- Feed small, frequent amounts of pureed or soft foods.
- Avoid spicy, salty, acidic, sticky, and extremely hot or cold foods.
- Keep head of bed elevated for 30 min after eating. If possible, feed patient sitting upright.
- Instruct patient to wear dentures and to chew thoroughly.
- Use suction machine when necessary.
- Have speech therapist conduct a bedside swallowing assessment to develop techniques for mouth positioning, swallowing techniques, assistive equipment, and correct consistency of food and beverages.
- For painful mucositis: Do not use magic mouthwash.[CW] Use frequent and consistent oral hygiene; salt or soda mouth rinses.
- For chronic or intractable hiccups: limited evidence for breath holding, small sips of fluids, eating sweet or sour food, acupuncture. Medications to treat include baclofen, gabapentin, chlorpromazine, methylphenidate, metoclopramide, amantadine, nifedipine, benzodiazepines, and haloperidol; or combination.

Pharmacotherapy

- For oral candidiasis: clotrimazole 10-mg troches, 5 doses/d, ***or*** fluconazole 150 mg po followed by 100 mg/d po × 5 d.
- For severe halitosis: antimicrobial mouthwash; fastidious oral and dental care; treat putative respiratory tract infection with broad-spectrum antibiotics.

Dyspnea (p 309)

Nonpharmacologic Interventions

- If prognosis of months to years and not on hospice, pulmonary rehabilitation (p 310).
- Teach positions to facilitate breathing, elevate head of bed or sitting position leaning on table, pursed lips breathing with COPD.
- Teach relaxation techniques.
- Eliminate smoke and allergens.
- Ensure brisk air circulation (facial breeze) with a room fan if helpful to patient (or beneficial long-term effect); oxygen is indicated only for symptomatic hypoxemia (ie, SaO_2 <90% by pulse oximetry) or if comfort perceived by patient.
- Do not administer supplemental oxygen to relieve dyspnea in patients with cancer who do not have hypoxia.[CW]
- Noninvasive positive pressure ventilation (NPPV) is helpful to some patients.
- Use olive oil or swabs, and humidified oxygen, for dry mouth.

Pharmacotherapy

- Opioids: oral morphine concentration (20 mg/mL: 1/4 to 1/2 mL sl, po; repeat in 15–30 min prn) ***or*** morphine tabs 5–10 mg po q2h; if oral route not tolerated, nebulized morphine 2.5 mg in 2–4 mL NS ***or*** fentanyl 25–50 mcg IV in 2–4 mL NS; ***or*** morphine 1 mg IV or equivalent IV opioid q5–10min.
- Bronchodilators (**Table 122**).
- Diuretics, if evidence of volume overload (**Table 22**).

- Anxiolytics (eg, lorazepam 0.5–2 mg po, sl, SC q2–4h or prn); titrate slowly to effect.
- Corticosteroids (eg, dexamethasone) can reduce pulmonary edema and dyspnea, with improvement in days.
- Guaifenesin *(Robitussin)* or nebulized saline to loosen thick secretions.

Excessive Secretions

Pooling of saliva and retention of secretions can cause gurgling, crackling, and rattling (often referred to as death rattle). Disturbing to caregivers and family because this sounds like choking. Educate that no evidence suggests that this is a source of distress to the patient.

Nonpharmacologic Interventions

- Positioning to promote drainage and suctioning prn, although can cause discomfort to patient and deep secretions might not be accessible.
- Nebulized saline may help loosen thick secretions, but can trigger coughing.

Pharmacotherapy

- Glycopyrrolate 0.1–0.4 mg IV, SC q4h prn ***or*** scopolamine 0.3–0.6 mg SC prn ***or*** transdermal scopolamine pch q72h ***or*** atropine 1% ophthalmic drops, 1–2 gtt sl q1–2h prn

Existential Suffering

- Often present in terminal illness and associated with reduced quality of life, depression, anxiety, suicidal ideation, and desire for hastened death.
- Descriptions include lack of meaning and purpose, loss of connectedness to others, thoughts about dying process, difficulty finding sense of self, loss of hope, autonomy, or temporality.
- It is helpful to know patient's spiritual beliefs using questions based on the *FICA* Spiritual History Tool to gather information on **f**aith and belief, **i**mportance, **c**ommunity, and **a**ddress in care (smhs.gwu.edu/gwish/clinical/fica/spiritual-history-tool).
- Symptom interventions (eg, antidepressants, CBT) work in palliative-care setting, as well.
- Clarify new-onset symptoms, such as insomnia, for evidence of anxiety and existential suffering that require a broader approach.
- Assist patients to see that many things haven't changed since diagnosis and help reframe (eg, relationship with children changing from giving care to receiving care).
- Support family member distress from losing loved one and caregiving roles.
- Adjust tx boundaries to communicate connectedness or caring (eg, hold hand of dying patient, gentle hand on shoulder).
- Recommend formalized interventions such as meaning-centered psychotherapy, dignity tx, and other manualized therapies for existential distress.
- Help patients find a silver lining (eg, still alive, time to explore relationships and beauty).

Nausea, Vomiting (p 153)

Determine cause to select appropriate antiemetic based on pathway-mediating symptoms and neurotransmitter involved (**Table 67**). For refractory nausea and vomiting (ie, not amenable to other tx), a trial of dexamethasone (2 mg IV q8h) can be tried; risks are dyspepsia, altered mental status. Taper when discontinued.

Do not use topical lorazepam *(Ativan)*, diphenhydramine *(Benadryl)*, haloperidol *(Haldol)* ("ABH") gel for nausea.[CW]

However, in palliative care, haloperidol is commonly prescribed to treat nausea. Initial dose of 1 mg po (or pr) or 0.5 mg SC (or IV) 2–3×/d; may need to be increased significantly.

Olanzapine for chemotherapy-induced nausea (see Gastrointestinal Diseases, p 144).

Renal Failure

Decreased renal perfusion leads to renal failure and progressive uremia. Signs to note include decreased urine output, eventual oliguria or anuria, altered level of consciousness.

Management

- With primary kidney disease and end-stage renal insufficiency, discuss decision to stop dialysis and parenteral hydration.
- With secondary renal insufficiency, symptom management deals with dry mouth, dry mucous membranes, and unpleasant mental status (eg, may experience euphoria or progressive sedation).
  - Administering fluids typically will not reverse circulatory shutdown and can worsen cases of fluid overload.
  - Ensure peaceful, dignified dying consistent with patient and family goals of care.

Skin Failure

An event in which the skin and underlying tissue die due to hypoperfusion that occurs concurrent with severe dysfunction or failure of other organs

See Skin Ulcers (p 330) for Chronic Wound Assessment.

Management

- Interdisciplinary approach focused on resident-centered and caregiver-centered outcomes
- Engage in frank discussions regarding prognosis, tx of symptoms, and goals of care
- Manage pain determining if acute pain associated with debridement, associated with care routines, or chronic
- Repositioning to off-load pressure
- Dietary consultation regarding amount of calories and fluid to promote healing, if healing is considered possible
- Avoid wet-to-dry dressings, which can increase bacterial burden and infection
- Recommended dressings: nonadhesive, absorptive, and odor-controlling that prevent desiccation of wound bed, protect periwound from maceration, and can be left in place for longer periods (eg, hydrogels, foams, polymeric membrane foams, silicones, alginates)
- Control odor by removing necrotic debris and using antimicrobials, activated charcoals, and external odor absorbers

Weakness, Fatigue

Nonpharmacologic Interventions

- Modify environment to decrease energy expenditure (eg, placement of phone, bedside commode, drinks).
- Adjust room temperature to patient's comfort.
- Educate on sleep hygiene and reordering tasks to conserve energy (eg, eating first, resting, then bathing).
- Modify daily procedures (eg, sitting while showering rather than standing).

Pharmacotherapy

- Treat remediable causes such as pain, medication toxicity, insomnia, anemia, cachexia, dehydration or electrolyte imbalance, infection or fever, and depression.
- Consider psychostimulants (eg, dextroamphetamine [Avoid[BC]] 2.5 mg po qam or q12h, methylphenidate 2.5 mg po qam or q12h to start titrate upward to 3×/d or 4×/d prn, or

modafinil *[Provigil]* 200 mg po qam); monitor for signs of psychosis, agitation, or sleep disturbance. Prescribe doses before noon especially for ER to avoid insomnia.

PROPORTIONATE PALLIATIVE SEDATION (PPS)

- PPS is the use of progressively higher levels of sedation using opioids to relieve intractable and distressing physical symptoms at the end of life. PPS can lead to unconsciousness. It is not intentionally ending life or hastening death, but relieving uncontrollable suffering.
- Legal in all states in the US; most patients are imminently dying (typically within 2 wk).
- Conditions for which PPS might be initiated include agitated terminal delirium; unrelenting nausea, vomiting, dyspnea; and intractable pain.
- If rapid sedation to unconsciousness is the best approach, involve experts in palliative care and ethics.
- Obtain patient or surrogate decision-makers verbal or written consent before tx.
- Encourage patient and family to say goodbyes before initiating PPS.
- Document the clinical decision-making, including the nature of the intractable suffering, other tx tried and failed, consultations obtained, and consent from patient, family, or surrogate decision-maker.

PHYSICIAN-ASSISTED DYING AND ACTIVE EUTHANASIA

- Evaluate requests for hastened death to clarify what patients are asking for, support patient and family in your commitment to find solution to suffering, evaluate decision-making capacity, and ensure that efforts to address suffering have been addressed with intensified tx, if possible.
- Seek ethics consultation to resolve patient request based on clinician's inability to address intolerable suffering and personal and ethical principles without abandoning the patient.

Physician-assisted Dying

Although not recognized or promoted as acceptable palliative-care practice, providers need to be aware of the status of physician-assisted dying (also called aid in dying, death with dignity, right to die, compassionate dying, assisted suicide) to respond to a request from patients. Physician-assisted dying is the patient's intentional, willful ending of their own life with the assistance of another; it may involve providing knowledge, means, or both, to end one's life, including counseling about lethal doses of drugs, prescribing such lethal doses, or supplying the drugs; a criminal offense in most states.

- In states where legal (CA, CO, DC, HI, NJ, OR, VT, WA), eligibility must be established and may include: (1) aged 18 y or older, (2) resident of the state, (3) capable of making and communicating healthcare decisions for oneself, and (4) diagnoses with terminal illness that will lead to death within 6 mo.
- The patient must verbally request the medication at least twice and contribute to at least 1 written request.
- Physician must notify the patient of alternatives (eg, palliative care, hospice, pain management).
- Finally, physician is to request—but not require—that the patient notify their next of kin about the request of a prescription for a lethal dose of medication.

Active Euthanasia

Direct intervention, such as lethal injection intended to hasten a patient's death (also called mercy killing), is a criminal act of homicide in all states in the United States.

PREOPERATIVE CARE

Surgical Decision Making

- With the prospect of potential surgery, the patient's tx goals should be determined before surgical consultation.
- Goal setting is predicated on decision-making capacity, patient preferences, and life expectancy (see *Goal-Oriented Care, Life Expectancy, and Medical Decision Making and Informed Decision Making and Patient Preferences for Life-Sustaining Care,* p 7).
- Cognitive impairment, functional dependence, malnutrition, and frailty are risk factors for adverse outcomes of surgery (eg, mortality, functional decline, institutionalization).
- If surgery is determined to be a potential option that is in accordance with tx goals, additional cardiac, pulmonary, cognitive, functional, nutritional, and metabolic assessments should be conducted to further estimate surgical risk (see next 3 sections).

Cardiac Risk Assessment in Noncardiac Surgery (2014 ACC/AHA Guidelines)

- Risk of perioperative cardiac complications (eg, MI, death) is related to patient characteristics and type of surgery.
  - Major patient-related risk factors include active HF, LV dysfunction, CAD, and valvular disease.
  - Other patient-related factors include age, renal dysfunction, DM, and poor functional status.
  - Low-risk surgeries (<1% perioperative risk of MI or death) include cataract, endoscopic, breast, dermatologic, and superficial procedures.
  - Medium-risk surgeries (≥1% to <5%) include intraabdominal, major orthopedic, otolaryngology, major GU, and neurologic procedures.
  - High-risk surgeries (≥5%) include vascular, intrathoracic, and transplant surgeries.
- Several tools are available for formal assessment of cardiac risk, including:
  - Revised Cardiac Risk Index (RCRI): score 1 point each for: Cr ≥2 mg/dL, HF, DM, hx of stroke or TIA, CAD, and undergoing intrathoracic, intraabdominal, or suprainguinal vascular surgery. Total score ≥2 confers increased risk.
  - A risk calculator from the National Surgical Quality Improvement Program of the American College of Surgeons is available at https://riskcalculator.facs.org/RiskCalculator/index.jsp. This risk calculator generates estimates of numerous surgical outcomes, including geriatric outcomes such as delirium, functional decline, new mobility aid use, and pressure ulcers.
- **Figure 11** shows a suggested algorithm for assessment of cardiac risk.
- Obtain a preoperative ECG for patients with known CAD, arrhythmia, PAD, prior stroke or TIA, or other structural heart disease. ECG is not indicated in patients undergoing low-risk surgery.

Choosing Wisely Recommendations for Preoperative Cardiac Assessment

- Don't perform stress cardiac imaging or advanced noninvasive imaging as a preoperative assessment in patients scheduled to undergo low-risk noncardiac surgery.[CW]
- Patients who have no cardiac hx and good functional status do not require preoperative stress testing before noncardiac thoracic surgery.[CW]
- Don't perform routine preoperative testing before low-risk surgical procedures.[CW]

Figure 11. Assessing Cardiac Risk in Noncardiac Surgery (adapted from 2014 ACC/AHA Guidelines)

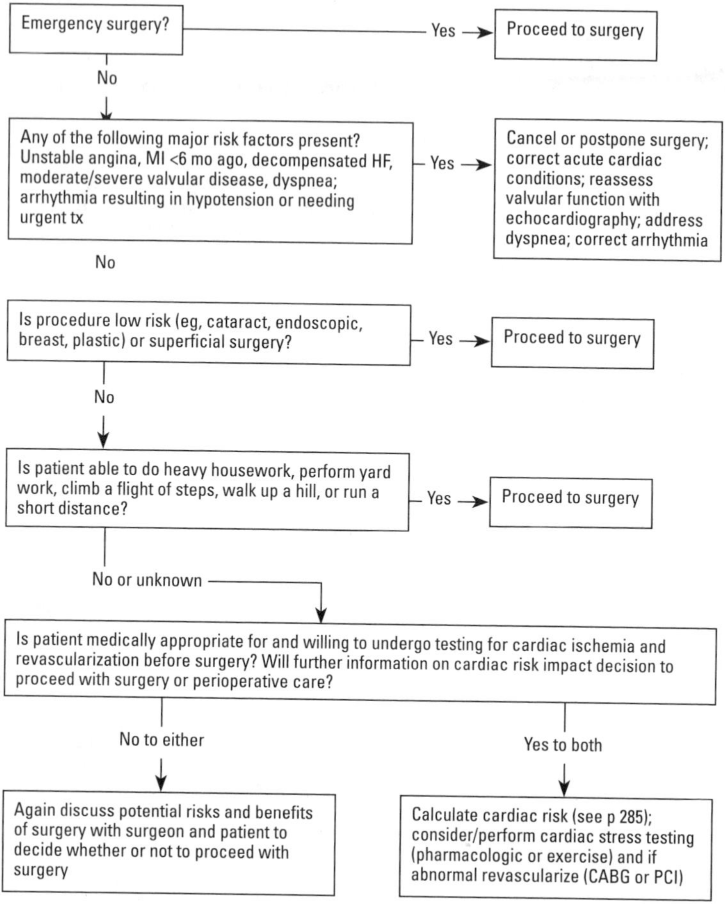

- Don't perform preoperative medical tests for eye surgery unless there are specific medical indications.[CW] See Eye chapter (p 126).
- Avoid echocardiograms for preoperative/perioperative assessment of patients with no hx or symptoms of heart disease.[CW]
- Don't order coronary artery calcium scoring for preoperative evaluation for any surgery, irrespective of patient risk.[CW]
- Don't initiate routine evaluation of carotid artery disease before cardiac surgery in the absence of symptoms or other high-risk criteria.[CW]

Pulmonary Risk Assessment

Major risk factors for postoperative pulmonary complications:

- COPD
- ASA Class II–V (I – healthy; II – mild systemic disease; III – moderate/severe systemic disease; IV – life-threatening systemic disease; V – moribund)
- ADL dependence
- HF
- Prolonged (>3 h) surgery; abdominal, thoracic, neurologic, head and neck, or vascular surgery; AAA repair; emergency surgery
- General anesthesia
- Serum albumin <3.5 mg/dL

Minor risk factors:

- Confusion/delirium
- Weight loss >10% in previous 6 mo
- BUN >21 mg/dL or Cr >1.5 mg/dL
- Alcohol use
- Current cigarette use
- Sleep apnea
- PH

Reducing risk of postoperative pulmonary complications:

- Smoking cessation 6–8 wk before surgery
- Before cardiac surgery, there is no need for PFTs in the absence of respiratory symptoms.[CW]
- Preoperative training in incentive spirometry, active-cycle breathing techniques, and forced-expiration techniques
- Postoperative incentive spirometry, chest PT, coughing, postural drainage, percussion and vibration, suctioning and ambulation, intermittent positive-pressure breathing, and/or CPAP
- Nasogastric tube use for patients with postoperative nausea or vomiting, inability to tolerate oral intake, or symptomatic abdominal distention

Other Preoperative Assessments

Screen for Conditions Associated with Postoperative Complications

- Cognitive impairment: Mini-Cog (p 2)
- Depression: PHQ-2
- Delirium risk factors: p 77
- Alcohol and substance abuse: CAGE questionnaire (p 354)
- Functional impairment: ADLs, IADLs
- Malnutrition: BMI <18.5 kg/m^2, >10% unintentional weight loss in past 6 mo, serum albumin <3.0 g/dL
- Frailty syndrome: at least 3 of the following: ≥10 lb unintentional weight loss in past year (shrinkage), decreased grip strength (weakness), self-reported poor energy and endurance (exhaustion), low weekly energy expenditure (low physical activity), slow walking (slowness)

Routine Lab Tests for Medium- and High-Risk Procedures

- Recommended: Hb, Cr, BUN, albumin
- Not routinely recommended as should be obtained selectively according to the patient's conditions: electrolytes, CBC, platelets, ABG, PT, PTT
- Avoid admission or preoperative CXRs for ambulatory patients with unremarkable hx and physical exam.[CW]

- Don't obtain preoperative chest radiography in the absence of clinical suspicion for intrathoracic pathology.[CW]

Advance Directives: Establish or update.

Cataract Surgery: Routine lab testing or cardiopulmonary risk assessment is unnecessary for cataract surgery performed under local anesthesia. If patient is on anticoagulation tx, it should not be interrupted. Use of α_1 blockers for BPH (p 296) within 14 d of cataract surgery is associated with increased risk of complications (intraoperative floppy iris syndrome), but it is unknown if cessation of α_1 blockers before surgery lowers risk.

Preoperative Medication Management

Cessation of Medications Before Surgery

- For low-risk surgeries, most medications do not need to be withheld before the procedure.
- See **Table 105** for withholding medications before medium- and high-risk surgeries.

Table 105. **Stopping Medications and Agents Before Medium-Risk and High-Risk Surgery**

Day Before Surgery	Agent to Stop	Comments
5–9	Antiplatelets	D/C for surgeries at high risk of bleeding (eg, CABG, intracranial surgery, prostate surgery)
7	Herbal agents	There is no evidence that herbal agents improve surgical outcomes, and many common herbal agents—including echinacea, ephedra, garlic, ginkgo, ginseng, kava, St John's wort, and valerian—have been associated with conditions that could produce adverse surgical outcomes.
5	Warfarin	D/C before surgery that is assessed to be of significant bleeding risk.[1] See below for bridging tx with LMWH. Resume warfarin 12–24 h after surgery if adequate hemostasis.
3	PDE-5 inhibitors SGLT2 inhibitors	Resume 12–24 h after surgery.
1–3	Dabigatran	D/C before surgery that is assessed to be of significant bleeding risk.[1] Stop 2–4 d before surgery if CrCl <50 mL/min. Resume 12–24 h after surgery if adequate hemostasis.
1–2	Apixaban Rivaroxaban	D/C before surgery that is assessed to be of significant bleeding risk.[1] Resume 12–24 h after surgery if adequate hemostasis.
1	ACEIs ARBs	Recommendation for stopping on day before surgery based on observational studies; RCTs needed to confirm benefit.
0	Diuretics	Withhold on day of surgery

[1] Abdominal, thoracic, or orthopedic surgery; spinal puncture; liver or kidney biopsy; TURP; or placement of spinal or epidural catheter

Anticoagulation Bridging Therapy When Withholding Warfarin Before Surgery

- Bridging tx with LMWH is based on VTE risk (**Table 106**). DVT tx doses of LMWH (**Table 17**) should be used for bridging tx. Begin LMWH 3 d before surgery; give last preoperative LMWH dose at one-half of total daily dose 24 h before surgery of oral anticoagulation tx before surgery that is assessed to be of significant bleeding risk (eg, port abdominal, thoracic, or orthopedic surgery, spinal puncture, liver or kidney biopsy, TURP, or placement of spinal or epidural catheter):
- Resumption of warfarin anticoagulation tx after surgery:
  - If bridging, resume LMWH 24 h after surgery, longer (48–72 h) with major surgical procedures or difficulty with hemostasis.

- Minor dental procedures: stop warfarin 2–3 d before procedure and recommend administration of prohemostatic agent (eg, tranexamic acid) by dentist.

Table 106. Indications for Perioperative Anticoagulation Bridging Therapy (ACCP Guidelines)

Thromboembolic Risk	Patient Conditions Determining Risk	Recommendations for LMWH Bridging Therapy
Low	• No VTE in past 12 mo • AF without prior TIA/stroke and 0–2 SRF[1] • Bileaflet mechanical aortic valve without AF, prior TIA/stroke, or SRF	Not recommended
Intermediate	• VTE in past 3–12 mo • Recurrent VTE • Active malignancy • AF without prior TIA/stroke and with 3–4 SRF[1] • Bileaflet mechanical aortic valve with AF, prior TIA/stroke, or any SRF	Optional according to individual thrombotic and bleeding risk
High	• VTE within past 3 mo • TIA/stroke within 3 mo • Rheumatic heart disease • AF with prior TIA/stroke and 3–4 SRF1 • Mechanical mitral valve or ball/cage mechanical aortic valve	Recommended

ACCP, American College of Chest Physicians; SRF, stroke risk factors: age ≥75, HTN, DM, HF.

[1] Recent data have called into question the benefit of bridging tx for patients with AF, showing low rates of thromboembolism (<0.5%) in whom warfarin was discontinued 5 d and DOACs discontinued 1–4 d before surgery without bridging tx, and increased risk of bleeding with bridging tx.

Patients With Coronary Stents (Bare Metal or Drug-Eluting) on Dual Antiplatelet Therapy:

- If possible, postpone surgery until at least 3 mo after stent placement, ideally after 6 mo.
- If surgery cannot be delayed until dual antiplatelet tx duration has been completed:
  - For most surgeries, which are at low risk of bleeding, continue dual antiplatelet tx.
  - For surgeries at intermediate risk of bleeding, D/C clopidogrel or prasugrel 5–7 d before procedure and maintain ASA tx. Because the platelet inhibition of ticagrelor is reversible, it should be stopped 1 d before procedure.
  - For surgeries at high risk of catastrophic bleeding (intracranial, spinal canal, or posterior chamber eye surgery), D/C clopidogrel or prasugrel 5 d before procedure, D/C ticagrelor 1 d before procedure, and consider D/C of ASA 5 d before procedure. Stopping ASA is an individual decision based on patient's risk factors for stent thrombosis and on assessed bleeding risk.
  - If both antiplatelet agents need to be stopped, consider bridging tx (requires admitting patient 2–4 d before surgery) with tirofiban or eptifibatide (**Tables 11** and **17**) in patients felt to be at very high risk of stent thrombosis (consult with cardiology).
  - If antiplatelet tx is discontinued, resume it the day of the surgical procedure.

NSAIDs: despite its common practice, there is no direct evidence to support cessation of NSAIDs before surgery. Coordinate decision to maintain or discontinue NSAID with surgeon.

SSRIs: SSRIs increase risk of bleeding with surgery, but discontinuing them before surgery is not recommended unless routine medication review indicates no tx need.

β blockers*:* if chronically stable on β blocker, continue perioperatively at usual dose. In patients with intermediate- or high-risk myocardial ischemia found on stress testing or with RCRI score >3 (p 285), consider initiating long-acting β blocker days to weeks before surgery (target HR=60) and continuing throughout postoperative period.

Statins: continue as usual dosage for patients already on a statin. Strongly consider prescribing a statin for all patients undergoing vascular surgery or for patients with multiple cardiac risk factors undergoing non–low-risk surgery.

Antibiotics: for endocarditis prophylaxis, see p 294

PRINCIPLES OF GERIATRIC CO-MANAGEMENT OF COMPLEX PATIENTS

- Both geriatrician and other specialist write orders with clearly demarcated areas of responsibility; care is co-managed.
- Both geriatrician and other specialist see patient daily.
- Patient goals are elucidated and shared with co-managing teams.
- Standard protocols are used as much as possible.
- In surgical cases, geriatrician performs/facilitates comprehensive preoperative assessment.
- Geriatrician often manages medical regimen to minimize ADRs.

POSTOPERATIVE DELIRIUM (also Delirium, p 77)

Epidemiology and Risk Factors

- Occurs after 15–50% of surgeries depending on type of procedure.
- Most episodes occur in first 2 postoperative days.
- Occurrences after postoperative day 2 are usually due to surgical complications or alcohol/sedative withdrawal.
- Major risk factors:
  - age ≥80
  - dementia
  - recent or unresolved delirium
  - major cardiac, open vascular, major abdominal surgery
  - emergency surgery
  - major surgical complication (eg, cardiogenic shock, prolonged intubation)
  - postoperative ICU stay ≥2 d
- Minor risk factors include MCI, poor functional status, significant comorbidity, general or IV-sedation regional anesthesia, poorly controlled pain, or taking opiates, sedatives, or anticholinergic drugs

Diagnosis and Management

- Systematic **preoperative** assessment and risk-lowering interventions have been shown to reduce the rate of postoperative delirium. This can be accomplished through proactive geriatrics team consultation/co-management, staff education regarding delirium prevention and detection, nurse-run programs to detect and prevent delirium, and the Hospital Elder Life Program (HELP) intervention (https://help.agscocare.org/).
- See p 77 for delirium diagnosis (CAM) and management.
- If workup finds bacteriuria, do not automatically ascribe a UTI as the cause of the delirium as asymptomatic bacteriuria is very common in older adults (p 181).

PREVENTIVE TESTS AND PROCEDURES

Table 107. Recommended Primary and Secondary Disease Prevention for People Aged 65 and Older

Preventive Strategy	Frequency/Indication
USPSTF Grade A/B[1] or CDC[1] Recommendations for Primary Prevention	
BMD (women)	at least once after age 65
Breast cancer risk-reducing medications (tamoxifen, raloxifene, or aromatase inhibitors)	offer to prescribe to women at increased risk of breast cancer
COVID-19 vaccination	full series for all adults
Diphtheria, pertussis, and tetanus vaccination	every 10 y
DM screening	every 3 y in people aged 40–70 who are overweight or obese
Exercise	adults aged ≥65 at increased risk of falls
Hepatitis A vaccination	at least once in adults at high risk (Section 12 of cdc.gov/vaccines/schedules/hcp/imz/adult-conditions.html)
Hepatitis B vaccination	at least once in adults at high risk (Section 13 of cdc.gov/vaccines/schedules/hcp/imz/adult-conditions.html)
Herpes zoster vaccination	after age 50 with RZV (*Shingrix*)[2]
HTN screening/BP measurement	yearly
Influenza vaccination	yearly
Lipid disorder screening	every 5 y, more often in CAD, DM, PAD, prior stroke
Pneumonia vaccination	once at age 65 with PCV20 pneumococcal conjugate vaccine; or PCV15 followed 1 y later by PPSV23 pneumococcal polysaccharide vaccine[3]
Smoking cessation	at every office visit
Weight management multicomponent intensive behavioral tx	Offer to or refer for adults with BMI ≥30
USPSTF Grade A/B[1] Recommendations for Secondary Prevention	
AAA ultrasonography	once between age 65–75 in men who have ever smoked
Alcohol abuse screening	unspecified but should be done periodically
Depression screening	yearly
Fecal immunochemical test (FIT), fecal occult blood test (FOBT), FIT-DNA test, CT colonography sigmoidoscopy, sigmoidoscopy combined with FIT, or colonoscopyidoscopy	Yearly for FOBT and FIT; every 1–3 y for FIT-DNA; every 5 y for CT colonography and sigmoidoscopy; every 10 y for colonoscopy or sigmoidoscopy with yearly FIT from age 50 to age 75 (age 76–85 is a USPSTF Grade C recommendation); see **Table 107** for follow-up testing; do not repeat colorectal cancer screening (by any method) for 10 y after a high-quality colonoscopy that does not detect neoplasia[CW]
Hepatitis B screening	at least once in adults at high risk (uspreventiveservicestaskforce.org/uspstf/recommendation/hepatitis-b-virus-infection-screening)

(cont.)

Table 107. Recommended Primary and Secondary Disease Prevention for People Aged 65 and Older (cont.)

Preventive Strategy	Frequency/Indication
Hepatitis C screening	at least once in adults aged 18–79
HIV screening	at least once in persons aged ≥65 with risk factors for HIV
Low-dose CT scanning for lung cancer	yearly in persons aged 50–80 with ≥20 pack-y of smoking and currently smoke or have quit in the past 15 y
Mammography[4]	every 2 y in women aged 50–74
USPSTF C/I[1] or Other[5] Recommendations for Primary Prevention	
Calcium (1200 mg) and vitamin D (≥800 IU) to prevent osteoporosis/fractures	daily
Falls prevention: risk assessment and management	at least once after age 65
Measurement of serum CRP	at least once in people with one CAD risk factor
Obesity/undernutrition screening	yearly
Omega-3 fatty acids to prevent MI, stroke	at least 2×/wk (see MI care, p 64)
USPSTF Grade C/I[1] or Other[5] Recommendations for Secondary Prevention	
Skin exam	yearly
Cognitive impairment screening	yearly
Glaucoma screening	yearly
Hearing impairment screening	yearly
TSH, especially in women	yearly
Visual impairment screening	yearly

[1] USPSTF (uspreventiveservicestaskforce.org/Page/Name/grade-definitions) grade recommendations: A = recommended, substantial benefit; B = recommended, moderate benefit; C = selectively offer based on professional judgment and patient preferences; I = evidence is inconclusive regarding benefits and harms of service. CDC recommendations: cdc.gov/vaccines/schedules/hcp/adult.html

[2] *RZV (Shingrix) is* administered in 2 doses 2–6 mo apart. It may be given in persons who have already received live zoster vaccine (*Zostavax)* (wait at least 8 wk after *Zostavax* to give first *Shingrix* dose). In a minority of patients, *Shingrix* can cause side effects (pain and swelling at injection site, muscle aches, fatigue, and/or mild fever for 2–3 d). Patients with hx of herpes zoster infection may be vaccinated.

[3] For older adults who have already received PPSV23, give either PCV15 or PCV20 ≥1 y later. For older adults who have already received PCV13, give PPSV23 ≥1 y later.

[4] Mammograms to age 70 are almost universally recommended; many organizations recommend that mammography should be continued in women over 70 who have a reasonable life expectancy.

[5] Not endorsed by USPSTF/CDC for all older adults, but recommended in selected patients or by other professional organizations.

For individualized age- and sex-specific USPSTF prevention recommendations, see ahrq.gov/professionals/clinicians-providers/guidelines-recommendations/guide.

Colonoscopy Finding	Time Till Next Colonoscopy
Normal	10 y
1–2 tubular adenomas <10 mm	7–10 y
3–4 tubular adenomas <10 mm	3–5 y
5–10 tubular adenomas <10 mm	3 y
Adenoma ≥10 mm	3 y
Adenoma with tubulovillous or villous histology	3 y
Adenoma with high-grade dysplasia	3 y
>10 adenomas on single exam	1 y
Piecemeal resection of adenoma ≥20 mm	6 mo

Table 108. Screening Colonoscopy Follow-up (2019 US Multi-Society Task Force Recommendations)

USPSTF GRADE D RECOMMENDATIONS (against performing preventive activity)

Against screening in asymptomatic older adults for:

- Asymptomatic bacteriuria
- Asymptomatic carotid artery stenosis
- Bladder cancer
- CAD with ECG, exercise treadmill test, or electron-beam CT in people with few or no CAD risk factors
- Cervical cancer in women aged ≥65 who have had adequate prior screening and are not otherwise at high risk for cervical cancer (includes those who have had a hysterectomy for benign disease)
- Colon cancer in people aged ≥85. Screening may be modestly beneficial in people aged 76–85 with long life expectancy and no or few comorbidities.
- COPD
- Ovarian cancer
- Pancreatic cancer
- Prostate cancer in men aged 70 and over
- Thyroid cancer
- Don't use PET/CT for cancer screening in healthy individuals.[CW]

Also against:

- Beta-carotene or vitamin E supplementation to prevent CVD or cancer
- Use of estrogen/progestin to prevent chronic conditions
- Vitamin D supplementation to prevent falls in community-dwelling older adults

CANCER SCREENING AND MEDICAL DECISION MAKING

- Many decisions about whether or not to perform preventive activities are based on the estimated life expectancy of the patient. Refer to **Table 3** for life expectancy data by age and sex.
- Most cancer screening tests do not realize a survival benefit for the patient until after 10 y from the time of the test. Cancer screening should be discouraged or very carefully considered in patients with ≤10 y of estimated life expectancy.
- Don't recommend screening for breast or colorectal cancer, or prostate cancer (with the PSA test), without considering life expectancy and the risks of testing, overdiagnosis, and overtreatment.[CW]

ENDOCARDITIS PROPHYLAXIS (2017 AHA Guidelines)

Antibiotic Regimens Recommended (Table 80)

Table 109. Endocarditis Prophylaxis Regimens

Situation	**Regimen** (single dose 30–60 min before procedure)[1]
Oral	Amoxicillin 2 g po
Unable to take oral medication	Ampicillin 2 g, cefazolin 1 g, or ceftriaxone 1 g IM or IV
Allergic to penicillins or ampicillin	Cephalexin 2 g, clindamycin 600 mg, azithromycin 500 mg, or clarithromycin 500 mg po
Allergic to penicillins or ampicillin and unable to take oral medication	Cefazolin 1 g, ceftriaxone 1 g, or clindamycin 600 mg IM or IV

[1] For patients undergoing invasive respiratory tract procedures to treat an infection known to be caused by *Staph aureus*, or for patients undergoing surgery for infected skin, skin structures, or musculoskeletal tissue, regimen should include an antistaphylococcal penicillin or cephalosporin.

Cardiac Conditions Requiring Prophylaxis (all others do not)

- Prosthetic cardiac valve
- Previous infective endocarditis
- Cardiac transplant recipients who develop cardiac valvulopathy
- Unrepaired cyanotic congenital heart disease
- Repaired CHD with residual defects at the site or adjacent to the site of a prosthetic patch or device
- CHD completely repaired with prosthetic material or device (prophylaxis needed for only the first 6 mo after repair procedure)

Procedures Warranting Prophylaxis (only in patients with cardiac conditions listed above)

- Dental procedures requiring manipulation of gingival tissue, manipulation of the periapical region of teeth, or perforation of the oral mucosa (includes extractions, implants, reimplants, root canals, teeth cleaning during which bleeding is expected)
- Invasive procedures of the respiratory tract involving incision or biopsy of respiratory tract mucosa
- Surgical procedures involving infected skin, skin structures, or musculoskeletal tissue

Procedures Not Warranting Prophylaxis

- All dental procedures not listed above
- All noninvasive respiratory procedures
- All GI and GU procedures

ANTIBIOTIC PROPHYLAXIS FOR PATIENTS WITH TOTAL JOINT REPLACEMENTS

(TJR; 2012 AAOS/ADA Guidelines)

Procedures/Conditions Prompting Consideration of Antibiotic Prophylaxis

- The American Academy of Orthopedic Surgeons in conjunction with the American Dental Association recommend that clinicians consider discontinuing the practice of routine antibiotic prophylaxis in patients with prior TJR who are undergoing dental procedures (orthoguidelines.org/topic?id=1002).
  - Bacteremias are produced not just by dental procedures, but also by common daily activities such as tooth brushing.
  - Although antibiotic prophylaxis reduces bacteremia after dental procedures, there is no evidence that withholding antibiotics or dental procedures themselves are associated with prosthetic knee or hip infections.

- Antibiotic prophylaxis should be considered for patients with prior TJR, regardless of when joint was replaced, who are undergoing ophthalmic, orthopedic, vascular, GI, head and neck, gynecologic, or GU procedures.
- Additional risk factors for considering prophylaxis in patients with prior TJR: immunocompromised state; disease-, radiation-, or drug-induced immunosuppression; inflammatory arthropathies; malnourishment; hemophilia; HIV infection; type 1 DM; malignancy; megaprostheses; comorbidities (eg, DM, obesity, smoking)
- Conditions not requiring prophylaxis: patients with pins, plates, or screws

Suggested Prophylactic Regimens

- Dental procedures (see those listed above for endocarditis): amoxicillin, cephalexin, or cephradine 2 g po 1 h before procedure
- Prophylactic antibiotic recommendations for other types of procedures vary by procedure (see Bratzler DW et al. *Am J Health-Syst Pharm.* 2013;70:195–283).

EXERCISE PRESCRIPTION

Before Giving an Exercise Prescription

Screen patient for:

- Musculoskeletal problems: decreased flexibility, muscular rigidity, weakness, pain, ill-fitting shoes
- Cardiac disease: consider stress test if older adult is beginning a vigorous exercise program and is sedentary with symptoms of active CVD (eg, angina, HF, PAD), DM, ESRD, or chronic lung disease.

Individualize the Prescription

- Older adults should be encouraged to decrease sedentary time—"move more, sit less" during the day.
- Exercise ideally should consist of varied components, addressing aerobic, strength, flexibility, and balance activities.
- Initiating low-intensity (rated 1–4 on a 10-point scale by the patient) to moderate-intensity (rated 5–6 on a 10-point scale) exercise is generally safe in older adults with multiple chronic conditions. Guidelines below should be adjusted according to patient's ability to tolerate each activity. Specify short- and long-term goals; include the following components (CDC and American College of Sports Medicine/AHA recommendations):

Aerobic: Moderate-intensity activity, at least 150 min/wk, preferably ≥30 min ≥5×/wk

- Moderate-intensity activities such as brisk walking are those that increase HR and would be rated 5–6 on a 10-point intensity scale by the patient.
- It is never too late to start exercising. Brisk walking in previously sedentary older adults significantly lowers risk of disability.
- Using pedometers to record the number of steps in a walking program has been demonstrated to increase physical activity, lower BMI, and lower BP.

Strength: Weight (resistance) training at least 2×/wk, 10 exercises on major muscle groups, 10–15 repetitions per exercise

Flexibility: Static stretching, at least 2×/wk for ≥10 min of flexibility exercises, 10–30 sec per stretch, 3–4 repetitions of major muscle/tendon groups

Balance: Balance exercises are recommended for people with mobility problems or who fall frequently.

Patient information: See nia.nih.gov/health/exercise-physical-activity. See also Assessment and Management of Falls, **Figure 6**.

BENIGN PROSTATIC HYPERPLASIA (BPH)

Lower urinary tract symptoms (LUTS; increased frequency of urination, nocturia, hesitancy, urgency, and weak urinary stream) may or may not be associated with enlarged prostate gland, bladder outlet obstruction (eg, urinary retention, recurrent infection, renal insufficiency), or histological BPH.

Evaluation

Evaluation of the severity of symptoms (International Prostate Symptom Score for BPH): Detailed medical hx focusing on physical exam of the urinary tract, including abdominal exam, digital rectal exam, and a focused neurologic exam; UA and culture if pyuria or hematuria. Postvoid residual (PVR) if neurologic disease, prior procedure that can affect bladder or sphincter function, UI, reports of incomplete emptying, and before initiating antimuscarinic tx or surgical tx (below). Before surgery, consider uroflowmetry and pressure flow studies (AUA). Measurement of PSA is controversial, but should not be measured if life expectancy is <10 y. Don't order Cr or upper tract imaging for BPH.[CW]

International Prostate Symptom Score (IPSS) Symptom Index for BPH

Questions to be answered (circle one number on each line)	**Not at all**	**Less than 1 time in 5**	**Less than half the time**	**About half the time**	**More than half the time**	**Almost always**
1. Over the past month or so, how often have you had a sensation of not emptying your bladder completely after you finished urinating?	0	1	2	3	4	5
2. Over the past month or so, how often have you had to urinate again less than 2 hours after you finished urinating?	0	1	2	3	4	5
3. Over the past month or so, how often have you found you stopped and started again several times when you urinated?	0	1	2	3	4	5
4. Over the past month or so, how often have you found it difficult to postpone urination?	0	1	2	3	4	5
5. Over the past month or so, how often have you had a weak urinary stream?	0	1	2	3	4	5
6. Over the past month or so, how often have you had to push or strain to begin urination?	0	1	2	3	4	5
7. Over the last month, how many times did you most typically get up to urinate from the time you went to bed at night until the time you got up in the morning?	none	1 time	2 times	3 times	4 times	>5 times

AUA Symptom Score = sum of responses to questions 1–7 =___.

0–7 points	Mild symptoms
8–19 points	Moderate symptoms
20–35 points	Severe symptoms

Management

Mild Symptoms: (eg, AUA IPSS <8;) watchful waiting with monitoring q6–12mo

Moderate to Severe Symptoms: (eg, AUA score ≥8) watchful waiting, medical or surgical tx

Nonpharmacologic Interventions: Reduce caffeine and alcohol, and avoid fluids before bedtime, anticholinergic drugs, antihistamines, TCAs, muscle relaxants. Double voiding to empty bladder completely, voiding in sitting position (if LUTS). If obstruction causing urinary retention who are not surgical candidates, clean intermittent catheterization can be used.

Pharmacotherapy: If mild to moderate symptoms, can start with α_1 blockers alone. Combining drugs from different classes may have better long-term effectiveness than single-agent tx. If overactive bladder symptoms without evidence of bladder outlet obstruction or high PVR, consider beginning with antimuscarinics or combination α blocker and antimuscarinic or β3 agonist. If large prostate (eg, >40 g) or severe symptoms, consider beginning with combined tx (α-adrenergic blockers and 5-α reductase inhibitors). No dietary supplements have been demonstrated to be effective.

- **α_1 Blockers** relax prostatic and bladder detrusor smooth muscle and work within days. Nonselective and selective agents are equally effective. Do not start in men with planned cataract surgery until after surgery is completed. Nonselective drugs appear to have lower rates of intraoperative floppy iris syndrome. Use of PDE5 inhibitors (tadalafil, sildenafil, vardenafil) with α_1 blockers can potentiate hypotensive effect. All have generic formulations.
  - **Nonselective** (more likely to cause orthostatic hypotension and dizziness)
    - Terazosin: increase dosage as tolerated: days 1–3, 1 mg/d po hs; days 4–7, 2 mg/d po; days 8–14, 5 mg/d po; day 15 and beyond, 10 mg/d po. Avoid use as antihypertensive or in patients with syncope.[BC]
    - Doxazosin: start 0.5 mg po with max of 16 mg/d po. Avoid use as antihypertensive or in patients with syncope.[BC]
  - **Selective for prostatic α_1 receptor** (less likely to cause hypotension or syncope, also benefits hematuria; more likely to cause ejaculatory dysfunction)
    - Tamsulosin: 0.4 mg po 30 min after the same meal each day and increase to 0.8 mg po if no response in 2–4 wk; decreases ejaculate volume; increases risk of retinal detachment, lost lens or lens fragment, or endophthalmitis if taken within 14 d before cataract surgery
    - Silodosin: 8 mg/d po or 4 mg/d po in moderate kidney impairment; not recommended in severe kidney or liver impairment, may have more sexual AEs (decreased ejaculate volume; retrograde ejaculation in ~30%)
    - Alfuzosin ER: 10 mg po after the same meal every day
- **5-α Reductase Inhibitors** (reduce prostate size and are more effective with large [>40 g] glands; do not use in the absence of prostate enlargement; tx for 6 mo may be needed before symptoms improve) may help prostate-related bleeding. Can decrease libido, ejaculation, and erectile function. Reduce the incidence of prostate cancer, but may lead to higher incidence of high-grade tumors in later years. Increased risk of depression and self-harm. Check PSA 6 mo after starting tx for new baseline and monitor for rises. All have generic formulations.
  - Finasteride 5 mg/d po
  - Dutasteride 0.5 mg/d po
- **Antimuscarinic Agents** (bladder relaxants) may have additional benefit beyond α_1 blockers on urinary frequency and urgency (**Table 74**); use with caution if PVR >250 mL. Maximum benefit within 1–2 wk. All have generic formulations.

- **β3 Adrenergic Agonists** (bladder relaxants) mirabegron and vibegron may have additional benefit when added to α_1 blockers in reducing number of micturitions per day and volume per micturition but not on overall symptom severity (**Table 74**). Neither have generic formulations.
- **Phosphodiesterase-5 (PDE5) Inhibitors** (**Table 125**) may improve symptoms of BPH/LUTS in men with or without erectile dysfunction but do not improve flow rates. Maximum symptom benefit occurs after about 1 mo. Do not use daily if CrCl <30 mL/min. Tadalafil has been approved for BPH. May be used as initial tx if concomitant ED. No added benefit when combined with other BPH drugs.
- **Surgical Management**: Indicated if recurrent UTI, recurrent or persistent gross hematuria, recurrent bladder stones, hydronephrosis, refractory urinary retention, or renal insufficiency secondary to BPH or as indicated by severe symptoms refractory to other tx (AUA). For men with moderate symptoms (AUA scores 8–15), surgical tx is more effective than watchful waiting, but the latter is a reasonable alternative. Single-dose antibiotic prophylaxis (eg, cefazolin, sulfamethoxazole/trimethoprim): Options vary by local urologist and availability of procedures:
  - TURP (transurethral resection of the prostate): standard tx, best long-term outcome data; 1% risk of UI and no increased risk of sexual dysfunction
  - For patients at high surgical risk, minimally invasive surgical tx can be performed in office under local anesthesia:
    - PUL (prostatic urethral lift): sutures that hold the prostate away from the urethra; has evidence for up to 5 y benefit and preserves sexual function; ~6% per year require surgical retreatment; less effective than TURP; should not be used in glands >80 g or if obstructing middle lobe.
    - Water-vapor thermal (steam) tx *(Rezūm)* if gland <80 g, 50% reduction in IPSS scores by 3 mo, sustained at 4 y; preserves sexual function.
  - For patients at high risk of surgical bleeding:
    - HoLEP (holmium laser enucleation of the prostate): using laser as a knife
    - PVP (photoselective vaporization of the prostate): laser procedure; effects on symptoms have been maintained for up to 2 y with complication rates similar to TURP
    - ThuLEP (thulium laser enucleation of the prostate): using laser as a knife

PROSTATE CANCER

USPSTF recommends that for men aged 55–69, periodic PSA-based screening should be an individual decision; recommends against PSA-based screening in men aged ≥70. Offer only after engaging in shared decision-making.[CW] Don't offer if <10 y life expectancy.[CW]

Evaluation

Predicting the extent of disease:

- Digital rectal exam
- PSA (p 296) should be obtained before biopsy
  - Age 60–69 y normal is 0.0–4.5 ng/mL
  - Age 70–79 y normal is 0.0–6.5 ng/mL
  - Free/total PSA ratio. Higher percentage indicates less likely to be prostate cancer.
  - PSA. 50 ng/mL probably indicates carcinoma.
  - African American men with and without cancer have higher PSA levels than other racial groups.
- Biopsy (Gleason primary and secondary grade). MRI before biopsy and MRI-targeted biopsies are superior to transrectal ultrasonography-guided biopsies
- If life expectancy ≤5 y and asymptomatic, workup only if high or very high risk

- Bone scan if symptomatic or high risk for occult metastasis by NCCN risk group (see below) unfavorable intermediate, high, very high
- CT or MRI abdomen and pelvis if intermediate, high, or very high or symptomatic, and nomogram-predicted probability of lymph-node involvement >10%. Don't perform PET, CT, or radionuclide bone scan in the staging of early prostate cancer at low risk of metastasis.[CW]
- Nomograms may help provide individualized estimates of biochemical (PSA-only) recurrence and prostate cancer–specific survival (https://www.mskcc.org/nomograms/prostate)

Histology

- Gleason score ≤6 has low 15- to 20-y morbidity and mortality; watchful waiting is usually appropriate.
- Gleason score ≥7, higher PSA, and younger age are associated with higher morbidity and mortality; best tx strategy (surgery, radiation tx, ADT, etc) is not known.

Grading system that incorporates Gleason score

- Grade Group 1 (Gleason score 3+3)
- Grade Group 2 (Gleason score 3+4)
- Grade Group 3 (Gleason score 4+3)
- Grade Group 4 (Gleason score 4+4, 3+5, or 5+3)
- Grade Group 5 (Gleason score 4+5, 5+4, or 5+5); worse prognosis than Grade Group 4

Staging

T1 = Clinically inapparent tumor, neither palpable nor visible by imaging
  a. Incidental finding <5% of tissue
  b. Incidental finding >5% of tissue
  c. Identified by needle biopsy (eg, because of increased PSA)

T2 = Tumor confined within prostate
  a. <1/2 of 1 lobe
  b. >1 lobe
  c. Both lobes

T3 = Tumor extends through the prostate capsule
  a. Unilateral or bilateral extracapsular extension
  b. Invading seminal vesicle

T4 = Tumor is fixed or invades adjacent structures other than seminal vesicles

N = Regional nodes indicating Stage IV disease

M = Distal metastasis indicating Stage IV disease

Risk stratification: NCCN very low, low, intermediate favorable, intermediate unfavorable, high, or very high based on grade, number of positive biopsy cores, PSA, and staging ***(www.nccn.org/professionals/physician_gls/pdf/prostate.pdf)***

Management

Don't treat low-risk clinically localized prostate cancer without discussing active surveillance as part of the shared decision-making process.[CW]

NCCN tx guidelines can be found at www.nccn.org/professionals/physician_gls/pdf/prostate.pdf

Modalities

- Radical prostatectomy reduces short- and long-term overall and disease-specific mortality, metastasis, and local progression compared with watchful waiting in men aged <65 with early disease, regardless of histology and PSA, including those who are at low risk. UI and sexual dysfunction are more common at 5 y compared to EBRT. Irritative urinary symptoms are less than radiation tx or active surveillance.
- Radiation tx may cause transient PSA increase that does not reflect cancer recurrence. Bloody stools after 12 mo are more common compared to prostatectomy.
  - EBRT is associated with acute worsening of urinary and bowel obstructive symptoms but tend to resolve over 24 mo.
  - Brachytherapy (radioactive seed implantation) has greater effect on prostate than EBRT.
- Proton-beam tx should not be recommended outside of a prospective clinical trial or registry.[CW]
- Hormonal androgen deprivation tx (ADT) is reserved for locally advanced or metastatic disease.
  - Monotx can be either bilateral orchiectomy or a GnRH agonist.
  - Combined androgen blockade (GnRH agonist plus antiandrogen) is used to avoid "flare" phenomenon (ie, increased symptoms early in tx), but survival benefit is uncertain and side effects are greater than with monotx.
  - Hormonal tx is commonly associated with hot flushes, nausea, edema, headaches, fatigue.
- Active surveillance includes monitoring no more frequently than q6mo and may include PSA, digital rectal exam, MRI, and prostate biopsies with the expectation to intervene with curative attempt if the cancer progresses.
- Observation includes monitoring no more frequently than q6mo and may include tests but usually not biopsies and continues until symptoms develop or are imminent, at which time palliative ADT is begun.

Monitoring and Lifestyle Modifications for Prostate Cancer Survivors

After surgery or radiation tx, PSA should be <0.1 ng/mL or undetectable. Monitor PSA q6–12mo for 5 y (q3mo if high risk), then every year. Digital rectal exam yearly but may be omitted if PSA undetectable. If nodal disease on ADT or localized on observation, physical exam and PSA q6 mo and bone imaging for symptoms and as often as q6–12mo. If undetectable PSA after radical prostatectomy and subsequent detectable PSA that increases on ≥2 determinations, workup for distant metastasis. A PSA doubling time of 3–12 mo in the absence of clinical recurrence indicates a higher risk of developing systemic disease and cancer-specific death.

Therapy for PSA-only Recurrence (no evidence of other disease)

- If after radical prostatectomy and no evidence of distant metastasis, EBRT ± ADT or observation. If distant metastasis, then systemic tx.
- If after radiation tx and life expectancy >10 y, then radical prostatectomy with pelvic lymph node dissection, or cryotherapy, or high-intensity focused ultrasound, or brachytherapy, or observation. If life expectancy ≤10 y or transrectal ultrasound biopsy negative and no distant metastasis, observation or ADT.

Lifestyle Modifications

- Dietary modifications that are micronutrient- and phytochemical-rich fruits and vegetables, low saturated fat, 600 IU vitamin D daily
- Physical activity or exercise: ≥150 min/wk moderate intensity exercise or 75 min/wk of vigorous intensity exercise
- Smoking cessation: smoking increases the risk of recurrence

Late Complications of Prostate Cancer

- CVD (controversial) due to effects of ADT on cardiac risk factors (obesity, lipids, decreased insulin sensitivity)
- GI, especially proctitis, from radiation, most common in first 3 y after tx
- Urinary frequency, urgency, stress incontinence, dysuria, stricture, retention, hematuria
- Erectile dysfunction, orgasmic dysfunction, penile fibrosis
- Hypogonadism (consider replacement if in remission and not receiving ADT)
- DM
- Osteoporosis as a result of ADT and RT. BMD is recommended.
- Secondary malignancies in field of radiation (bladder, rectal)
- Psychosocial (fatigue, depression)

PROSTATITIS

Definition

Acute or chronic inflammation of the prostate secondary to bacterial (usually gram-negative organisms) and nonbacterial causes

Symptoms and Diagnosis

Acute: fever; chills; dysuria; obstructive symptoms; tender, tense, or boggy on examination (exam should be minimal to avoid bacteremia); Gram stain and culture of urine (usually caused by gram-negative organisms, especially *E coli* or *proteus*). Passage of catheter through urethra is contraindicated.

Chronic: recurrent UTIs, especially with same organism; obstructive or irritative symptoms with voiding, perineal pain (may include chronic pelvic pain syndrome). Exam often indicates hypertrophy, tenderness, edema, or nodularity, but may be normal. Compare first void or midstream urine with prostatic secretion or postmassage urine: bacterial if leukocytosis and bacteria in expressed sample (typically caused by gram-negative organisms, especially *E coli*), nonbacterial if sample sterile with leukocytosis

Pharmacotherapy (Table 80)

Antibiotic tx should be based on Gram stain and culture. Begin tx for acute prostatitis empirically to cover likely organisms (gram-negative) while culture is pending. If occurs after transrectal prostate biopsy, more likely to be due to drug-resistant organisms. Do not insert Foley catheter in acute prostatitis. If urinary retention, consult a urologist.

Acute prostatitis (recommend tx for 4–6 wk)

- Trimethoprim-sulfamethoxazole[BC] DS 1 po q12h, ***or***
- Ciprofloxacin[BC] 500 mg po or 400 mg IV q12h, ***or***
- Ofloxacin 400 mg po 1×, then 300 mg q12h, ***or***
- Third-generation cephalosporin or aminoglycoside IV if unable tolerate po, septic, or bacteremic

Chronic prostatitis (fluoroquinolones have good penetration of inflamed prostate and are generally considered first choice for initial and recurrent infections)

- Ciprofloxacin[BC] 500 mg po q12h × at least 6 wk, ***or***
- Levofloxacin 500 mg po q24h × at least 6 wk, ***or***
- Ofloxacin 200 mg po or IV q12h × 3 mo, ***or***
- Trimethoprim-sulfamethoxazole[BC] DS 1 po q12h × 2–4 mo
- If resistant to other antibiotics doxycycline, fosfomycin 3 g po q24h for 1 wk followed by q48h for 6–12 wk, or both.
- α blockers may help chronic prostatitis in combination with antibiotics. Less consistent benefits have been demonstrated with anti-inflammatory agents and finasteride.

PSYCHOTIC DISORDERS

DIFFERENTIAL DIAGNOSIS

- Bipolar affective disorder
- Late-life delusional (paranoid) disorder
- Major depressive disorder with psychotic features
- Early-onset schizophrenia (symptoms manifest age 20–30); late-onset schizophrenia (symptoms after age 40); very late–onset schizophrenia (symptoms appear after age 60)
- Schizoaffective disorder
- In addition to the primary psychiatric disorders listed above, secondary etiologies of psychosis are much more common in older adults than younger adults, often requiring more extensive medical workup. These include:
    - Delirium
    - Dementia
    - Medications/drugs: eg, antiparkinsonian agents, anticholinergics, benzodiazepines or alcohol (including withdrawal), stimulants, corticosteroids, cardiac medications (eg, digitalis), opioid analgesics
    - Physical disorders: hypo- or hyperglycemia, hypo- or hyperthyroidism, sodium or potassium imbalance, Cushing syndrome, Parkinson disease, B_{12} deficiency, sleep deprivation, AIDS
    - Pain, untreated
    - Structural brain lesions: tumor or stroke
    - Seizure disorder (eg, temporal lobe)

Risk Factors for Psychotic Symptoms in Older Adults: chronic bed rest, cognitive impairment, female sex, sensory impairment, social isolation

MANAGEMENT

- Establish a trusting therapeutic relationship with the patient; focus on empathizing with the distress that symptoms cause rather than reality orientation.
- Encourage patients to maintain significant, supportive relationships.
- Alleviate underlying physical causes.
- Address identifiable psychosocial triggers.
- For *DSM-5*, rate presence and severity (most severe in last 7 d) of psychotic symptoms (eg, hallucinations, delusions, disorganized speech) on a 5-point scale ranging from 0 (not present) to 4 (present and severe).
- Before using an antipsychotic to treat behavioral symptoms of dementia, carefully assess and quantify (eg, using the Neuropsychiatric Inventory Questionnaire [NPI-Q]) psychotic features (ie, delusions and hallucinations) and if psychotic symptoms are severe, frightening, or may affect safety.
- Aripiprazole, olanzapine, quetiapine, risperidone are first choice because of fewer AEs (TD extremely high in older adults taking first-generation antipsychotics). See **Table 110** and **Table 111** for AEs of second-generation antipsychotics.

- Caution if hx of falls and fractures due to potential hypotension.[BC]
- Start at low dose and go slow with dose titration.
- All antipsychotics are associated with increased mortality in older adults.[BC]
- Parkinson disease hallucinations and delusions: Pimavanserin *(Nuplazid)*, an inverse agonist at the 5HT2A receptor, has been specifically approved. Same warning for risk of QTc prolongation as for antipsychotics (**Table 94**). Alternatives are quetiapine and clozapine. See Dementia and Cognitive Impairment chapter.

Table 110. Representative Medications for Managing Psychosis

Class, Medication	Dosage, mg/d	Comments (Metabolism)
Second-generation Antipsychotics		Avoid for behavioral problems of dementia
✓Aripiprazole *(Abilify)*	2–5 mg (1) po initially; max 30 mg/d po or IM	Wait 2 wk between dosage changes (CYP2D6, -3A4) (L)
(Abilify Maintena)	300–400 mg IM q30d	Deltoid or gluteal injection. Ensure adequate muscle mass. Adjust dose for CYP2D6 and -3A4 interactions. Not for complications of dementia.
Aripiprazole lauroxil *(Aristada)*	400–6620 mg IM q30d; 882 mg IM q4–6wk 1064 mg IM q2mo	441-mg deltoid or gluteal injection; 662-mg, 882-mg, and 1064-mg gluteal-only injections. Ensure adequate muscle mass. Adjust dose for CYP2D6 and -3A4 interactions. Not for complications of dementia.
Asenapine *(Saphris)*	5–10 mg sl q12h	Do not swallow (L)
(Secuado)	3.8 mg/24 h pch 5.7 mg/24 h pch 7.6 mg/24 h pch	First transdermal patch for schizophrenia; provides sustained concentration over 24 h; potential skin irritation at patch site.
Brexpiprazole *(Rexulti)*	Initial 1 mg/d; 2–4 mg/d	Max dose CrCl <60: 3 mg/d
Clozapine	25–150 mg IM q4wk (1)	May be useful for parkinsonism and TD; significant risk of neutropenia and agranulocytosis; weekly CBCs × 6 mo, then biweekly; may cause significant constipation and bowel obstruction (L)
Iloperidone *(Fanapt)*	Initial: 1 mg po q12h, increase by ≤2 mg po q12h to 6–12 mg po q12h; max 24 mg/d po	Very limited geriatric data (CYP2D6), inhibits 2C19 and 3A4 (L)
Lumateperone *(Caplyta)*	42 mg po 1×/d	CYP3A4 interactions; regulatory trials did not include any patients aged ≥65
Lurasidone *(Latuda)*	40 mg po 1×/d	Very limited geriatric data Dose should not exceed 80 mg/d in renal impairment (CrCl <50)
✓Olanzapine	2.5–10 mg po or IM (1)	Weight gain (L)
Paliperidone *(Invega)*	3–12 mg IM (1)	CrCl = 51–80, max 6 mg/d; CrCl ≤50, max 3 mg/d; very limited geriatric data (K)

(cont.)

Class, Medication	Dosage, mg/d	Comments (Metabolism)
Pimavanserin *(Nuplazid)*	34 mg po q24h	Approved for Parkinson disease psychosis (**Table 94**). Avoid in combination with CYP3A4 inducers. Use cautiously with CYP3A4 inhibitors; use 10 mg q24h with strong CYP3A4 inhibitors. (L)
✓Quetiapine	25–800 mg po or IM (1–2)	(L, K)
✓Risperidone	0.25–1 mg IM (1–2)	Dose-related EPS; IM not for acute tx; do not exceed 6 mg (L, K)
Ziprasidone	20–80 mg po or IM (1–2)	May increase QTc; very limited geriatric data (L)

Table 110. Representative Medications for Managing Psychosis (cont.)

✓ = preferred for treating older adults but does not imply low risk; mortality may be increased in patients with dementia.

CrCl unit = mL/min.

Table 111. Adverse Events of Preferred Second-generation Antipsychotics

Adverse Event	Aripiprazole	Olanzapine	Quetiapine	Risperidone
Cardiovascular				
Hypotension	?	+	+++	+
QTc prolongation[1]	0	++	++	++
Endocrine/Metabolic				
Weight gain	+	+++	++	++
DM	?	+++	++	++
Hypertriglyceridemia	0	+	0	?
Hyperprolactinemia	0	+	0	+++
Gastrointestinal				
Nausea, vomiting, constipation	0	0	?	?
Neurologic				
EPS	+	+	+	+++
Seizures	?	?	?	ND
Sedation	+	++	++	+
Systemic				
Anticholinergic	0	++	+	0
Neuroleptic malignant syndrome	ND	ND	ND	+

ND = no data; ? = unpredictable effect; 0 = no effect; + = mild effect; ++ = moderate effect; +++ = high risk of effect

[1] QTc upper limit of normal = 440 millisec

Table 112. Management of Adverse Events of Antipsychotic Medications		
AE	**Management**	**Comment**
Drug-induced parkinsonism	Reduce dosage or change drug or drug class	Often dose related; avoid anticholinergic agents[BC]
Akathisia[1] (motor restlessness)	Consider adding β-blocker (eg, propranolol 20–40 mg/d po or IV) or low-dose benzodiazepine (eg, lorazepam 0.5 mg po, IV, or IM q12h)	Also seen with second-generation antipsychotics; more likely with traditional agents
Hypotension	Slow titration; reduce dosage; change drug class	More common with low-potency agents
Sedation	Reduce dosage; give hs; change drug class	More common with low-potency agents
TD	Stop drug (if possible); consider second-generation antipsychotic (eg, aripiprazole, quetiapine) with lower potential for EPS[2]	Increased risk in older adults; may be irreversible

Note: Periodic (q4mo) reevaluation of antipsychotic dosage and ongoing need is important (see CMS guidance on unnecessary drugs in the nursing home: www.cms.hhs.gov/transmittals/downloads/R22SOMA.pdf). Older adults are particularly sensitive to AEs of antipsychotic drugs. They are also at higher risk of developing TD. Periodic use of an AE scale such as the Abnormal Involuntary Movement Scale (AIMS) is highly recommended.

[1]Akathisia can be assessed with the Barnes Akathisia Scale (https://qxmd.com/calculate/calculator_808/barnes-akathisia-ratin).

[2] Should EPS develop, they can quantified with the Simpson Angus Scale (www.sciencedirect.com/topics/medicine-and-dentistry/simpson-angus-scale).

Tardive Dyskinesia (TD)

TD, a polymorphous, hyperkinetic movement disorder, is commonly orofacial but can be truncal and in severe cases can be disabling. Caused by exposure to dopamine-receptor antagonists, especially first-generation antipsychotics, risk increases after age 65. Postmenopausal women at highest risk. AIMS is the gold standard for monitoring (https://cpnp.org/aims).

Valbenazine *(Ingrezza)*, deutetrabenazine *(Austedo)*, and tetrabenazine *(Xenazine)* are VMAT2 inhibitors approved to treat patients with TD. No dosage adjustment for age. SAEs: somnolence, QTc prolongation. Drug interactions: MAOIs, strong CYP3A4 and -2D6 inhibitors, digoxin.

Neuroleptic Malignant Syndrome (NMS)

NMS is a life-threatening idiosyncratic reaction to antipsychotic drugs (see Delirium, **Table 34**). Although uncommon, NMS may occur within 1–2 wk after starting or changing doses of an antipsychotic and should be considered for patients presenting with fever, altered mental status, muscle rigidity, and autonomic dysfunction. Tx includes immediately stopping the antipsychotic and implementing supportive measures.

RESPIRATORY DISEASES

COUGH

Among the most common presenting symptoms in office practice; consider likely diagnosis based on duration of symptoms and treat the specific disorder (**Table 113**). **Table 114** lists agents sometimes used in symptomatic management of cough.

Table 113. Diagnosis and Management of Cough by Duration of Symptoms

Cause	Preferred Management
Acute cough: duration up to 3 wk	
The common cold, acute rhinosinusitis	Sinus irrigation or nasal ipratropium (*Atrovent NS 0.06%*, **Table 117**). Not recommended: sedating antihistamines (dry mouth, urinary retention, confusion); oral pseudoephedrine[BC] (HTN, tachycardia, urinary retention). Don't routinely treat uncomplicated rhinosinusitis or bronchitis with antibiotics.[CW]
Acute bronchitis	Criteria for antibiotics: Illness >1 wk; high-risk patients; HF, COPD, asthma Antibiotic choice: amoxicillin, doxycycline, erythromycin for 5 d; depending on local resistance patterns third-generation cephalosporin or macrolide Criteria for bronchodilators: troublesome cough, bronchospasm, wheezing, FEV_1 <80% Criteria for antitussives: (**Table 114**) cough causing discomfort
Allergic rhinitis	p 310
Bacterial sinusitis	Oxymetazoline nasal spr × 5 d; antibiotic against *Haemophilus influenzae* and streptococcal pneumonia (eg, amoxicillin-clavulanate or doxycycline) × 7–10 d.
Pertussis	Macrolide or trimethoprim-sulfa antibiotic × 6 wk (age >65)
Other: pneumonia, HF, asthma, COPD exacerbation, COVID-19	Pneumonia, p 178; HF, p 64; asthma, p 316; COPD, p 313
Subacute cough: duration 3–8 wk	
Postinfectious	Inhaled ipratropium; systemic steroids tapered over 2–3 wk; if protracted, dextromethorphan with codeine; use bronchodilators if there is bronchospasm (**Table 117**)
Subacute bacterial sinusitis	Obtain imaging with coronal CT, culture, and treat with antibiotics for 3 wk
Asthma	p 316
Pertussis	Macrolide or trimethoprim-sulfa antibiotic × 2 wk; may need to treat as above for postinfectious cough
Chronic cough: duration >8 wk	25% of patients have more than 1 cause requiring concurrent tx; see Stepwise Approach, p 308
Perennial/allergic rhinitis	Tx for 2–4 wk for reduction/resolution, p 310
Chronic rhinosinusitis sinusitis (usually inflammation, not infection)	Imaging with coronal CT and consider ENT referral; cultures may show colonization; may need a course of nasal steroids
Asthma or cough-variant asthma	Tx for 6–8 wk for reduction/resolution, p 316
Reflux esophagitis	Treat for up to 3 mo for reduction/resolution using a PPI q12h

(cont.)

Table 113. Diagnosis and Management of Cough by Duration of Symptoms (cont.)	
Cause	**Preferred Management**
ACEIs	Stop ACEI
Smoking	Stop smoking (cough may persist for 4 wk)
Occupational exposure	Eliminate/minimize occupational exposure
Aspiration	Dysphagia, p 144. Evaluate with modified barium swallow
Sleep apnea	May present as cough that is also present at night (see Sleep chapter, p 342)
Eosinophilic bronchitis	Eosinophils in sputum, but no reversible airway obstruction on spirometry; treat with inhaled glucocorticoids (p 310) for 3–4 wk
External ear disease	Tx according to etiology
Bronchiectasis (purulent sputum)	Cyclic antibiotics often needed
Pulmonary fibrosis/Sarcoidosis	Pulmonary consultation
Idiopathic refractory cough	See Stepwise Approach, below

Stepwise Approach to Evaluating Chronic Cough

- Step 1: Hx and physical exam, medication review, red flags (hemoptysis or weight loss); obtain CXR, spirometry. If CXR and spirometry are normal, common causes are perennial/allergic rhinitis, reflux, cough-variant asthma.
- Step 2: Assess bronchial hyperresponsiveness with methacholine challenge, sputum eosinophil count (cough-variant asthma).
- Step 3: Consider rarer causes: refer to ENT for nasendoscopy; high-resolution chest CT (pulmonary fibrosis); bronchoscopy; refer to cough clinic.
- Step 4: Consider neuromodulatory tx for idiopathic refractory chronic cough.
  - Speech and language tx
  - Pharmacotherapy: low-dose slow-release morphine sulfate 5 mg po 2×/d, or gabapentin or pregabalin titrated to effect (reduce gabapentin/pregabalin dose if CrCl <60 mL/min[BC]). Amitriptyline[BC] 10 mg po hs is superior to codeine + guaifenesin.

Management

- Do not suppress cough in stable COPD.
- Medications used in acute or subacute cough have very limited efficacy, and all act centrally for cough suppression (**Table 114**).

Table 114. Antitussives and Protussives	
Medication	**Comments and Adverse Events (Metabolism)**
Benzonatate[1]	Antitussive, inconsistent evidence of benefit. AEs: CNS stimulation or depression, headache, dizziness, hallucination, constipation (L)
Dextromethorphan	Antitussive, inconsistent evidence of benefit. AEs: mild drowsiness, fatigue; interacts with SSRIs and SNRIs; combination may cause serotonin syndrome (L)
Guaifenesin[1]	Protussive (increases secretions); use best established in chronic cough. AEs: none at low dosages; high dosages cause nausea, vomiting, diarrhea, drowsiness, abdominal pain (L)

(cont.)

Table 114. Antitussives and Protussives (cont.)	
Medication	**Comments and Adverse Events (Metabolism)**
Codeine phosphate/ Guaifenesin	Antitussive and protussive; do not exceed 20 mg codeine/dose or 120 mg/24 h. AEs: sedation, constipation (L)
Hydrocodone/ Homatropine	Antitussive, inconsistent evidence of benefit. Do not exceed 30 mL or 6 tabs in 24 h AEs: sedation, constipation, confusion (L)

[1] Benzonatate 100 mg plus guaifenesin 600 mg may be effective for acute viral cough.

DYSPNEA

Definition

A subjective experience of breathing discomfort that consists of qualitatively distinct sensations that vary in intensity (ATS).

- **Acute dyspnea** develops over hours to days; almost always due to MI, PE, acute COPD or asthma exacerbation, pneumonia
- **Chronic dyspnea**: when symptoms present for >4–8 wk

Considerations in Chronic Dyspnea

- Age >65: occurs in 17% at rest at least occasionally; in 38% when hurrying on level ground or on slight hill
- Hx: consider if level of dyspnea is appropriate to level of exertion (vs suggests pathology)
  - Consider age, peers, usual activities, level of fitness
  - Ask, "What activities have you stopped doing?"
- Associated symptoms: cough, sputum, wheezing, chest pain, orthopnea, paroxysmal nocturnal dyspnea

Evaluation

Hx and physical exam should suggest organ system; then evaluate for cause (**Table 115**). Also check for anemia and hypothyroidism.

- Exertional dyspnea that develops after walking 50–100 ft suggests HFpEF or PH.
- Exercise-induced asthma begins about 3 min into exercise and peaks at 10–15 min.
- Intermittent dyspnea suggests asthma or PEs; dyspnea of HF waxes and wanes but has some baseline level of symptoms.

Table 115. Diagnosis of Dyspnea		
Suspected System	**Diagnostic Strategy**	**Diagnosis**
Cardiac	Chest radiograph, ECG, echocardiogram, radionuclide imaging, BNP or NT-proBNP (p 65)	Ischemic or other form of heart disease
Lung	Spirometry	Asthma, COPD, or restriction
	Diffusing capacity	Emphysema or interstitial lung disease
	Echocardiogram	Pulmonary HTN

(cont.)

Table 115. Diagnosis of Dyspnea (cont.)		
Suspected System	**Diagnostic Strategy**	**Diagnosis**
Respiratory muscle dysfunction	Inspiratory and expiratory mouth pressures	Neuromuscular disease (eg, myasthenia gravis)
Deconditioning/obesity vs psychological disorders	Cardiopulmonary exercise test	Deconditioning shows decreased maximal oxygen consumption but normal cardiorespiratory exercise responses.

Management

Nonpharmacologic Interventions

- Exercise reduces dyspnea and improves fitness in almost all older adults regardless of cause; physical conditioning reduces dyspnea during ADLs and exercise, and is primary tx for deconditioning.
  - Use low-impact, indoor activity
  - Base intensity on HR or symptom of dyspnea
  - Recommend 20–30 min on most days
- Indications for pulmonary rehabilitation include the following:
  - Dyspnea during rest or exertion
  - Hypoxemia, hypercapnia
  - Reduced exercise tolerance or a decline in ADLs
  - Worsening dyspnea and a reduced but stable exercise tolerance level
  - Pre- or postoperative lung resection, transplantation, or volume reduction
  - Chronic respiratory failure and the need to initiate mechanical ventilation
  - Ventilator dependence
  - Increasing need for emergency department visits, hospitalization, and unscheduled office visits

Pharmacotherapy: See specific diseases elsewhere in this chapter.

ALLERGIC RHINITIS

Description

- The most common atopic disorder; may be seasonal, episodic or perennial; in older adults, most often perennial.
- Symptoms include rhinorrhea, sneezing, and irritated eyes (Allergic Conjunctivitis, p 132), nose, and mucous membranes; the presence of at least 2 of these symptoms suggests allergic rhinitis.
- Postnasal drip, mainly from chronic rhinitis, is the most common cause of chronic cough.

Management

Nonpharmacologic Interventions: Avoid allergens, eliminate pets and their dander, dehumidify to reduce molds; reduce outdoor exposures during pollen season; reduce house dust mites by encasing pillows and mattresses. Arachnocides reduce mites. Saline and sodium bicarbonate nasal irrigation (eg, using a neti pot) are helpful as primary or adjunctive tx; use sterile (not tap) water when mixing home solutions to avoid risk of amoebic meningoencephalitis.

Pharmacotherapy: Target tx to symptoms and on whether symptoms are intermittent or persistent, agents listed in preferred order below; and agents are listed in **Table 116** and **Table 117.**

- Intermittent mild
  - oral second-generation antihistamine or nasal antihistamine
  - oral second-generation antihistamine + pseudoephedrine for major congestion
  - nasal steroid
- Intermittent moderate or severe
  - oral second-generation antihistamine or nasal antihistamine
  - nasal steroid
  - nasal antihistamine/nasal steroid combination or intranasal antihistamine+ nasal steroid
  - oral second-generation antihistamine + pseudoephedrine
- *Persistent mild*
  - nasal steroid
  - oral second-generation antihistamine or nasal antihistamine
  - oral second-generation antihistamine + pseudoephedrine for major congestion
  - *nasal cromolyn sodium*
- *Persistent moderate or severe*
  - nasal antihistamine/nasal steroid combination or nasal antihistamine + nasal steroid
  - *nasal steroid*
  - *nasal antihistamine*

Refractory symptoms: Consider other causes of chronic rhinosinusitis, refer to ENT; refer to allergist/immunologist for immunotherapy; consider omalizumab (refer to asthma or allergy specialist) or a short course of oral steroids.

Ocular symptoms: Occur in most patients with allergic rhinitis. Nonpharmacologic approaches include avoidance, hand washing after exposure, cool compresses, avoiding contact lenses during symptoms. Oral H_1 antihistamine or topical ophthalmic H_1 antihistamine are drugs of choice (allergic conjunctivitis, p 132 and **Table 116**). Nasal steroids also reduce eye symptoms.

Table 116. Choosing Medication for Allergic Rhinitis or Conjunctivitis

Medication or Class	Rhinitis	Sneezing	Pruritus	Congestion	Eye Symptoms
Nasal steroids[1]	+++	+++	++	++	++
Ipratropium, nasal[1]	++	0	0	0	0
Antihistamines[2,3]	++	++	++	+	+++
Pseudoephedrine[4]	0	0	0	++++	0
Phenylephrine nasal[5]	0	0	0	+++	0
Cromolyn, nasal[3]	+	+	+	+	0
Leukotriene modifiers[6]	+	+	+	+	++

0 = drug is not effective; the number of "+"s grades the degree of effectiveness.

[1] Effective in seasonal, perennial, and vasomotor rhinitis.

[2] Better in seasonal than in perennial rhinitis; nasal, ocular, and oral forms; ocular form effective only for eye symptoms, but nasal form may help ocular symptoms.

[3] Start before allergy season.

[4] Use for more than a few days causes rebound symptoms (rhinitis medicamentosa) when stopped; tx for rhinitis medicamentosa is taper of decongestant and addition of nasal steroids

[5] Topical tx rapid in onset but results in rebound if used for more than a few days; enhances effectiveness of nasal steroids and improves sleep during severe attacks.

[6] Montelukast (FDA approved for this indication) is no longer recommended due to neuropsychiatric disturbances documented in children; many allergists consider that this is a concern for adults.

Table 117. Medications for Allergic Rhinitis	
Type, Medication	**Adverse Events/Comments**
Second-Generation Antihistamines	*Class AEs:* bitter taste, nasal burning, sneezing (nasal preparations); eye burning, stinging, injection (ocular preparations) (K, L) *Onset 60 min;* adding to nasal steroids is not better than nasal steroid monotx
Oral	
Cetirizine^OTC^	Sedating at recommended doses; lower dose; avoid in dry eye (K)
Desloratadine	Sedating above recommended doses
✓Fexofenadine^OTC^	Nonsedating even at higher than recommended doses; fruit juice reduces absorption, so take 4 h before or 1–2 h after ingestion of juice; combination product containing pseudoephedrine is ***not*** recommended
Levocetirizine	Sedating at recommended doses; pharyngitis, fatigue, dry eye
✓Loratadine^OTC^	Sedating above recommended doses. Avoid in dry eye; combination product containing pseudoephedrine is ***not*** recommended
Nasal	
✓Azelastine	Dysgeusia, dysosmia, epistaxis, headache
✓Olopatadine	Dysgeusia, epistaxis (nasal), burning, stinging, headache blurry vision (ocular)
Oral Decongestants	
Pseudoephedrine (also in combination preparations^OTC^)	Arrhythmia, insomnia^BC^, anxiety, restlessness, elevated BP, urinary retention in men
Phenylephrine (has replaced pseudoephedrine in many combination products^OTC^)	Bradycardia, HTN, MI, HF, insomnia^BC^ In oral combination products, not more effective than placebo Use for >3 d causes rhinitis medicamentosa
Nasal Steroids	*Class AEs:* nasal burning, sneezing, bleeding, sore throat, headache; septal perforation (rare); fungal overgrowth (rare); ulceration; increased IOP (rare)
Second generation (systemic bioavailability <1% or undetectable); patients who fail to respond to 1×/d may respond to 2×/d dosage; reduce to daily when symptoms controlled. Onset of effect within 12 h maximum effect seen at >7 d.	
✓Fluticasone propionate^OTC^	2 spr/d or 1 spr 2×/d, 1 spr/d maintenance
Fluticasone furoate^OTC^ *(Flonase Sensimist)*	2 spr/d, 1 spr/d maintenance
Mometasone	2 spr/d
Ciclesonide *(Omnaris)* *(Zetonna)*	2 spr/d 1 spr/d
First generation (systemic bioavailability 10–50%) Same as Class AEs plus systemic ADRs from absorbed steroids	
Beclomethasone *(Beconase AQ)* *(Qnasl)*	1–2 spr q12h 2 spr/d
Triamcinolone *(Nasacort Allergy 24* ^OTC^, *Nasacort AQ)*	2 spr/d
Budesonide^OTC^	1 spr/d
Flunisolide	2 spr 2×/d

(cont.)

Table 117. Medications for Allergic Rhinitis (cont.)	
Type, Medication	**Adverse Events/Comments**
Mast Cell Stabilizer	
Cromolyn[OTC]	1 spr q6–8h Nasal irritation, headache, itching of throat; begin 1–2 wk before exposure to allergen
Leukotriene Modifiers (montelukast, zafirlukast, zileuton, p 322)	Mildly synergistic with antihistamines; ADRs include neuropsychiatric disturbances; use only after other tx fails.
Other	
Ipratropium	2 spr q6–12h (use 0.3% for allergies, ***not*** 0.6%) Epistaxis, nasal irritation, dry nose and mouth, pharyngeal irritation Caution: Do not spray in eyes, may increase IOP; 0.3% for rhinitis; 0.6% for viral nasal symptoms
Azelastine-Fluticasone *(Dymista)*	2 spr/d May improve adherence when both are required. More effective than either one alone.

✓ = preferred for treating older adults; [BC] Avoid; CrCl unit of measure = mL/min.

CHRONIC OBSTRUCTIVE PULMONARY DISEASE

Diagnosis

Consider COPD if any of these factors are present in an individual over age 40. The greater the number of factors, the more likely is the diagnosis. 10% of people aged >65 are affected.

- **Dyspnea:** that is progressive, worse with exercise, and persistent
- **Chronic cough:** with or without sputum production
- **Hx of exposure to risk factors:** tobacco smoke, smoke from heating fuels, occupational dust, smog, and chemicals
- Spirometry is required to establish a diagnosis. Assess airflow limitation based on spirometry measures after bronchodilators. COPD is diagnosed when $FEV_1/FVC < 0.70$ or perhaps 0.65 (in patients over age 65) or $FEV_1/FEV_6 < 0.70$ in patients over age 65 or those with severe disease.

Management

- Should be based on 3 factors: symptoms, airflow limitation, and frequency of exacerbations
- Assess **symptoms** using quantitative scale, eg, The Modified Medical Research Council Dyspnea Scale (mMRC) shown below:
  0 "I only get breathless with strenuous exercise"
  1 "I get short of breath when hurrying on the level or walking up a slight hill"
  2 "I walk slower than people of the same age on the level because of breathlessness or have to stop for breath when walking at my own pace on the level"
  3 "I stopped for breath after walking about 100 yards or after a few minutes on the level"
  4 "I am too breathless to leave the house" or "I am breathless when dressing"

mMRC 0–1, indicates fewer symptoms; mMRC ≥2, indicates more symptoms

- Then determine stage of **airflow limitation** by FEV_1 after bronchodilators in patients with $FEV_1/FVC < 0.7$.
- Finally, classify frequency of **exacerbations** as follows: low risk ≤1 exacerbation/y and no hospitalization, high risk ≥2 exacerbations/y or ≥1 exacerbation/y with ≥1 hospitalizations.

- The goals of pharmacotherapy and nonpharmacologic interventions are to minimize both symptoms and exacerbations and improve quality of life. The degree of airflow limitation should not be the sole determinant of tx.

General Approach

- For all patients:
  - Smoking cessation is essential at any age (p 356).
  - Pulmonary rehab increases exercise tolerance and decreases dyspnea and fatigue (p 310).
  - As needed short-acting bronchodilators (SABA or anticholinergic); the combination of the 2 gives greater acute relief. If the patient is taking a LAMA, use SABA for acute relief.
  - Low-dose CT screening for lung cancer if current or former smokers (Prevention, p 291)
- Many patients prefer 1×/d LAMA to 2×/d LABA.
- Mucolytic tx can be considered for patients with chronic productive cough; continue if reduced cough and sputum is more readily expectorated during a trial. Example tx: guaifenesin long-acting 600 mg po q12h (**Table 114**) or N-acetyl cysteine 600 mg 2×/d.
- Adding nutritional support promotes weight gain and fat-free mass; improves physical activity and general health.
- O_2 for all patients with chronic resting hypoxia (**Table 120**)

Stepped Approach to Pharmacotherapy

- Add agents when symptoms or exacerbations are inadequately controlled; D/C medication if no improvement. Assess improvement in symptoms, ADLs, exercise capacity, rapidity of symptom relief (**Table 118**).
- Consider de-escalation if symptoms improve while providing close follow-up.
- If symptoms do not improve, consider switching agents or mode of delivery.
- Long-term tx with LAMAs and LABAs, slows the loss of FEV_1 and reduces the number of exacerbations and hospitalization.
- Inhaled corticosteroids (ICS) combined with LABA or LAMA is additionally helpful for these outcome measures in patients with high eosinophil counts. For acute exacerbations, see **Table 119**.

Table 118. Pharmacotherapy for COPD

COPD Severity	Initial Therapy	Patient Response and Therapy Escalation
FEV_1 : ≥60% predicted mMRC score: 0–1 Exacerbations: ≤1 outpatient and 0 requiring hospitalization	Preferred: SAMA + SABA Alternative: SAMA or SABA	Medication used >2–3×/wk **Then:** Preferred: LAMA; Alternative: LABA
FEV_1 : <60% predicted mMRC score: 0–1 Exacerbations: ≤1 outpatient and 0 requiring hospitalization	Preferred: LAMA Alternative: LABA	Uncontrolled symptoms or further exacerbations **Then:** Preferred: LAMA + LABA; Alternative: LAMA
FEV_1 : Any % mMRC score: ≥2 Exacerbations: ≤1 outpatient and 0 requiring hospitalization	Preferred: LAMA + LABA Alternative: LAMA	Uncontrolled symptoms and elevated eosinophils **Then:** LAMA +LABA +ICS[1]

(cont.)

Table 118. Pharmacotherapy for COPD (cont.)

COPD Severity	Initial Therapy	Patient Response and Therapy Escalation
FEV_1 : Any % mMRC score: Any Exacerbations: ≥2 outpatient or ≥1 requiring hospitalization Eosinophils: ≤100 cells/μL	Preferred: LAMA + LABA Alternative: LAMA + LABA +ICS[1]	Any further exacerbations **Consider** roflumilast if FEV_1 <50%, BMI >21, and symptoms of bronchitis **Consider** azithromycin if patient is not smoking[2]
FEV_1 : Any % mMRC score: Any Exacerbations: ≥2 outpatient or ≥1 requiring hospitalization Eosinophils: Elevated	Preferred: LAMA + LABA + ICS[1] Alternative: LAMA + LABA	Any further exacerbations **Consider** roflumilast if FEV_1 <50%, BMI >21, and symptoms of bronchitis **Consider** azithromycin if patient is not smoking[2]

ICS, inhaled corticosteroids; LABA, long-acting β_2 agonist; LAMA, long-acting muscarinic receptor antagonist; mMRC, modified Medical Research Council; SABA, short-acting β_2 agonist; SAMA, short-acting antimuscarinic.

[1] Consider osteoporosis prophylaxis.

[2] Azithromycin is ineffective at reducing exacerbations in smokers. Check ECG; assess QT; if >450 millisec, not recommended.

Table 119. Outpatient Management of COPD Exacerbation

Stage and Evaluation	Management
COPD Exacerbation (Assess cardinal symptoms: increased dyspnea, sputum volume, and sputum purulence; check oximetry)	
Mild exacerbation (1 cardinal symptom; no resting dyspnea or respiratory distress; able to perform ADLs)	Increase dosage and/or frequency of SABA or SABA + SAMA with spacer or by nebulizer; no antibiotics; monitor for worsening
Moderate or severe exacerbation (2 or 3 cardinal symptoms; assess pulse oximetry; obtain CBC, CXR, ECG, ABG [if acute or acute on chronic hypercapnia]; consider BNP and D-dimer and rapid flu test or other respiratory virus)	**Add steroid** (eg, prednisone 40 mg po 1×d for 3–7 d) **Start antibiotic:** if <3 mo antibiotic exposure, use alternative class. Base choice on whether COPD is complicated or uncomplicated (see below) **Titrate O_2** to 88–92% sat; if new O_2 requirement consider hospital stay Nutritional supplement
• **Complicated COPD** (1 or more of: age >65, FEV_1 <50%, ≥2 exacerbations/y, cardiac diagnosis). Reassess 48–72 h after start of antibiotic tx • If improved, continue antibiotics for 3–5 d. • If unimproved, obtain sputum culture; reassess bronchodilators, steroids, and for HF, pneumonia, pneumothorax.	Fluoroquinolone (moxifloxacin, levofloxacin) or amoxicillin-clavulanate If at risk for pseudomonas (FEV_1 <30%, chronic systemic steroids, isolation or colonization in past 12 mo, bronchiectasis, broad spectrum antibiotic in last 3 mo), use levofloxacin or ciprofloxacin and obtain sputum culture.

Other Considerations for Patients with COPD

- Anxiety or major depression: seen in up to 40% of patients and should be treated.
- Palliative and end-of-life care. Offer discussion of these issues for patients with severe COPD. In particular, if the patient should become critically ill, verify that ICU care is consistent with goals of care and if the patient is willing to accept the burdens of such care.

Long-term Oxygen Therapy

- **Table 120** provides indications for oxygen use. Assess patients with FEV_1 <30%, cyanosis, edema, HF for resting hypoxia. Assess dyspnea on exertion by an exercise test.
- Tx for resting hypoxia improves survival, hemodynamics, polycythemia, exercise capacity, lung mechanics, and cognition. Tx of exertional hypoxia improves symptoms in most patients (not survival).
- Patients with COPD and normal daytime SaO2 may desaturate at night and require studies for sleep apnea.
- Portable devices should weigh <5 lb; flow rates up to 15 L/min are provided by liquid oxygen (more expensive).

Table 120. Indications for Long-term Oxygen Therapy[1,2]

PaO_2 Level	SaO_2 Level At Rest	Other
≤55 mm Hg	≤88%	>15 h/d for benefit[1], greater if 20 h/d
55–59 mm Hg	≥89%	Signs of tissue hypoxia (eg, cor pulmonale by ECG, HF, hematocrit >55%); or nocturnal desaturation, sats <90% for >30% of the time
≥60 mm Hg	≥90%	Desaturation with exercise
		No desaturation with exercise, but with dyspnea and ventilatory abnormalities during exercise; supplemental oxygen may permit greater exertion; exercise endurance improves up to an inspired oxygen fraction of 50% or flow rate of 6 L/min. May not be covered by Medicare.
		Desaturation with sleep apnea not corrected by CPAP
		Nocturnal SpO2 ≤88% or decreases >5% with signs or symptoms of nocturnal hypoxemia (eg, impaired cognitive function, morning headaches, restlessness, insomnia). Not covered by Medicare.

[1] Titrate O_2 saturation to ~90% higher flow rates may be needed at night and with exercise. Patients can titrate during exercise if they have an accurate oximeter (check home oximeter against one used in clinic).

[2] For patients recently discharged home on supplemental oxygen after hospitalization for acute illness, don't renew oxygen without reassessing need.[CW]

ASTHMA

Definition

- A heterogeneous disease usually characterized by airway inflammation. It is defined by the hx of respiratory symptoms such as wheezing, shortness of breath, chest tightness, and cough that vary over time and intensity together with variable airflow limitation on spirometry.

Diagnosis in Older Adults

- Half of older people with asthma have not been diagnosed. Prevalence of 7% >65 y is about the same as children.
- Atopy and nocturnal symptoms are ***less*** common.
- Diagnosis is based on symptoms and requires spirometry.[CW]
  - Aging causes a decline in lung function through reduction in both respiratory muscle function and elastic recoil that produces a pattern of irreversible fixed obstruction; this effect is greater in less active persons.

- ◦ Aging reduces FEV_1/FVC and may result in the overdiagnosis of COPD. This results in the misdiagnosis of COPD in some older adults with asthma.
- ◦ Suspect asthma in the presence of any of these symptoms: wheezing, cough, shortness of breath, chest tightness, or when these symptoms are brought on by viral illness.
- ◦ If FEV_1/FVC is ≤0.65 and the diffusing capacity of carbon dioxide is reduced, COPD is likely. The diffusing capacity of carbon dioxide is normal in asthma.
- ◦ If a SABA does not reverse airflow obstruction during PFTs (asthma is not excluded), do one of the following:
  - ▪ Perform bronchial provocative testing with methacholine (induce obstruction); but note that aging increases bronchial hyperresponsiveness to methacholine and the test may be less reliable **or**
  - ▪ Repeat testing after 2 wk of oral steroids to determine if obstruction seen in the initial test is reversible.
    Note: The component of age-related irreversible obstruction will persist.

Asthma-COPD Overlap

- More than half of people aged >65 with reversible airflow obstruction have both COPD and asthma (overlap syndrome); inhaled glucocorticoids must be part of tx.
- Tx is the same as for asthma through Step 3 (**Table 121**). If no IgE elevation, consider roflumilast or chronic macrolides as in COPD.

Additional Considerations

- Age of onset: Some older adults have had asthma from a young age; others develop asthma for the first time after age 65. Second peak in incidence after age 65; 5–10% after age 65 are affected and account for two-thirds of asthma deaths.
- Those with long-standing asthma develop fixed obstruction (reduced FEV_1/FVC that is not reversed by bronchodilators) as an effect of both the disease and aging.
- Cough is a common presentation for asthma in those aged >65.
- Symptoms may be confused with those of HF, COPD, GERD, or chronic aspiration.
- Typical triggers: aeroallergens (eg, cats, dust mites, cockroaches), irritants (eg, smoke, paint, household aerosols), viral URI, GERD, allergic rhinitis, metabisulfate ingestion (eg, wine, beer, food preservatives), medications (eg, ASA, NSAIDs, nonselective β blockers).
- About 95% of patients with asthma also have perennial rhinitis and tx of both improves asthma outcomes.

Management

Nonpharmacologic Interventions

Avoid triggers. Atopy and indoor environmental exposures are common triggers, especially dampness-related agents, possibly even in nonsensitized individuals. Use dehumidifiers and encase pillows and mattresses to reduce exposure to dust mites. Educate patients on disease management. Peak flow meters are less helpful in monitoring older adults; aging decreases peak flow and increases variability.

Pharmacotherapy

- Evidence on best tx for older adults with asthma is lacking because most clinical trials exclude people >65 y and those with comorbidities or a hx of smoking >10 pack-years. No guidelines for treating older patients with asthma have been published. What is given below is based on guidelines for the general adult population with asthma.

- While ICS are the backbone of tx for asthma with eosinophilic inflammation (younger-onset asthma), neutrophilic inflammation is more common in older adults, and ICS may be less effective but still recommended.
- LAMAs are effective as add-on tx in patients up to age 75.
- LTRAs are effective in older patients, although less so than in younger patients.
- Mepolizumab and omalizumab are effective in older patients with asthma that have circulating or sputum eosinophilia.
- SABAs are no longer preferred rescue tx in asthma. Studies show better outcomes when combination LABA and ICS are used as needed for acute symptoms.
- Oral vitamin D_3 supplementation (especially for persons with levels <25 nmol/L) reduces the risk of acute exacerbations that would require systemic steroids.

Stepped Approach

- The **number of the following symptoms** that were present in **the last 4 wk** determines the level of symptom control:
  - Daytime symptoms >2×/wk?
  - Limitations of activities due to asthma?
  - Nighttime waking due to asthma?
  - Reliever needed more than 2×/wk?
- Asthma is "Well controlled" if 0 (zero) symptoms, "Not well controlled" with 1–2 symptoms, and "Very poorly controlled" with 3–4 symptoms.
- Any exacerbation should prompt review of maintenance tx to ensure that it is adequate.
- By definition, an exacerbation in any week makes that an uncontrolled asthma week.
- If control is not achieved, step up, but first review inhaler technique, adherence, and avoidance of triggers (**Table 121**).
- When symptoms are controlled for 3 mo, try stepwise reduction (eg, step down from 2×/d ICS and LABA combination to 1×/d).
- LABAs should not be used unless given in combination with an ICS. LABAs as monotx are associated with increased mortality and are contraindicated as monotx.

Table 121. Asthma Therapy for Older Adults

Step[1]	Preferred	Other Controller Options
Step 1	Low-dose ICS/formoterol prn	Low-dose ICS whenever SABA is taken
Step 2	Daily low-dose ICS or prn low-dose ICS/ formoterol	Low-dose ICS whenever SABA is taken or LTRA
Step 3	Low-dose ICS + LABA Consider specialist consultation	Medium-dose ICS **or** low-dose ICS + LTRA
Step 4	Consult asthma specialist Medium-dose ICS + LABA	High-dose ICS, tiotropium mist inhaler is add-on or add on LTRA

(cont.)

Table 121. Asthma Therapy for Older Adults (cont.)		
Step[1]	**Preferred**	**Other Controller Options**
Step 5	Consult asthma specialist for phenotypic assessment-eosinophilic or neutrophilic High-dose ICS + LABA add-on tx (eg, tiotropium). For severe allergen-associated disease, monoclonal antibodies to IgE (omalizumab), IL-5 (mepolizumab, resilizumab), IL-5 receptor (benralizumab), IL-4 receptor (dupilumab). For severe uncontrolled asthma of any cause: Tezepelumab-ekko	Add low-dose oral corticosteroids but consider side effects
Reliever/ Rescue tx	Low-dose ICS/formoterol prn	LABA (caution in heart disease)

ICS, inhaled corticosteroid; LABA, long-acting β agonist; LTRA, leukotriene modifier; SABA, short-acting β agonist.

[1] Go to next step if symptoms not controlled. After 3 mo of stability, try reduction but do not stop ICS.

Source: Adapted from ginasthma.org.

Office Management of Acute Exacerbations in Primary Care

- **Assess severity.**
  - **Mild to moderate attacks**
    - **Symptoms/signs:** Talks in phrases, prefers sitting to lying, not agitated, RR increased, HR 100–120; O_2 sats 90–95%
    - **Pharmacotherapy:** Begin SABA 4–6 puffs by metered-dose inhaler (MDI) or nebulizer with ipratropium q20min × 1 h, then 2–4 puffs q3–4h for 24–48 h. Prednisolone 1 mg/kg; oxygen to keep sats 93–95%. Monitor hourly for worsening. Ready for home discharge when not needing SABA, O_2 sats >94% on room air, and home resources adequate. Continue prednisolone for 5–7 d. Step up controller tx; check inhaler technique and adherence.
  - **Severe attack or life-threatening attacks**
    - **Symptoms and signs:** speaks in words, sits hunched forward, agitated, uses accessory muscles, HR >120, O_2 sats <90%. **Life-threatening:** drowsy, confused, or silent chest.
    - **Therapy:** Urgent transfer to hospital. While waiting: inhaled SABA and ipratropium, O_2, systemic steroids.

DELIVERY DEVICES FOR ASTHMA AND COPD

All of these devices have 10–14 steps to achieve correct drug delivery; all patients should be observed initially and periodically for adequacy of technique.

Metered-dose inhalers (MDIs): prescribed as number of puffs.

- Spacers (require a separate prescription) improve drug delivery and should be used for essentially all older patients. One type (valve holding chamber) has a one-way valve to regulate inspiratory flow and prevent exhalation into the device.
- A Z-stat mask (adult size) affixed to a spacer further improves delivery when patient ability to take and hold breath is limited.
- Use separate spacers for steroids. Wash spacers monthly. *Potential errors in use:* failure to shake canister before use; difficulty depressing canister.

Dry powder inhalers (DPIs): prescribed as caps or inhalations; require moderate to high inspiratory flow. DPIs are not used correctly by 40% of people aged >60 and 60% of those aged >80. Instructions should be repeated and reinforced for proper use and effective tx.

Potential errors in use: All: Inadequate inspiratory flow rate: *Ellipta:* forget to open cover until it clicks. *Diskus:* dose counter is difficult to read. *HandiHaler* and *Neohaler:* difficulty removing capsules from foil; greater number of steps.

Soft mist inhalers (SMIs): prescribed as inhalations. Less dependent on inspiratory flow rates. Drug delivery to lung is similar to MDI with spacer, however proper technique can be complex for patients.

Potential errors in use: Device assembly; requires some coordination of inhalation; difficulty in twisting inhaler

Nebulizers

- Prescribed as milligrams or milliliters of solution. Consider for patients with disabling or distressing breathlessness on maximal tx with inhalers. Often the best choice for patients with cognitive impairment or when patients cannot manage SMIs, DPIs, or MDIs. *Pitfalls:* Less portable, require frequent cleaning, require more frequent dosing.
- See **Table 122** for nebulized products: ipratropium, albuterol, arformoterol, levalbuterol, budesonide, and glycopyrrolate.
- Caution when patients with glaucoma use nebulized antimuscarinics; the mask should fit well or a T-type delivery device should be used. Ultrasonic and jet nebulizers are available; the latter can be used with supplemental oxygen.

Table 122. Asthma and COPD Medications

Medication Class/Agent [Delivery Device] (frequency)	AEs (Metabolism, Excretion, Comment)
Short-acting Antimuscarinics (SAMAs)	
✓ Ipratropium *(Atrovent)* [MDI, nebulizer] (q6h)	Dry mouth, urinary retention, possible increase in cardiovascular mortality (lung, poorly absorbed; F)
Long-acting Antimuscarinics (LAMAs)	
Aclidinium *(Tudorza Pressair)* [DPI] (q12h)	Bronchospasm, nasopharyngitis, cough, diarrhea, and ADRs seen with ipratropium (lung, poorly absorbed; F)
Tiotropium *(Spiriva)* [DPI] (q24h) *(Spiriva Respimat Spray)* [SMI (1.25, 2.5)] (q24h)	Same as ipratropium except good data on cardiovascular safety (14% K, 86% F)
Umeclidinium *(Incruse Ellipta)* [DPI] (q24h)	Nasopharyngitis, URI, cough, arthralgia, AF <1% in trials
Glycopyrrolate *(Seebri Neohaler)* [DPI] (q12h)	Cough, nasopharyngitis (K)
Short-acting β 2-Agonists (SABAs)[1]	*Class AEs:* tremor, nervousness, headache, palpitations, tachycardia, cough, hypokalemia. *Caution:* use half-doses in patients with known or suspected coronary disease. (L)
✓ Albuterol *(Ventolin, Proventil, ProAir)* [MDI] (q4–6h) [nebulizer] (q6h)	max 12 puffs/d
(ProAir RespiClick) [DPI] (q4–6h)	max 12 inhalation/d
Levalbuterol *(Xopenex)* [nebulizer (q6–8h), MDI (q4–6h)]	No advantage over racemic albuterol (intestine, L)

(cont.)

Table 122. Asthma and COPD Medications (cont.)	
Medication Class/Agent [Delivery Device] (frequency)	**AEs (Metabolism, Excretion, Comment)**
Long-acting β-Agonists (LABA)	*Class AEs:* tremor, nervousness, headache, palpitations, tachycardia, cough, hypokalemia; do not use in asthma without an ICS.
Arformoterol *(Brovana)* [nebulizer] (q12h)	*Caution:* use half-doses in patients with known or suspected coronary disease; not for acute exacerbation.
✓ Salmeterol *(Serevent Diskus)* [DPI] (q12h)	
✓ Formoterol *(Foradil)* [DPI, nebulizer] (q12h)	Onset of action 1–3 min (L, K)
Indacaterol *(Arcapta)* [DPI] (q24h)	Greater bronchodilator effect than other LABAs, also greater risk of cough after inhalation, HTN
Olodaterol *(Striverdi Respimat)* [SMI] (q24h)	Pharyngitis
Corticosteroids: Inhaled	*Class AEs:* nausea, vomiting, diarrhea, abdominal pain; oropharyngeal thrush; dysphonia; dosages >1 mg/d may cause adrenal suppression, reduce calcium absorption and BMD, and cause bruising (L)
✓ Beclomethasone *(QVAR)* [MDI] (q6–12h)	
✓ Budesonide [DPI, nebulizer] (q12h)	
Ciclesonide *(Alvesco)* [SMI] (q12h)	
✓ Flunisolide *(Aerospan)* [SMI] (q12h)	
✓ Fluticasone propionate *(Flovent Diskus)* [DPI] (q12h)	
✓ Fluticasone furoate (*Arnuity Ellipta*) [DPI] (q24h)	
Mometasone *(Asmanex HFA)* [SMI] (q12h)	
(Asmanex Twisthaler) [DPI] (q12h)	
Corticosteroids: Oral	
Prednisone [po] (q12–24)	Leukocytosis, thrombocytosis, sodium retention, euphoria, depression, hallucination, cognitive dysfunction; other effects with long-term use (L)
Methylxanthines Long-acting theophyllines[BC] (eg, *Theo-Dur, Slo-Bid*) [po] (q12h) (eg, *Theo-24*) [po] (q24h)	*Class AEs:* atrial arrhythmias, seizures, increased gastric acid secretion, ulcer, reflux, diuresis; clearance ↓ by 30% after age 65; initial dosage ≤400 mg/d, titrate using blood levels; 16-fold greater risk of life-threatening events or death after age 75 at comparable blood levels (L)

(cont.)

Table 122. Asthma and COPD Medications (cont.)	
Medication Class/Agent [Delivery Device] (frequency)	**AEs (Metabolism, Excretion, Comment)**
Leukotriene Modifiers (LTRAs) *Class AEs:* drowsiness, dizziness, headache, fatigue, and possibly neuropsychiatric disturbances, GI AEs	
✓ Montelukast [po] (q24)	(L)
Zafirlukast [po] (q6h)	Fever; monitor LFTs and coumarin anticoagulants (L, reduced by 50% if age >65)
Zileuton-*CR* [po] (q12h 1 h pc)	Monitor LFTs, myalgia, and coumarin anticoagulants; other drug interactions; inhibits synthesis of leukotrienes less studied, least preferred in the class (L)
PDE4 Inhibitor	
Roflumilast *(Daliresp)* [po] (q24h)	For severe COPD (FEV_1 <50%) associated with chronic bronchitis but not emphysema. Weight loss, nausea, headache, back pain, influenza, insomnia; do not use if acute bronchospasm or moderate or greater liver impairment; caution in patients with depression (suicidality); inhibits CYP3A4 and -1A2 (eg, erythromycin) (L)
Combination: Long-acting β-Agonists + Inhaled Corticosteroids	
Vilanterol-Fluticasone *(Breo Ellipta)* [DPI] (q24h)	Same as LABAs and ICSs
✓ Budesonide-Formoterol [MDI] (q12h)	Same as individual agents (L, K)
✓ Formoterol-Mometasone *(Dulera)* [MDI] (q12h)	Nasopharyngitis, sinusitis, headache
✓ Salmeterol-Fluticasone [DPI] (q12h)	approved for asthma and COPD
Salmeterol-Fluticasone [DPI] (q12h)	approved for asthma
Combination: Long-acting β-Agonists + Long-Acting Anticholinergics	
Tiotropium-Olodaterol *(Stiolto Respimat)* [SMI] (q24h)	Same as LABAs and tiotropium (L, K)
Umeclidinium-Vilanterol *(Anoro Ellipta)* [DPI] (q24h)	Same as LABAs; see also Umeclidinium. Not for use in asthma. (L, K)
Glycopyrrolate-Indacaterol *(Utibron Neohaler)* [DPI] (q12)	Same as LABAs and glycopyrrolate (K, L)
Other Medications and Combinations	
✓ Albuterol-Ipratropium [nebulizer] (q6h)	Same as individual agents (L, K)
✓ *(Combivent Respimat)* [SMI] (q6h)	Not to exceed 6 inhalations in 24 h
Cromolyn sodium [nebulizer] (q6h)	Cough, throat irritation (L, K); used in stable asthma
Fluticasone furoate-umeclidinium-vilanterol *(Trelegy Ellipta)* [DPI] (q24h)	Same as individual agents
Albuterol and budesonide *(Airsupra)* inhaler	Same as individual agents

✓= preferred for treating older adults

[1] Older nonselective β_2 agonists such as isoproterenol, metaproterenol, or epinephrine are not recommended and are more toxic.

RESTRICTIVE LUNG DISEASE (RLD)

- Up to 11% of people over age 75 meet criteria for RLD. In old age, RLD is often due to disorders outside of the lung itself. RLD can be disabling, progressive, and sometimes treatable.
- RLD is more likely to produce ADL disability (RR = 9.0; 95% CI: 3.1–26.6) than is moderate COPD (RR = 2.3; 95% CI: 0.7–4.5).
- These disorders are characterized by reduced total lung capacity (TLC). However, TLC is not part of routine pulmonary function tests (PFTs). In practice, FVC is used as a surrogate for TLC.

Diagnosis and Staging

- Patients present with exertional dyspnea, which often has insidious onset. PFTs show decreased lung volumes (FVC <80% of the lower limit of normal [LLN]), an FEV_1/FVC ratio >85–90%, and flow volume curve shows a complex profile.
- Disease severity is based on the degree of reduction of FVC; FVC 60–80% of LLN = mild, 50–60% = moderate, <50% = severe.

Differential Diagnosis

The many disorders that cause RLD can be grouped as shown in **Table 123** along with differentiating characteristics and some common causes in the older population.

Table 123. Common Causes of Restrictive Lung Diseases in Older Adults

Category (Mechanism)	Differentiating PFT Findings	Common Causes
Intrinsic lung diseases (inflammation or scarring of the lung tissue)	Abnormal DLCO	Idiopathic pulmonary fibrosis Postinflammatory lung fibrosis Radiation Drug induced Connective tissue diseases (RA, etc) Chronic HF
Extrinsic disorders (mechanical compression of lungs or limitation of expansion)	Normal DLCO	Kyphosis/Kyphoscoliosis Obesity Ankylosing spondylitis Pectus excavatum or carinatum
Neuromuscular disorders (decreased ability of the respiratory muscles to inflate/deflate lungs)	Normal DLCO Reduced maximal inspiratory and/or expiratory pressures	ALS Thyroid and adrenal disorders Vitamin D deficiency Postpolio syndrome
CNS disorders	Normal DLCO	Parkinson disease Multisystem atrophy Progressive supranuclear palsy Multiple sclerosis

DLCO, diffusing capacity of the lung for carbon monoxide.

Management

- Follows the underlying cause. Because many of these disorders are outside of the lung itself, diagnosis and management often falls to geriatric healthcare providers.
- For RLD from kyphosis including hyperkyphosis:
  - Exercise focused on postural alignment, flexibility, core strengthening, back extensor muscle strengthening
  - Other: spinal orthosis, postural taping, manual tx; surgery only for severe pulmonary impairment

SEXUALITY

CHANGES IN SEXUAL FUNCTION WITH AGING

Men

- Between age 60–70, 50–80% of men engage in any sexual activity, and that decreases to 15–20% for those aged ≥80.
- Factors influencing decreased activity include poor health, social issues, partner availability, decreased libido, and ED (see below).
- Changes in the sexual response cycle with age include:
  - *Excitement phase:* delay in erection, decreased tensing of the scrotal sac, loss of testicular elevation
  - *Plateau phase:* prolonged time in phase, reduced pre-ejaculatory secretion
  - *Orgasm* is reduced in intensity and duration.
  - *Refractory period* between erections is prolonged.

Women

- Between age 75–85, 17% of women report sexual activity, and of those, over half report sexual activity 2–3×/mo.
- Among women with a spouse or other partner, factors reported to reduced sexual activity include partner's or their own physical health problems.
- Changes in the sexual response cycle after menopause and which are attributed to decline in estrogen include:
  - *Excitement phase:* clitoris requires longer direct stimulation, reduced and delayed vaginal lubrication
  - *Plateau phase:* less expansion and congestion of the vagina
  - *Orgasm:* fewer and weaker contractions, but multiple orgasm can occur.
  - *Resolution phase:* vascular congestion lost more rapidly.

A reliable resource to assist older men and women in addressing these changes can be found at aarp.org/home-family/sex-intimacy/

Low Libido

- Libido declines with age in sexually active men and women. Libido is associated with satisfaction with the primary partner and happiness. Low libido is associated with low physical and emotional sexual satisfaction and low general happiness. Also consider drug-induced causes (see below).
- In men also consider:
  - Hypogonadism (see below)
  - Strong association with LUTS (see Prostate chapter) and other sexual and voiding disorders.

DRUG-INDUCED SEXUAL DYSFUNCTION

The following drugs and drug classes are believed to sometimes cause sexual dysfunction in both men and women. In cases of suspected drug-induced sexual dysfunction, improvement after drug withdrawal provides the best evidence for the adverse effect. Tx with a drug from an alternative class to treat an underlying condition may be necessary.

- Antidepressants: SSRIs (see below) reduce libido and delay orgasm; lithium causes ED; MAOIs may cause ED or anorgasmia.

- Antipsychotics: olanzapine produces less loss of libido or ED than risperidone, clozapine, and oral and depot first-generation agents.
- Antihypertensives: any agent may cause ED related to reduced genital blood flow.
  - Spironolactone has antiandrogen effect.
  - Centrally acting sympatholytics (eg, clonidine) produce relatively high rates of sexual dysfunction (ED and loss of libido).
  - Peripherally acting sympatholytics, eg, reserpine (ED and loss of libido).
- Digoxin: possibly related to reduced T levels
- Lipid-lowering agents: fibrates (gynecomastia and ED) and many statins (eg, lovastatin, pravastatin, simvastatin, atorvastatin) are the subject of case reports of both ED and gynecomastia. Statins affect the substrate for sex hormones and have been shown to reduce total and sometimes also bioavailable T.
- Acid-suppressing drugs: The H2RA cimetidine and the PPI omeprazole can cause gynecomastia. Famotidine has caused hyperprolactinemia and galactorrhea.
- Metoclopramide: induces hyperprolactinemia
- Anticonvulsants: phenobarbital, phenytoin, carbamazepine, primidone; all increase metabolism of androgen.
- Anticholinergics and antihistamines produce vaginal dryness.
- Alcohol: high dosages reduce libido.
- Opioids: reduce libido and produce anorgasmia related to reduced T levels.

IMPOTENCE (ERECTILE DYSFUNCTION OR ED)

Definition

Inability to achieve sufficient erection for intercourse. Prevalence nearly 70% by age 70.

Causes

Often multifactorial; >50% of cases arterial, venous, or mixed neuropathic/vascular cause (**Table 124**).

Pharmacotherapy

An at-home trial of a PDE5 inhibitor (**Table 125**) is both diagnostic of ED and therapeutic for the common causes of ED (vascular, neuropathic, mixed); these agents are also effective for ED after most prostate cancer tx and in DM2. All should be taken on an empty stomach. Agents differ in onset of action; taper up if dose is ineffective; taper down if ADRs. Alternate tx (devices, injections) are included in **Table 125**. Refer to urology for injectable products.

Table 124. Causes of Erectile Dysfunction (ED) in Older Men

Causes (in order of frequency)	Associated Findings/Risk Factors	Onset
Vascular	Vascular risk factors; femoral bruits; poor pedal pulses. Venous vascular disease suggested by penile plaques (Peyronie disease).	Gradual
Neuropathic	DM; hx of pelvic trauma, surgery, irradiation; spinal injury or surgery; Parkinson disease, multiple sclerosis; alcoholism; loss of bulbocavernosus reflex or orthostatic BP changes	Gradual
Drug induced (p 331)	Loss of sleep-associated erections	Sudden
Psychogenic, including bereavement	Sleep-associated erections or erections with masturbation are intact	Sudden

(cont.)

Causes (in order of frequency)	Associated Findings/Risk Factors	Onset
Hypogonadism[1]	Decreased libido >ED; low T, small testes, gynecomastia; 1/3 of patients with DM2 have low T.	Gradual
Other Endocrine	Hyper-/hypocortisolism, hyper-/hypothyroidism, hyperprolactinemia	Gradual

Table 124. Causes of Erectile Dysfunction (ED) in Older Men (cont.)

[1] Don't prescribe testosterone (T) for men with ED and normal T levels.[CW]

Table 125. Management of Erectile Dysfunction

Therapy	Comments
PDE5 Inhibitors	
All Agents: Effective in 60–70% of men with ED of various etiologies. Ocular ADRs include ocular surface abnormalities, increased IOP and glaucoma, uveitis, non-arteritic anterior ischemic optic neuropathy, chorioretinopathy, retinal occlusion, and visual field changes. PDE5 inhibitors potentiate the hypotensive effects of α blockers. Potent CYP3A4 inhibitors reduce metabolism of all PDE5 inhibitors and increase risk of toxicity. *Common ADRs:* headache, flushing, rhinitis, dyspepsia. *Other ADRs:* priapism, low-back pain. Start lowest dose and titrate prn. *All should be taken on an empty stomach to maximize absorption.*	
Avanafil *(Stendra)*	More rapid onset; take 30 min before sexual activity; use not recommended in severe renal or hepatic impairment.
Sildenafil	Take 1 h before sexual activity. *Other AEs:* increased sensitivity to light, blurred vision, bluish discoloration of vision; 20-mg tabs least expensive option; safety uncertain in renal and hepatic impairment.
Vardenafil *(Levitra)*	Take 1 h before sexual activity. *Other AEs:* Avoid using in congenital or acquired QT prolongation and in patients taking class IA or III antiarrhythmics; not recommended in hemodialysis and or severe liver impairment.
Tadalafil *(Cialis)*	Take 30–60 min before sexual activity. Longer duration of action (up to 36 h). More effective in complete ED. *Other AEs:* myalgia, pain in limbs; 2.5 mg/d may be as effective as taking higher doses prn; daily dosing not recommended in severe renal or liver impairment. Visual color distortion < than with sildenafil.
Devices	
Vacuum tumescence devices (eg, *Osbon-Erecaid*)	*Rare:* ecchymosis, reduced ejaculation, coolness of penile tip. Good acceptance in older population; intercourse successful in 70–90% of cases.
Penile prosthesis	*Complications:* infection, mechanical failure, penile fibrosis
Other	
Prostaglandin E (alprostadil) and combination injectable products available through urology	
Trazodone for psychogenic ED	Take 25–100 mg po hs. May also help for premature ejaculation; below dose needed to treat depression. ADRs: sedation, orthostasis

Diagnosis of Hypogonadism in Middle-aged and Older Men

- Hypogonadism is more closely associated with libido than with ED.
- Diagnose T deficiency only in men with consistent symptoms and unequivocally low T levels.
- Ask the following questions from the European Male Aging Study Sexual Function Questionnaire. If the answers to **all 3 questions** are the responses in **bold**, hypogonadism is likely present.

- How often did you think about sex? This includes times of just being interested in sex, daydreaming, or fantasizing about sex, as well as times when you wanted to have sex.
  - **2 or 3 times or less in the last month**
  - Once/wk or more often
    - It is common for men to experience erectile problems. This may mean that one is not always able to get or keep an erection that is rigid enough for satisfactory activity (including sexual intercourse and masturbation).
- In the last *month*, are you:
  - Always able to keep an erection that would be good enough for sexual intercourse, or usually able to get and keep an erection that would be good enough for sexual intercourse?
  - **Sometimes or never able to get and keep an erection that would be good enough for sexual intercourse?**
- How frequently do you awaken with full erection?
  - **Once in the last month or less often**
  - 2 or 3 times or more often in the last month

- Morning fasting total T level <264 ng/dL that remains <275 ng/dL on 1–2 repeat tests using CDC's accuracy-based Hormone Standardization (HoSt) program.
- If T is low, check LH/FSH to determine primary or secondary. If secondary, evaluate other pituitary functions.

Management of Hypogonadism

- Prescribe T only when there is clear evidence of moderate to severe deficiency.[CW, BC]
- Other symptoms and signs of low T: low BMD, depression, decreased body hair.
- The T trials of men aged ≥65 with unequivocally low T levels (<275 pmol/L) and either low libido, mobility limitations, mild anemia, and/or low vitality, treated for 1 y with normalization of T levels show:
  - Improved libido, sexual activity, erectile function; higher Hb, BMD, better mood; possible improved walking distance.
  - Cognition was not improved, and CAD plaque increased.
- Testosterone is not recommended with breast or prostate cancer, prostate nodule or induration, PSA >3 ng/dL, or significant prostate obstructive symptoms.
- Testosterone is not recommended if hematocrit >48%, untreated sleep apnea, or HF.
- Monitor AEs and response q3mo. *AEs:* polycythemia, fluid retention, liver dysfunction.
- Recheck PSA at 3–6 mo of tx and follow-up levels if rising; check hematocrit at 6 mo and 12 mo.
- Probably effective in the tx of opioid-induced androgen deficiency.

Options for Testosterone Replacement

During tx, check serum T concentration and adjust dose to achieve level 300–400 ng/dL; check midway between injections (except undecanoate: check before next injection); all other preparations, check manufacturer's recommendation for monitoring levels and adjusting dose.

Injectable (route/frequency)

- Testosterone enanthate (SC 1×/wk; IM q2–4wk)
- Testosterone undecanoate *(Aveed)* (IM q10wk)
- Testosterone cypionate (IM q2–4wk)
- Testosterone pellets *(Testopel)* (SC q3–6mo)

Transdermal (all topically 1×/d)

- *Androderm*
- *Fortesta*
- *AndroGel*
- *Testim*

Buccal

- *Striant* q12h

Intranasal

- *Natesto* 3×/d

Oral: *Testosterone undecanoate (Jatenzo)* 2×/d. Not recommended for age-related decline in testosterone; risks exceed benefits; MI, stroke, and cardiovascular death.

FEMALE SEXUAL DYSFUNCTION

Definition: a sexual problem that is persistent or recurrent and causes distress or interpersonal problems; cause is often multifactorial.

Evaluation

- Ask about problems (eg, changes in libido, partner's function, and health issues).
- Ask about absence or significantly reduced sexual interest/arousal.
- Screen for depression.
- Ask about incontinence.
- Eliminate medications contributing to sexual dysfunction (see *Drug-Induced Sexual Dysfunction*).
- When dyspareunia is reported:
  - Ask about onset, associated symptoms, pain location, and triggers.
  - Perform pelvic exam (see **Table 126**).

Management

Dyspareunia

Table 126. Evaluation and Management of Dyspareunia (Pain with Intercourse)

Type	Management	Comment
Superficial pain (Introital)		
Localized vulvar (provoked pain at introitus)	Estrogen or estrogen + testosterone[1]; topical precoital lidocaine; pelvic floor PT	Testosterone is off label in US.
Regional neuropathic	Pelvic floor PT; see neuropathic pain tx (Pain chapter)	Distribution is along nerve pathways
Localized skin disorders	**Table 138**	eg, lichen planus, lichen sclerosis
Vulvovaginal infection	Antifungals, antibiotics, antivirals	
Genitourinary syndrome of menopause (GSM)	Vaginal estrogen replacement, vaginal DHEA, ospemifene, topical precoital lidocaine	See GSM below and **Table 127**

(cont.)

Table 126. Evaluation and Management of Dyspareunia (Pain with Intercourse) (cont.)		
Type	**Management**	**Comment**
Deep Pain		
Myofascial pain (muscle spasm, trigger points)	Pelvic floor PT	
Chronic pelvic pain disorders (pain on bladder filling, IBS)	GU or GI referral	
Chronic systemic pain disorders	Systemic pain control	Pain clinic referral

[1] Also improves desire, arousal, and orgasmic response in most studies

Other Therapies for Sexual Dysfunction

- Counseling for one or both partners; sex and couples therapy are often helpful.
- Treat UI, FI, or both (see Incontinence chapter).
- Studies of sildenafil have not consistently shown effectiveness.

Genitourinary Syndrome of Menopause (GSM)

- GSM, also known as vulvovaginal atrophy or atrophic vaginitis, is due to loss of estrogen.
- Dyspareunia is a symptom of GSM.
- Other symptoms of GSM include burning, pruritis, dryness, vaginal bleeding, dysuria, urinary frequency, urethral discomfort, and recurrent UTI.
- First-line tx for dryness or discomfort, vaginal moisturizers or lubricants (worth a trial for dyspareunia).
- Vaginal moisturizers (eg, *Replens, Feminease, K-Y Liquibeads*) are used routinely 2–3 d/wk.
- Vaginal lubricants (eg, *K-Y Jelly, Astroglide, Pjur*) are added for intercourse.
- If dyspareunia or other symptoms of GSM are uncontrolled by moisturizers or lubricants, tx with topical estrogens (**Table 127**) may be used if no other contraindications; these produce minimal systemic levels.

Table 127. Pharmacotherapy for Genitourinary Syndrome of Menopause[1]	
Estradiol ring	Insert intravaginally and change q90d
Estradiol vaginal tablet	Insert 4 mcg/d or 10 mcg/d intravaginally × 2 wk, then 2×/wk
Estradiol cream	0.5–4 g/d intravaginally × 2 wk, then 0.5–1 g 2–3×/wk
Conjugated estrogen cream	0.5 g/d intravaginally × 2 wk, then 0.5–2 g 2–3×/wk
Prasterone insert (DHEA)	6.5 mg/d intravaginally hs
Ospemifene oral tablets	60 mg po 1×/d with food[1]

[1] Vaginal estrogens are first-line and preferred tx.

Note: For women with a uterus, consider concomitant progestin tx. Contraindications: stroke, MI, DVT, or PE, estrogen-dependent neoplasia, and genital bleeding.

CHRONIC WOUND ASSESSMENT AND MANAGEMENT

Wound Assessment

Evaluation of chronic wounds should include (**Table 128** for wound characteristics specific to wound type):

- Wound hx (onset, recurrence, contributing factors such as trauma, etc) and impact on quality of life
- Location
- Wound size and shape: length, width, depth. Consistent measurement is important for evaluating tx effectiveness. Use a centimeter ruler to measure length and width, and a cotton-tipped swab to measure depth, tunneling, and undermining. Include photo in medical record.
- Stage (pressure ulcer), grade (diabetic foot ulcer)
- Wound edges and bed: color, presence of slough, necrotic tissue, granulation tissue, epithelial tissue, undermining, or tunneling
  - Darkly pigmented skin may appear blue, purple, or just darker. Can be difficult to identify Stage 1 pressure injuries and deep-tissue pressure injuries, and other dermatitis. Palpate for temperature and consistency.
- Exudate: purulent vs nonpurulent (serous, serosanguineous, sanguineous)
- Periwound skin and soft tissue: warmth, erythema, induration
  - Note warmth, capillary refill, and presence of pulses, edema, anasarca, and lymphedema
- Presence of pain at rest and with wound care procedures
- Signs of wound infection:
  - Worsening wound (increased necrotic tissue, drainage, enlargement, purulence)
  - Lack of healing despite appropriate wound care and offloading of pressure (for wounds exposed to pressure)
  - Odor dependent on microbe present. gram-negative and anaerobic, foul odor; pseudomonas, sweet.
  - Purulent exudate
  - Surrounding erythema
  - Increasing pain
  - Local swelling, warmth
  - Cellulitis may be present, as well as systemic signs of infection.
  - Reduced or loss of function of affected limb
- A swab culture of wound surface exudates is of no value in diagnosing infection due to wound contamination. Educate staff not to collect cultures of wound slough or pus; encourage use of Levine technique for culture.
  - Levine technique (cleanse with NS followed by rotating a swab over a 1-cm square area of viable wound tissue [not necrotic] with sufficient pressure to express fluid from the wound tissue beneath the wound surface)
  - Biopsies are relatively invasive, costly, require skilled operators, and potentially exacerbate infection, but may be needed if antibiotic resistance is suspected.
  - Consider imaging if deep infection or osteomyelitis are suspected.

- Test wound fluid samples for elevated protease activity for human neutrophil-derived elastase (HNE) and matrix metalloproteases (MMP). Chronic wounds having values of HNE >5, MMP ≥13, or both, should be considered wound healing impaired (*WoundChek Protease Status* test kit).
- Ongoing documentation of wound hx, characteristics, rate of healing (measurements and photographs) in the patient's health record.

Table 128. Typical Wound Characteristics by Wound Type

	Arterial	Diabetic	Pressure	Venous
Location	Distal location, areas of trauma	Plantar surface of foot, especially over metatarsal heads, toes, and heel	Over bony prominences (eg, trochanter, coccyx, ankle)	Gaiter area (between ankle and knee), particularly medial malleolus
Size and shape	Shallow, well-defined borders	Wound margins with callus	Variable length, width, depth depending on stage (staging system, p 339)	Edges may be irregular with depth limited to dermis or shallow subcutaneous tissue
Wound bed	Pale or necrotic	Granular tissue unless PAD present	Varies; bright red, pale pink. Can be shallow erosion to deeper ulceration with slough and necrotic tissue; tunneling and undermining	Ruddy red; yellow slough may be present; undermining or tunneling uncommon
Exudate	Minimal amount due to poor blood flow	Variable amount; serous unless infection present	Serous or serosanguinous. May be purulent, becoming serous as healing progresses; foul odor with infection	Copious; serous unless infection present
Surrounding skin	Halo of erythema or slight fluctuance indicates infection	Normal; may be calloused	Normal; may have erythema, edema, induration if infected. Wound edges may be distinct, diffuse, or rolled under.	May appear macerated, crusted, or scaly; presence of stasis dermatitis, hyperpigmentation
Pain	Cramping or constant deep aching	Variable intensity; none with advanced neuropathy	Painful, unless sensory function impaired or with deep, extensive tissue necrosis	Variable; may range from absent to severe, dull or aching in character.

Principles of Wound Management

- Establish wound care goals, considering advance directives and patient's values and preferences to determine tx.
- Address risk factors for poor healing and manage comorbidities (eg, malnutrition, DM, smoking, immunosuppression, vascular disease, pressure or shear force, chronic moisture).
  - Protein (1.25–1.5 g/kg/d) and calories (30–35/kg/d) unless contraindicated because of impaired renal function
    - If dietary intake inadequate, consider nutritional support using other routes.
  - Correct deficiencies of vitamins A, C, E, and zinc if suspected.

- Arginine-containing nutritional supplements (4.5 g/d); amino acid supplements
- Avoid exposure to cold; vasoconstriction reduces blood flow to wound.
- Avoid smoking to prevent vasoconstriction that reduces blood flow to wound.
- Ensure adequate hydration with oral or parenteral fluid.

- Treat wounds based on etiology with local wound care and surgery, if indicated.
- Treat high levels of proteolytic activity with protease modulator dressing to facilitate wound closure. Retest until protease levels are normal (≤1×/wk).
- Remove debris and necrotic tissue.
  - Cleanse wound using NS or Lactated Ringer's potable water (with or without soap), or commercially available wound cleaner with each dressing change. Avoid antiseptics because of cytotoxicity.
  - Irrigate using 4–15 psi to cleanse adherent debris. Can be achieved through various methods (eg, a 19-gauge IV catheter on a 35-mL syringe, an irrigation cap, manufactured devices). Whirlpool tx not recommended.
  - Consider combining autolytic or topical enzyme debridement methods with sharp debridement to facilitate more rapid removal of necrotic tissue, by an experienced clinician or a licensed podiatrist.
    - Sharp debridement
    - Autolytic methods (eg, moisture-retaining dressings or hydrogels, *MediHoney*)
    - Mechanical (eg, hydrotherapy, irrigation)
    - Biological (maggot debridement tx)
    - Chemical (eg, topical enzymes such as collagenase anacaulase *[Nebrid]*)
  - Debridement provides a brief (24–48 h) opportunity for bacterial susceptibility to antimicrobials.
- Document rate of wound healing based on weekly decreases in wound area measurements.
- Referral for surgical evaluation if warranted
- Control pain associated with wound care procedures by offering pain medication 30 min before procedure. Choose least painful tx option.
  - *Mepitel* two-side wound contact layer to minimize pain and trauma at dressing change. Does not adhere to moist wound and allows secondary dressing change without disturbing wound bed to promote faster healing.
  - Use complementary approaches, such as massage, touch, high-intensity TENS.
  - Gauze-based negative-pressure wound tx (NPWT), rather than foam, less painful in older adults, those with bone and tendon exposure in wounds.
  - Topical lidocaine gel
  - For moderate to severe pain not managed by oral medications or with dose-limiting AEs, topical opioids may be used (eg, morphine sulfate mixed in a neutral water-based gel applied 2×/d). Can titrate to effect. Caution in ulcers with large surface area because of the risk of systemic absorption.
  - Treat cellulitis surrounding ulcer with a systemic gram-positive bactericidal antibiotic (cellulitis, p 101) unless gram-negative organisms are suspected and may require aggressive IV antibiotics.
  - If osteomyelitis is suspected, evaluate with X-ray, CT, MRI, or bone biopsy.
  - Referral for surgical evaluation if warranted.
- Control bacterial burden/infection.
  - Many chronic wounds may be covered with invisible biofilm that delays healing and require aggressive tx.

- Protect wound from contamination.
- Treat infected wounds by addressing underlying condition.
- Control odor with dressing (eg, charcoal, chlorophyllin dressings) or topical agents (eg, sodium hypochlorite, hypochlorous acid).
- Consider antimicrobial dressings to reduce bioburden (eg, silver-, chlorhexidine-, honey-, iodine-containing).
- If infection is suspected, assess type and quantity of bacteria by validated quantitative swab or tissue biopsy. Clinical signs and symptoms are not accurate in establishing infection or the need for antimicrobials or antibiotics, and point-of-care diagnostic tests to detect bacterial burden should be used.
- For ulcers with ≥1 million CFU/g of tissue or any tissue level of β-hemolytic streptococci, use a topical antimicrobial (eg, dressings with bioavailable silver, cadexomer iodine at concentrations up to 0.45%). Limit duration of use of topical antimicrobials to avoid cytotoxicity or bacterial resistance.
- Consider 2-wk trial of topical antibiotic for clean ulcers that are not healing after 2–4 wk of optimal care; antibiotic spectrum should include gram-negative, gram-positive, and anaerobic organisms (eg. mupirocin, neomycin, polymyxin B, and bacitracin).
- Systemic antibiotics are indicated for clinical infection, deep invasion, cellulitis, osteomyelitis, or systemic inflammatory response (**Table 129**). Bone biopsy for suspected osteomyelitis by MRI or tx if MRI positive and 6-wk antibiotic tx recommended; 8-wk antibiotic tx if MRSA.

Table 129. Empiric Antibiotic Therapy to Treat Infections in Chronic Wounds

Severity of Infection	Clinical Features	Empiric Medication Options	Duration of Treatment
Mild	Superficial, localized signs of inflammation or infection, without signs of a systemic response or osteomyelitis, and ambulatory management planned	Cephalexin Amoxicillin-clavulanate Clindamycin Levofloxacin or moxifloxacin Doxycycline or trimethoprim-sulfamethoxazole (for MRSA)	1–2 wk
Moderate	Superficial, nonlocalized infection or deep-tissue involvement (including osteomyelitis), without a systemic inflammatory response, and either planned ambulatory or inpatient management	Ceftriaxone or cefoxitin Ampicillin-sulbactam Levofloxacin or moxifloxacin Doxycycline, linezolid, or vancomycin (for MRSA)	1–8 wk (after surgical debridement, if indicated)
Severe	Superficial to deep-tissue involvement (including osteomyelitis), with a systemic response, or is life-/limb-threatening and requires inpatient care	Vancomycin, linezolid, or daptomycin (for MRSA) PLUS piperacillin-tazobactam Vancomycin, linezolid, or daptomycin (for MRSA) PLUS carbapenem	1–8 wk (after surgical debridement, if indicated)

- Provide moist wound environment and control exudates using appropriate dressings. Avoid wet-to-dry dressings and choose dressings that minimize friction, shearing, skin irritation, and additional pressure.
  - Select dressings appropriate to wound type and characteristics (**Table 130**).
    Note: Wound care products are classified by the FDA as medical devices (ie, exempt from the requirement to demonstrate efficacy), so little evidence-based support. Choices based on product availability, insurance coverage, cost, rationale for product type and goals of care (healing vs protection and comfort). See Common Dressings For Wound Management, pp 335–336.

- Fill dead space (tunnels, undermining) loosely with moistened gauze dressings or other wound fillers (eg, calcium alginate strips, hydroconductive wound dressings [*Drawtex*])
- Negative-pressure wound tx—high quality evidence of 25% reduction in wound size and time to healing
  - Indications: Stage 3 and 4 pressure ulcers, neuropathic ulcers, venous ulcers, dehisced incisions; also used over closed incisions and skin grafts.
  - Contraindications: presence of >20% nonviable or necrotic tissue in wound, untreated osteomyelitis, malignancy in wound
  - Avoid use in patients taking anticoagulants
  - Guidelines for use:
    - Dressing change regimen: variable whether using with or without silver
    - Specialized training in application and monitoring of tx are essential for successful outcomes.
- If wound does not show signs of healing over a 2-wk period of optimal tx, reevaluate wound management strategies and factors affecting healing.
- May require surgical intervention for complete closure of healing wounds; bacterial contamination >10^5 cfu/g cannot be readily closed with 50–100% dehiscence and persistent infection.
- For nonhealable or palliative wounds where the goals are protection and comfort, use products to reduce bioburden and control moisture, odor, and pain.
- Consult vascular surgery, plastic surgery, infectious disease, podiatry, wound nursing, and home care services, as indicated.

Table 130. Recommended Dressings by Wound Characteristics

Product	Superficial Skin Disruption	Eschar	Exudate	Granulating/ Epithelializing	Fibrinous Wound Bed/ Slough	Deep Wounds	Colonized/ Infected
Alginates			+			+	
Collagen			+				
Foams			+				
Gauze packing (with saline)			+			+	
Hydrocolloids		+		+	+	+	
Hydrogels		+		+	+		
Hydrofibers			+			+	
Polymeric membrane dressings	+	+	+	+		+	
Protease lowering dressings					+		
Silver/Iodide							+
Transparent films	+						

- Adjunctive tx to support wound healing process
  - Electrical stimulation may be an option to stimulate healing and reduce pain with dressing changes.
  - Ultrasound
    - Low frequency (22.5–35 kHz) noncontact ultrasound tx can help debride wound surface with minimal discomfort
    - Promotes healing with and without antibiotics in small clinical studies; larger RCTs needed.
  - Hyperbaric oxygen
  - Skin substitutes (eg, porcine collagen, cadaver dermal matrix, combo products, allogenic fibroblasts) can provide temporary wound coverage; used in specialty wound care settings; expensive
- Prevent further injury
  - Use pressure-reducing surfaces or chair cushions and suspend the heels (pillows under the calf and knee, offloading boots or devices, 5-layer preventive dressings) to keep pressure off toes
  - Avoid using doughnut-type devices because they increase venous congestion and edema.
  - Reposition q2h and avoid any pressure on the wound; avoid prolonged sitting.
  - Maintain head of bed at lowest elevation consistent with medical conditions and limit time elevated.
  - Use active support surface to distribute load when multiple pressure injuries or patient cannot vary positions in bed.
  - Manage moisture from incontinence, perspiration, wound drainage (premium absorbent underpads, topical barriers)

COMMON DRESSINGS FOR WOUND MANAGEMENT

Transparent film

Indications and Use: Protection from friction, superficial abrasions, promotion of autolytic debridement; apply skin barrier/protection to intact skin to protect from adhesive-related skin damage

Contraindications: Draining ulcers, suspicion of bacterial or fungal skin infection

Composites (2 or more physically distinct dressing products combined as a single dressing)

Indications and Use: Light, moderate, or heavy exudate; conform to skin surface shape; designed with adhesive border; easy application and removal; dressing change frequency dependent on wound type (follow package insert); apply skin barrier/protectant to intact skin from adhesive-related skin damage

Contraindications: Caution with fragile skin; adhesive may injure skin; some types may be contraindicated with wounds with dead space (refer to package insert)

Hydrogel

Indications and Use: Promotes autolytic debridement; provides moisture to dry wounds; available with and without silver; needs to be held in place with topper dressing

Contraindications: Avoid use in macerated areas; wounds with moderate to heavy exudate

Foam

Indications and Use: Light to moderate exudate; leave in place 3–5 d (periwound maceration likely if not changed when indicated); available with and without silver or adhesive border; can be applied over other dressing materials or other tx.

Contraindications: Excessive exudate; dry, crusted wound; dry eschar

Hydrocolloids

Indications and Use: Light to moderate drainage; autolytic debridement of slough; preventive for high-risk friction areas; leave in place 3–7 d (periwound maceration likely if not changed when indicated); can apply as window to secure transparent film or under-taping; can be applied over other dressing materials or other tx; apply skin barrier or protectant to intact skin to protect from adhesive-related skin damage; may produce odor during dressing change

Contraindications: Fragile skin; infected wounds; heavily draining wounds, sinus tracts

Collagen

Indications and Use: Light, moderate, or heavy exudate; chronic, nonhealing wounds; nonadherent, biodegradable gel; conforms to wound surface; may be combined with other topical agents; change dressing q1–3d (refer to package insert)

Contraindications: Sensitivity to collagen or bovine products; avoid use with necrotic wounds; rehydration may be needed

Gauze packing (moistened with saline)

Indications and Use: Light to heavy exudate; wounds with depth, especially those with tunnels, undermining; apply dressing within wound borders; may need to be remoistened at least q4h to maintain moist wound environment; may macerate periwound skin in higher exudating wounds

Contraindications: May be painful to remove; can traumatize tissue when removed

Calcium alginate

Indications and Use: Heavy exudate; sinus tracts, tunnels, or cavities; apply dressing within wound borders; must use skin prep to protect periwound skin; requires secondary dressing; change q24–48h

Contraindications: Dry or minimally draining wound; dry eschar

Silver

Indications and Use: Silver can be added to many dressings as bacteriostatic. It increases cost and has unknown efficacy. Consider in infected wounds; highly colonized wounds; may cause silver staining of tissue

Contraindications: Sensitivity to silver; avoid use with other topical medications (silver can inactivate enzymatic debriding agents); signs of systemic side effects, especially erythema multiforme; fungal proliferation.

PRESSURE INJURY

Definition

Localized damage to skin and/or underlying soft tissue usually over a bony prominence or related to a medical or other device. The injury can present as intact skin or an open ulcer and may be painful. The injury occurs as a result of intense or prolonged pressure or pressure in combination with shear. The tolerance of soft tissue for pressure and shear may also be affected by microclimate, nutrition, perfusion, comorbidities, and condition of the soft tissue (National Pressure Ulcer Advisory Panel; npiap.com).

Wound Assessment

- See Chronic Wound Assessment (p 330). Early identification—with at least weekly assessment—is important to healing.
- Look for pressure injuries under area subjected to constant pressure (ie, bony prominences, orthopedic devices, oxygen equipment, other medical devices).
- If ≥1 heel pressure injuries (HPIs), the following assessments are recommended:
  - Manual ankle-brachial index (ABI) test, including peroneal artery to evaluate leg ischemia
  - Transcutaneous oxygen ($TcPO_2$) applied to hindfoot to assess calcaneal ischemia and rule out orphan heel syndrome
- Determine extent of tissue injury by using Pressure Injury Staging System. Illustrations available at npiap.com/page/PressureInjuryStages:
  - **Stage 1 Pressure Injury**: nonblanchable erythema of intact skin (may appear differently in darkly pigmented skin). Presence of blanchable erythema or changes in sensation, temperature, or firmness may precede visual changes. Color changes do not include purple or maroon discoloration; these may indicate deep-tissue pressure injury (see below).
  - **Stage 2 Pressure Injury:** partial-thickness skin loss with exposed dermis only or clear blisters
  - **Stage 3 Pressure Injury:** full-thickness skin loss, not into muscle or bone
  - **Stage 4 Pressure Injury:** full-thickness loss of skin and tissue with exposed or palpable bone, tendon, or muscle
  - **Unstageable Pressure Injury:** obscured full-thickness skin and tissue loss prevents visualization of depth of involvement.
  - **Deep-Tissue Pressure Injury:** persistent nonblanchable deep red, maroon, or purple discoloration. Sacrum and heel are the most common areas for deep-tissue pressure injuries. May appear as blood-filled blister with tissue consistency changes.
  - **Medical Device–related Pressure Injury**: Injuries resulting from the use of devices designed and applied for diagnostic or tx purposes (eg, catheters, oxygen tubing). The resultant pressure injury generally conforms to the pattern or shape of the device and should be staged using the staging system.
  - **Mucosal Membrane**: Injury found on mucous membranes with hx of a medical device in use at the location of injury. Due to the anatomy of the tissue, these injuries cannot be staged.

Management

Refer to Principles of Wound Management, p 331, and Common Dressings for Wound Management, p 335.

Apply local wound care practices as directed by stage of pressure injury and wound condition.

Specific recommendations for HPI include:

- Heel ulcers do not need debridement if no signs of inflammation or infection (eg, edema, erythema, drainage) and if stable with dry eschar.
- In HPI Stages 2, 3, 4, and impaired vascular perfusion (ABI <0.5 and toe pressure <30 mm Hg and/or $TcPO_2$ <40 mm Hg), avoid occlusive moisture dressings.
- Use silicone dressing to prevent medical adhesive-related skin injuries.
- In HPI Stage 3 with normal limb perfusion and no signs of infection, NPWT should be started to promote healing and reduce complications.

- In HPI Stage 4, surgical intervention is recommended to support wound healing and prevent amputation.
- In HPI Stage 4 with bone infection involving surrounding soft tissue, surgical intervention is recommended.
- For heel suspected deep-tissue pressure injury and blood blisters, fluid should be aspirated.

Surgical referral may be warranted for Stage 4 pressure injury and for severely undermined or tunneled wounds.

- Consider prognosis where palliative local wound care may be more appropriate.
- Optimize glucose control in the perioperative period to reduce dehiscence and recurrence risk.
- Consider growth factor tx for pressure ulcers that are not responsive to comprehensive tx or before surgical repair.

ARTERIAL ULCERS

Definition

Any lesion caused by severe tissue ischemia secondary to atherosclerosis and progressive arterial occlusion

Wound Assessment (see PAD, p 73)

- See Chronic Wound Assessment (p 330). Most often located in distal areas of lower extremities, including toes, and the tops and outside edges of the feet. Typically pale wound bed with minimal exudate.
- Evaluate circulation to include:
  - Ankle-brachial index (ABI) test. Wound healing unlikely if ABI <0.5.
  - Exercise caution when relying only on the ABI due to high prevalence of hardened arteries that artifactually give normal or supernormal readings.
  - Diminished or absent distal pulses, pale skin, slow capillary refill are common.
  - Assess circulation using noninvasive tests such as pulse volume recording, toe pressures, and transcutaneous oxygen readings.
- Evaluate for ischemic pain.

Management (also PAD, p 73, Diabetes, p 115, Chronic Heart Failure, p 64, and Renal Failure, p 193)

Protect from Injury

- Avoid compression of arterial wounds when ABI is <0.8.
- Avoid friction and pressure by using lamb's wool or foam between toes.
- Use lamb's wool and a pressure offloading boot (eg, *Rooke Boot*) to insulate and protect limb from trauma.
- Suspend the heels (pillow under calf and knee, offloading boots or devices, 5-layer preventive dressings) and keep pressure off toes.

Local Wound Care

Tx dictated by adequacy of perfusion and status of wound bed:

- Avoid debridement of necrotic tissue until perfusion status is determined.
- Assess vascular perfusion and refer for surgical intervention if consistent with overall goals of care.

- If wound is infected, revascularization procedures, surgical removal of necrotic tissue, and systemic antibiotics are tx of choice.
- Topical antibiotics should not be used solely to treat infected ischemic wounds and may cause sensitivity reactions.
- If wound is not infected and dry eschar is present, maintain dry intact eschar as a barrier to bacteria. Application of an antiseptic may decrease bacterial burden on wound surface although evidence is lacking.
- If wound is not infected and soft slough and necrotic tissue are present, apply moisture-retaining dressings to promote autolytic debridement while allowing for frequent inspection of wound for signs of infection.

DIABETIC (NEUROPATHIC FOOT) ULCERS

Definition

Any lesion on the plantar surface of the foot caused by neuropathy and repetitive pressure on foot.

Wound Assessment

- See Chronic Wound Assessment (p 330). Usually occur in repetitive stress areas and often painless. Covered with fibrotic tissue or callus and may penetrate to bone.
- Assess for specific DM-related signs of infection:
  - Sudden increase in blood glucose
  - Wound can be probed to the bone—highly sensitive indicator of osteomyelitis
- Exclude arterial disease by assessing for palpable pedal pulses, ABI, a transcutaneous oxygen pressure of >30 mm Hg, or normal Doppler-derived wave form.
- Determine grade of ulcer (Wagner classification). Do not use National Pressure Ulcer Advisory Panel (NPUAP) staging system.

  Grade 0: Preulcerative lesions; healed ulcers present; bony deformity present
  Grade 1: Superficial ulcer without subcutaneous tissue involvement
  Grade 2: Penetration through subcutaneous tissue
  Grade 3: Osteitis, abscess, or osteomyelitis
  Grade 4: Gangrene of digit
  Grade 5: Gangrene of foot requiring disarticulation

Management (also Diabetes, p 115)

Local Wound Care

- In addition to recommendations under Chronic Wound Management (p 330):
- Debride devitalized tissue and callus: surgical debridement is method of choice for effective, rapid removal of nonviable tissue
- Avoid occlusive dressings to reduce risk of wound infection
- Offload pressure and stress from foot
  - Avoidance of pressure on foot essential to management of diabetic foot ulcer
  - Use orthotic that redistributes weight on plantar surface of foot when ambulating (eg, total contact cast, *DH Offloading Walker*)
- If ulcer does not reduce in size by ≥50% after 4 wk of tx, reassess tx and consider alternative options (eg, NPWT, growth factor tx, skin substitutes, extracellular matrix, hyperbaric oxygen tx).
  - Skin substitutes *(Apligraf, Dermagraft)* containing growth factors present in the skin may stimulate healing and decrease time to wound closure. Wound must be granular to be effective.

◦ Hyperbaric oxygen tx effective in promoting healing of complicated chronic diabetic foot ulcers is covered by Medicare and some insurance companies. Caution in patients with HF, advanced COPD, and those treated with anticancer drugs. Tx applied in chamber for 1.5–2 h/d for 20–40 d.

VENOUS ULCERS

Definition

Any lesion caused by venous insufficiency

Wound Assessment

- See Chronic Wound Assessment (p 330). Ulcer typically superficial with a moist pink-to-red bed and irregular edges. Edema, induration, and loss of hair are common. Skin around the ulcer is often darkened (due to hemosiderin staining) with variable drainage, depending on the presence of infection and edema.
- Assess lower-extremity edema.
- Assess pedal pulses (see Leg Edema in Cardiovascular chapter, p 67). Not uncommon to have combined venous/arterial disease.
- Order color duplex ultrasound for both supine and standing positions to confirm venous etiology (ie, abnormal venous reflux or obstruction)
- Nonhealing open venous ulcers (ie, no response to tx after 4 wk) should raise suspicion that etiology is not venous or tx needs reevaluation.
  - Biopsy for histological diagnosis (eg, malignancy, vasculitis, collagen-vascular disease, systemic diseases)
  - Culture for mycobacteria and/or fungi

Management (see Leg Edema, Cardiovascular p 67)

Compression Therapy

- Essential component of venous ulcer tx decreases healing time and pain
- Compression stockings should be used constantly and forever in healed or surgically repaired venous ulcers.
- Exercises can improve calf muscle pump function.
- Therapeutic level of compression is 30–40 mm Hg at ankle, decreasing toward knee
- Sclerotherapy may be useful as an adjunct to compression tx in venous ulcer tx.
- Pentoxifylline used in conjunction with compression tx improves ulcer healing.
- Oral tx with micronized purified flavonoid fraction (MPFF) may be a useful adjunct to compression tx.
- Types of compression tx:
  - Static compression device
    - Layered compression wraps *(PROFORE, DeRoyal Dewrap)*
    - Short-stretch wraps *(Comprilan)*
    - Paste-containing bandages *(Unna-Flex)*. For use in actively ambulating patient; support compression of calf muscle "pump".
  - Dynamic compression devices (indicated when static compression not feasible)
    - Pneumatic compression device (intermittent pneumatic pumps) that propels venous blood upward when applied to lower leg
  - Compression tx for long-term maintenance
    - Therapeutic compression stockings (eg, *Jobst, Juzo, Sigvaris);* some available with zippers or individual segment wraps

Local Wound Care

In addition to recommendations under Chronic Wound Management (p 330):

- Use exudate-absorbing dressings (eg, calcium alginate dressings, foam dressings).
- Use skin barrier or protectant to protect skin around wound from exudate.
- Infected venous ulcers should be treated with systemic antibiotics because of the development of resistant organisms with topical antibiotics.
- Electrical stimulation may reduce size of venous leg ulcers.
- Laser tx, phototherapy, and ultrasound tx have not been shown to improve venous ulcer healing.
- Refer to a wound specialist for the use of skin substitutes (eg, *Apligraf, Dermagraft, GammaGraft*) containing growth factors or surgical intervention.
    - Wounds must be granulating for skin substitute to be effective.
    - Minimize bacteria load to $\leq 10^5$ cfu/g of tissue, with no β-hemolytic streptococci in ulcer before attempting surgical closure.
    - Cultured epithelial autografts or allografts do not improve stable healing of venous ulcers.
    - Porcine small intestinal submucosal construct may enhance healing of venous ulcers.
    - NPWT helps remove fluid, assists in granulation tissue formation, decreases wound size, and helps promote graft take.

SKIN TEAR

Definition

Separation of skin layers resulting from shearing, friction, or blunt trauma (eg, wheelchair injuries, falls, transfer injury, tape removal)

Assessment

See Chronic Wound Assessment (p 330). Can be partial-thickness or full-thickness and appear as either a small linear split in the skin or peeled back skin. Use International Skin Tear Advisory Panel (ISTAP) classification system.

Type 1: skin tear without tissue loss
Type 2: partial loss of skin tear flap
Type 3: complete loss of epidermal flap

Management

- Preserve skin flap and protect surrounding tissue; encourage healing and prevent infection.
- Control bleeding with pressure and elevation of limb.
- Cleanse wound with warm tap water, saline, or wound cleanser.
- Approximate flap with gentle unfolding and smoothing over the wound.
- Use atraumatic dressing to keep flap in place. Leave for several days for flap to adhere to the wound bed.
- Monitor for signs of infection. If flap becomes necrotic, refer to a wound care specialist.
- Control pain.

SLEEP DISORDERS

CLASSIFICATION

- Circadian rhythm disorders (eg, jet lag)
- **Insomnia** (difficulty initiating or maintaining sleep, or poor quality sleep). *Note:* Phase advance (reduced sleep during early morning and peak sleepiness earlier in the evening) are normal aspects of aging and do not need to be treated. At least 7 h of sleep per night are recommended for older persons.
- Parasomnias (disorders of arousal from non-REM and REM sleep and isolated [eg, sleep talking], including sleep stage transition)
- Hypersomnia of central origin (eg, narcolepsy)
- **Sleep-related breathing disorders** (central and obstructive sleep apnea and sleep-related hypoventilation-hypoxia syndromes)
- **Sleep-related movement disorders** (eg, RLS, periodic limb movement disorder, leg cramps)

Bolded disorders are covered in this chapter.

INSOMNIA

Risk Factors and Aggravating Factors

Treatable Associated Medical and Psychiatric Conditions: adjustment disorders, anxiety, bereavement, cough, depression, dyspnea (cardiac or pulmonary), GERD, nocturia, pain, paresthesias, Parkinson disease, stress, stroke

Medications That Cause or Aggravate Sleep Problems: alcohol, antidepressants, β blockers, bronchodilators, caffeine, clonidine, corticosteroids, diuretics, L-DOPA, methyldopa, nicotine, phenytoin, progesterone, quinidine, reserpine, sedatives, sympathomimetics including decongestants

Evaluation

Self-Report Measures

- Insomnia Severity Index (ISI): https://www.myhealth.va.gov/mhv-portal-web/web/myhealthevet/insomnia-severity-index
- Athens Insomnia Scale: sleepontario.com/docs/scales/Athens-Insomnia-Scale/Athens-Insomnia-Scale-English.pdf

Don't perform polysomnography unless symptoms suggest a comorbid sleep disorder.[CW]

Consumer Sleep Tracking Devices and Actigraphy

Most wearables and nonwearables perform as well as actigraphy and have high sensitivity in detecting sleep, but low to medium specificity compared to polysomnography.

Management

For most patients, behavioral tx should be initial tx. Don't use benzodiazepines or other sedative hypnotics as first choice for insomnia.[CW] Despite benefits of hypnotics on sleep quality, total sleep time, and frequency of nighttime awakening, these are small compared to the risk of cognitive or psychomotor AEs. Combined behavioral tx and pharmacotherapy is more effective than either alone.

- Sleep improvements are better sustained over time with behavioral tx, including discontinuing pharmacotherapy after acute tx.

Nonpharmacologic Interventions

- Sleep hygiene (less effective as a standalone tx compared to CBT)
  - During the daytime
    - Get out of bed at the same time each morning regardless of how much you slept the night before.
    - Exercise daily (conventional or tai chi) but not within 2 h of bedtime.
    - Get adequate exposure to bright light during the day.
    - Decrease or eliminate naps, unless necessary part of sleeping schedule.
    - Limit or eliminate alcohol, caffeine, and nicotine, especially before bedtime.
  - At bedtime
    - If hungry, have a light snack before bed (unless there are symptoms of GERD or it is otherwise medically contraindicated), but avoid heavy meals at bedtime.
    - Don't use bedtime as worry time. Write down worries for next day and then don't think about them.
    - Sleep only in your bedroom.
    - Control nighttime environment (ie, comfortable temperature, quiet, dark)
      - Wear comfortable bedclothes.
      - If it helps, use soothing noise (eg, a fan or other appliance, a white-noise machine, or an app such as *myNoise* or *White Noise Free Sleep Sounds*).
      - Remove or cover the clock.
      - No television watching in the bedroom.
      - Avoid reading e-books or tablets with light-emitting device. *Uvex Skyper* safety eyewear eliminates almost all blue light. Standard *Kindle* does not emit light.
    - Maintain a regular sleeping time, but do not go to bed unless sleepy.
    - Develop a sleep ritual (eg, hot bath 90 min before bedtime followed by preparing for bed for 20–30 min, followed by 30–40 min of relaxation, meditation, or reading).
      - If unable to fall asleep within 15–20 min, get out of bed and perform soothing activity, such as listening to soft music or reading (but avoid exposure to bright light or computer screens).
- Stimulus control strengthens the association between the sleep environment and sleep and establishes consistent sleep patterns.
- Sleep restriction: reduce time in bed to estimated total sleep time (minimum 5 h) and increase by 15 min/wk when ratio of time asleep to time in bed is ≥90%. During the period of sleep restriction, daytime sleepiness may be increased and reaction time may be slower. Less effective than CBT, but more effective than sleep hygiene.
- CBT for insomnia (CBT-I) recommended initial tx for chronic insomnia. Combines multiple behavioral approaches (eg, sleep restriction, stimulus control, cognitive tx that targets maladaptive thoughts and beliefs about sleep); brief version includes only sleep restriction, stimulus control, and sleep hygiene. Face-to-face may be more effective but can be delivered effectively either by phone or online (sleepio.com, myshuti.com, freecbti.com, CBT-I Coach App, CBTforInsomnia.com), but the last have high attrition. A list of US providers is available at www.behavioralsleep.org/index.php/united-states-sbsm-members. CBT-I is the most effective option for maintaining long-term improvement of insomnia regardless of initial tx. Also effective if comorbid OA pain. Prevents incident and recurrent depression. Benefits may persist beyond the end of tx.

- Brief behavioral treatment for insomnia (BBTI) is shorter (eg, individualized behavioral instructions delivered in 2 intervention sessions and 2 phone calls) and does not include cognitive tx components. A small trial of older adults showed BBTI reduced self-reported sleep onset latency and time spent awake after sleep onset until getting out of bed for the final time and improved sleep efficiency and sleep quality.
- Relaxation techniques: physical (progressive muscle relaxation, biofeedback); mental (imagery training, mindfulness meditation, hypnosis)
- Bright light: 10,000 lux for 30 min/d upon awakening for difficulty initiating sleep; 2500 lux for 2 h/d in evening for difficulty maintaining sleep
- Auricular acupuncture with seed and pellet has weak evidence.
- Hot shower or bath (104–109°F) 1–2 h before bed

Pharmacotherapy—Meta-analysis indicates improved sleep quality, total sleep time, and less frequent awakenings, but 2–5× increase in AEs, including sleepwalking and sleep driving.

Principles of Prescribing Medications for Sleep Disorders

- Prescribe medications for short-term use (no more than 3–4 wk) or use intermittent dosing (2–4×/wk).
- D/C medication gradually. See Deprescribing (p 18) and deprescribing.org (Benzodiazepine & Z-Drug [BZRA] Deprescribing Algorithm).
- Combine with behavior tx rather than give medication alone.
- Use lowest effective dose.
- Be alert for rebound insomnia after discontinuation.
- No evidence supports the use of kava, valerian, chamomile.
- Do not use OTC antihistamines to treat insomnia in older adults.[BC]
- Do not use benzodiazepines, trazodone, or antipsychotics to treat chronic insomnia (VA-DoD).
- For patients with anxiety at bedtime, consider SSRIs or buspirone.
- For sleep-onset insomnia, use a shorter-acting agent (eg, zolpidem, zaleplon, suvorexant). For sleep-maintenance insomnia, use a longer-acting agent (eg, suvorexant, eszopiclone, zolpidem ER, low-dose doxepin).
- In clinical trials of hypnotics, there is a significant placebo effect on perceived sleep-onset latency, total sleep time, and global sleep quality, but not objective measures of sleep.
- All increase risk of falls. Zolpidem is also associated with traumatic brain injury and hip fractures due to falls.

Table 131. Useful Medications for Sleep Disorders in Older Adults

Class, Medication	Half-Life (Elimination)	Comments
Antidepressant, sedating		
Trazodone	12 h (L)	May improve perceived sleep quality and nocturnal awakenings; moderate orthostatic effects. AASM recommends against its use.
Doxepin	15.3 h	May cause next-day sedation; many potential drug interactions
Mirtazapine	20–40 h	Low dose 7.5–15 mg; not FDA approved for insomnia

(cont.)

Class, Medication	Half-Life (Elimination)	Comments
Benzodiazepines, intermediate-acting[BC,1]		Complex sleep-related disorders including sleepwalking, driving, eating, and other behaviors performed while not fully awake, increased risk of falls, may impair next-day performance, including driving; may cause aggressive behavior
Estazolam	12–18 h (K)	Rapidly absorbed, effective in initiating sleep; slightly active metabolites that may accumulate
Lorazepam	8–12 h (K)	Effective in initiating and maintaining sleep; associated with falls, memory loss, rebound insomnia
Temazepam	8–10 h[2] (K)	Daytime drowsiness may occur with repeated use; effective for sleep maintenance; delayed onset of effect (K)
Nonbenzodiazepines[BC,1] (benzodiazepine receptor agonists)		Avoid as first-line medications for older adults. Complex sleep-related disorders including sleepwalking, driving, eating, and other behaviors performed while not fully awake, increased risk of falls, may impair next-day performance, including driving
Eszopiclone	5–6 h (L)	CYP3A4 interactions; avoid administration with high-fat meal; not for tx of anxiety
Zaleplon	1 h (L)	Avoid taking with alcohol or food
Zolpidem	1.5–4.5 h[3] (L)	CYP3A4 interactions; confusion and agitation may occur but are rare
(Edluar)	2.8 h	
(Ambien CR)	1.6–5.5 h	Do not divide, crush, or chew. Avoid driving the day after taking.
(Zolpimist)	2–3 h	Spray over tongue; absorption more rapid
(Intermezzo)	2.4 h	sl: For middle-of-the-night insomnia
Dual Orexin Receptor Antagonists		
Suvorexant *(Belsomra)*	12 h	Metabolized by CYP34A; can impair next-day driving and cause REM-sleep behavior disorder
Daridorexant *(Quviviq)*	8 h	Metabolized by CYP34A
Lemborexant *(Dayvigo)*	17–19 h	CYP3A4 substrate; more effective than zolpidem ER on sleep onset and maintenance
Hormone and Hormone Receptor Agonists		
Melatonin	1 h	Beneficial effect on sleep latency and small effect on daytime sleepiness but not other measures, including sleep maintenance. May be best taken 2–5 h before bedtime; not regulated by FDA. *REMfresh* is an OTC continuous-release product.
Ramelteon *(Rozerem)*	Ramelteon: 1–2.6 h; active metabolite: 2–5 h (L, K)	Not helpful for sleep maintenance. Many potential drug interactions. Do not administer with or immediately after high-fat meal

Table 131. Useful Medications for Sleep Disorders in Older Adults (cont.)

[1] May cause severe allergic reactions and complex sleep-related behavioral disturbances

[2] Can be as long as 30 h in older adults

[3] 3 h in older adults; 10 h in those with hepatic cirrhosis

SLEEP DISTURBANCES IN DEMENTIA

In addition to age-related changes with sleep, persons with dementia have more disruptive sleep. Conversely, sleep disturbances are associated with increased risk for cognitive decline and dementia. In patients with Parkinson dementia and LBD, sleep disorders begin early in the disorder; they occur in later stages in persons in AD. Sleep architecture disturbances include more and longer awakenings, with increases in Stage 1 sleep and decreases in slow-wave sleep. Circadian rhythm disturbances are common, including sundowning (behavioral symptoms peak during late afternoon and evening).

Management

Nonpharmacologic Interventions

For patients with dementia, reducing insomnia risk factors and behavioral approaches are first line, including consistent wake-up and bedtimes, bright light tx in morning, maintaining nighttime darkness, and avoiding awakenings for medications.

Pharmacotherapy

In clinical trials, melatonin or ramelteon have not proved beneficial; trazodone confers only modest benefit. Suvorexant is more effective than placebo at 4 wk for patients with mild but not more severe dementia. Trazodone associated with 40 min more total sleep time.

SLEEP APNEA

Definition

Repeated episodes of apnea (cessation of airflow for ≥10 sec) or hypopnea (transient reduction [≥30% decrease in thoracoabdominal movement or airflow and with ≥4% oxygen desaturation, or an arousal] of airflow for ≥10 sec) during sleep with excessive daytime sleepiness or altered cardiopulmonary function. Predicts future strokes and cognitive impairment. HF (in men), and all-cause mortality (if severe).

Classification

Obstructive (OSA) (90% of cases): Airflow cessation as a result of upper airway closure in spite of adequate respiratory muscle effort. Older persons are more likely to have airway collapsibility as a cause.

- Mild apnea-hypopnea index (AHI): 5–15
- Moderate: AHI 15–30
- Severe: AHI: >30

Central (CSA): Cessation of respiratory effort

Mixed: Features of both obstructive and central

Risk Factors

Older age, male sex, family hx, Asian ethnicity, hx of hypothyroidism (in women), obesity, smoking, increased neck circumference, upper airway structural abnormalities (eg, soft palate, tonsils)

Associated Conditions

HTN; HF; AF; stroke and TIAs; Parkinson disease; hypothyroidism, chronic lung diseases including, COPD, asthma, pulmonary fibrosis, and PH; polycythemia; fibromyalgia; GERD, and Barrett esophagus, ESRD

Clinical Features

Excessive daytime sleepiness, loud snoring, choking or gasping on awakening, morning headache, nocturia

Evaluation

- STOP Questionnaire (oasyssleep.com/dentist-support/STOP-Questionnaire-for-Obstructive-Sleep-Apnea.pdf) and STOP-BANG questionnaire (stopbang.ca/osa/screening.php) are useful screens
- Epworth Sleepiness Scale (https://www.cdc.gov/niosh/emres/longhourstraining/scale.html) is useful for documenting and monitoring daytime sleepiness.
- Full night's sleep study (polysomnography) in sleep lab is indicated for those who habitually snore and either report daytime sleepiness or have observed apnea.
- Home sleep apnea testing can be used to diagnose moderate to severe OSA, but should not be used if patients have comorbid conditions (eg, HF) that predispose to a sleep-related breathing disorder or another sleep disorder.
- Results are reported as AHI, which is the number of episodes of apneas and hypopneas per hour of sleep.
- Medicare reimbursement threshold for positive airway pressure (PAP) based on a minimum of 2 h sleep by polysomnography is AHI (1) ≥15 or (2) ≥5 and ≤14 with documented symptoms of excessive daytime sleepiness, impaired cognition, mood disorders, or insomnia, or documented HTN, ischemic heart disease, or hx of stroke.
- No need for retitration if asymptomatic, adherent patients with stable weight.[CW]

Management

Nonpharmacologic Interventions

- Patient education including information about increased risk of motor vehicle crashes
- Weight loss with active lifestyle counseling is effective in mild and moderate OSA but does not normalize OSA parameters. When combined with aerobic exercise, sleep hygiene, and alcohol and tobacco cessation, can reduce AHI in middle-aged persons with moderate to severe OSA. Bariatric surgery (if BMI ≥35 who are intolerant of PAP) improves but does not cure moderate or severe OSA
- Avoidance of alcohol or sedatives
- CBT-I is effective in insomnia and moderate to severe OSA.
- Lying in lateral rather than supine position (if normalization of AHI in nonsupine position is confirmed by sleep study) but usually not sufficient as sole tx; may be facilitated by soft foam ball in a backpack or devices that use vibratory feedback.
- Moderate-intensity aerobic exercise (eg, 150 min/wk [4 d/wk]), even without weight loss, can improve symptoms.
- Oral appliances that keep the tongue in an anterior position during sleep or keep the mandible forward; less effective than PAP in reducing AHI score, daytime sleepiness, cognitive function, but better adherence and some benefits. Generally used in mild to moderate OSA (AHI <30) for patients who do not want PAP.
- For moderate sleep apnea (>15 and <30 AHI), PAP or oropharyngeal exercises, including tongue, soft palate, and lateral pharyngeal wall, performed daily improves symptoms and reduces AHI score.
- For clinically important sleep apnea (eg, AHI ≥15 events/h), PAP for ≥4 h/night is initial tx but there may be some benefit with shorter use. PAP may also improve HTN, HF outcomes, GERD, and the metabolic syndrome associated with OSA, and reduce the risk of recurrent AF. Don't retitrate if asymptomatic, adherent, and stable weight.[CW] Repeat testing if persistent or recurrent symptoms. PAP can be delivered through several modes:

- Continuous (CPAP) by nasal mask, nasal prongs, or mask that covers the nose and mouth is the simplest and most effective at reducing AHI. A short course (14 d) of eszopiclone may facilitate adherence when initiating CPAP.
  - Bilevel (BPAP) uses 2 preset (inspiratory and expiratory) levels of pressure.
  - Autotitrating (APAP) changes PAP in response to change in air flow, circuit pressure, or vibratory snore.
  - Nasal (EPAP) *(Provent)* is a 1-way valve inserted into each nostril that creates resistance during exhalation.

Pharmacotherapy (should not be used as primary tx)

- Stimulants (modafinil, armodafinil, solriamfetol, methylphenidate) may be helpful for excessive daytime sleepiness; use in addition to (not instead of) CPAP. High rate of AEs.
- Small studies suggest potential benefit of dronabinol but causes somnolence; more trials are needed. AASM recommends against the use of this or medical cannabis.

Surgical (referral if PAP declined or not tolerated for ≥1 mo, AASM)

- Palatal implants (for mild to moderate OSA)
- Tracheostomy (indicated for patients with severe apnea who cannot tolerate positive pressure or when other interventions are ineffective)
- Uvulopalatopharyngoplasty (curative in fewer than 50% of cases). Less invasive alternatives include laser-assisted uvulopalatoplasty, radiofrequency ablation, and maxillomandibular advancement. All decrease the AHI but have not been demonstrated to be superior to medical management in clinical trials.
- Multilevel surgery (modified uvulopalatopharyngoplasty and minimally invasive tongue reduction volume) may improve 6-mo outcomes in patients refractory to medical management
- Hypoglossal nerve stimulation with an implantable neurostimulator device *(Inspire, Sleep Therapy System)*. FDA eligibility criteria include moderate or severe OSA (eg, AHI 15–65/h), predominantly obstructive events, CPAP failure or intolerance, and no anatomical findings that would compromise performance of the device. At 1 y, insomnia and depression scores were similar to those receiving PAP at 3 mo.
- Maxillofacial surgery (rare cases)

SLEEP-RELATED MOVEMENT DISORDERS

Nocturnal Leg Cramps

- Must have muscle contraction, occur during time in bed, and be relieved by forceful stretching of affected muscles
- Most are idiopathic but may be due to hypocalcemia, extracellular volume depletion, neurologic disorders (eg, Parkinson disease, myopathies, neuropathies), lower extremity structural abnormalities, prolonged sitting, or working on concrete flooring.

Nonpharmacologic Interventions

- Treat acute cramps by:
  - Forcefully stretching affected muscle (eg, dorsiflexion of foot with knee extended to relieve calf cramp)
  - Walking or jiggling leg followed by elevating the leg
  - Ice massage
- Prevent recurrent leg cramps

- ◦ Daily stretching exercises (eg, feet flat on floor, legs straight, lean forward, arms above head on wall, and hold 10–30 sec up to 5×/night)
- Avoid dehydration.

Pharmacotherapy

- Despite evidence of effectiveness, quinine is not recommended for nocturnal leg cramps because of the potential for serious AEs.
- Magnesium oxide is ineffective.
- Small studies have supported the use of vitamin B complex, verapamil, and diltiazem. Gabapentin has been used but with little evidence to support its effectiveness.

Restless Legs Syndrome (the majority will also have periodic limb movement disorder)

Diagnostic Criteria

- A compelling urge to move the limbs, usually associated with paresthesias or dysesthesias
- Motor restlessness (eg, floor pacing, tossing and turning in bed, rubbing legs)
- Vague discomfort, usually bilateral, most commonly in calves
- Symptoms occur while awake and are exacerbated by rest, especially at night
- Symptoms relieved by movement—jerking, stretching, or shaking of limbs; pacing

Secondary Causes: Iron deficiency (ferritin <50 mcg/L or transferrin saturation <20%), spinal cord and peripheral nerve lesions, uremia, DM, Parkinson disease, venous insufficiency, medications/drugs (eg, TCAs, SSRIs, lithium, dopamine antagonists, caffeine)

Don't use polysomnography to diagnose RLS.[CW]

Nonpharmacologic Interventions

- Sleep hygiene measures (p 342)
- Avoid alcohol, caffeine, nicotine.
- Rub limbs.
- Use hot or cold baths, whirlpools.
- Complementary and alternative tx (eg, transcutaneous direct current stimulation, acupuncture, pneumatic compression devices, yoga)

Pharmacotherapy

- Exclude or treat iron deficiency (treat if ferritin <50 mcg/L; see Anemia and Myeloproliferative Disorders chapter), peripheral neuropathy.
- If possible, avoid caffeine, SSRIs, TCAs, lithium, and dopamine antagonists.
- Start at low dosage, increase as needed. If refractory to one class, can add a drug of the other class.
  - ◦ Alpha-2-delta calcium channel ligands (especially if comorbid pain, anxiety, or insomnia)
    - ▪ Gabapentin ER formulation, gabapentin enacarbil *(Horizant)* begin at 600 mg/d po at 5 PM, has been FDA approved for RLS; reduce dose when CrCl <60 mL/min.[BC]
    - ▪ Pregabalin *(Lyrica)* begin 50–75 mg/d at bedtime but may need up to 450 mg/d po; less augmentation compared to pramipexole; reduce dose when CrCl <60 mL/min.[BC]
  - ◦ Dopamine agonists (especially if very severe pain, comorbid depression, obesity); may cause augmentation (worsening symptoms with increasing dose); can be used prn if intermittent symptoms.
    - ▪ Pramipexole (begin at 0.125 mg/d 2–3 h before bedtime; most will require ≤0.5 mg/d po)
    - ▪ Rotigotine *(Neupro)* transdermal (1 mg/24 h daily to max 3 mg/24 h [**Table 95**])
    - ▪ Ropinirole (begin at 0.25 mg/d 1–3 h before bedtime; most will require 2 mg/d po, and some will require 4 mg/d po) 1 h before time of usual onset of symptoms

- Other drugs
  - Carbidopa-levodopa *(Sinemet)* 25/100 mg po 1–2 h before bedtime. Begin at 1/2 tab and can increase to 2 tab max. Symptom augmentation may develop earlier in the day (eg, afternoon instead of evening) and may be more severe with carbidopa-levodopa; tx may require reducing dosage or switching to dopamine agonist. Can be used prn if intermittent symptoms.
  - Low-dose opioids if other tx fail
  - Cabergoline *(Dostinex)* beginning 0.25 mg po 2×/wk; may also be effective but has potential for causing valvular heart disease.
  - Clonidine
  - Dipyridamole
- If refractory, can use combination tx.
- If augmentation, switch tx regimen.
- If symptoms are intermittent, can use dopamine agonist or L-DOPA prn.

Periodic Limb Movement Disorder (a minority will also have RLS)

Diagnostic Criteria

- Insomnia or excessive sleepiness
- Repetitive, highly stereotyped limb muscle movements (eg, extension of big toes with partial flexion of ankle, knee, and sometimes hip) that occur during non-REM sleep
- Polysomnographic monitoring showing >15 episodes of muscle contractions per hour and associated arousals or awakenings
- No evidence of a medical, mental, or other sleep disorder that can account for symptoms

Management: Indicated for clinically significant sleep disruption or frequent arousals documented on a sleep study.

- Nonpharmacologic interventions: See sleep hygiene measures, p 342.
- Pharmacotherapy: See RLS, Pharmacotherapy, p 349. Pramipexole may be more effective than pregabalin.

REM Sleep Behavior Disorder

- Loss of atonia during REM sleep (ranging from simple limb twitches to acting out dreams), exaggeration of features of REM sleep (eg, nightmares), and intrusion of aspects of REM sleep into wakefulness (eg, sleep paralysis)
- High risk (80–90%) of developing α-synuclein-mediated neurodegenerative disorder (eg, Parkinson disease, multisystem atrophy, LBD); conversion rate is approximately 50% every 10 y. Higher risk if subtle motor dysfunction, abnormal color vision, olfactory dysfunction.
- Can rarely be caused by antidepressant medications (eg, SSRIs, venlafaxine, mirtazapine), β blockers, anticholinergics, and pontine lesions.

Evaluation: If needed, in-laboratory video polysomnography

Nonpharmacologic Interventions: change sleeping environment to reduce risk of injury

Pharmacotherapy: high-dose melatonin 6–18 mg po or clonazepam 0.25–1 mg po hs; if associated with Parkinson disease, L-DOPA, or pramipexole

SLEEP DISORDERS IN LONG-TERM CARE FACILITIES

Risk Factors

- Medical and medication factors (see Insomnia, p 342)
- Environmental factors (eg, little physical activity, infrequent daytime bright light exposure, extended periods in bed, nighttime noise and light interruptions)

Nonpharmacologic Interventions

- Morning bright light tx >2500 lux for 30 min or longer
- Exercise (eg, stationary bicycle, tai chi) and social activity
- Reduction of nighttime noise and light interruptions
- Staff education and training
- Maintain a consistent schedule of meals and activities
- Multicomponent interventions combining the above and a bedtime routine
- Match roommates based on nighttime routine (eg, incontinence care, turnings)
- Mixed evidence for acupressure right before sleep and for melatonin

SCOPE OF THE PROBLEM

- *Alcohol:*
  - Misuse/abuse is the primary substance use disorder in people aged ≥50.
  - Higher blood concentrations per amount consumed is due to decreased lean body mass and total body water.
  - Many medical conditions (eg, dementia, HTN) interact with alcohol.
  - Many drugs interact with alcohol: APAP, anesthetics, antihypertensives, antihistamines, antipsychotics, narcotic analgesics, NSAIDs, sedatives, antidepressants, anticonvulsant medications, nitrates, β blockers, oral hypoglycemic agents, anticoagulants.
  - Baby boomers are likely to maintain higher alcohol consumption.
- *Illicit drugs:* Baby boomers have more frequent use of drugs such as cocaine, than previous cohorts of older people.
- *Marijuana and its derivatives* for medicinal and recreational purposes are also more common in baby boomers.
- *Smoking:* 10% of people aged >65 (12% of men, 8% of women) are current smokers.
- *Prescription drug misuse/dependence* is an important problem in the older population; in particular, opioids and benzodiazepines are a continuing problem.
- *Gambling addiction:* The only behavioral disorder considered an addiction in *DSM-5*. Older people are at high risk, especially those who are isolated after losses such as retirement, death of spouse or friends, etc.

SUBSTANCE USE DISORDERS

Evaluation and Classification

DSM-5 consolidates substance abuse with substance dependence and addresses each substance-related disorder (alcohol, opioid, tobacco, and sedative, hypnotic, anxiolytic) as separate disorders but uses 11 overarching criteria (see below) for diagnosis. The number of criteria met determines the severity of the disorder.

DSM-5 Criteria/Symptoms for Substance Use Disorders

- Continuing to use a substance despite negative consequences.
- Repeated inability to carry out roles (at work, home) on account of use.
- Recurrent use in physically hazardous situations.
- Continued use despite recurrent/persistent social/interpersonal problems during use.
- Tolerance, needing increased dose to achieve effect/diminished effect with same amount.
- Withdrawal syndrome or use of the drug to avoid withdrawal.
- Using more substance or using for a longer period than intended.
- Persistent desire to cut down use or unsuccessful attempts to control use.
- Spending a lot of time obtaining, using, or recovering from use.
- Stopping/reducing important occupational, social, or recreational activities due to use.
- Craving or strong desire to use.

DSM-5 Criteria for Diagnosis and Classification of Substance-related Disorders

Two or more symptoms (above) indicate a substance-related disorder; severity is determined by the number of symptoms.

- Mild disorder: 2–3 symptoms
- Moderate disorder: 4–5 symptoms
- Severe disorder: 6 or more symptoms

GAMBLING DISORDER

Definition

A persistent and recurrent urge to gamble that causes clinical distress or impairment in family, professional, or personal areas. Diagnosis follows *DSM-5* criteria. Older adults are at high risk due to retirement, social isolation, physical-mental diseases (eg, FTD), or the loss of a partner.

Prevalence: 0.1–5.8% of adults; lifetime prevalence 1.1–10.6%

Therapy: psychotherapeutic (data supports CBT and motivational interviewing), psychopharmacological (data limited on effectiveness), financial, educational, and self-help methods (ie, Gamblers Anonymous).

DSM-5 Criteria/Symptoms for Gambling Disorder

Exhibits four or more (of the following) in a 12-mo period and the gambling behavior is not better explained by a manic episode:

- Needs to gamble with increasing amounts of money to achieve the desired excitement.
- Is restless or irritable when attempting to cut down or stop gambling.
- Has made repeated unsuccessful efforts to control, cut back, or stop gambling.
- Is often preoccupied with gambling (eg, persistent thoughts of reliving past experiences, handicapping or planning the next venture, thinking of ways to get money to gamble).
- Often gambles when feeling distressed.
- After losing money, returns to get even ("chasing" one's losses).
- Lies to conceal the extent of gambling.
- Jeopardized or lost a significant relationship, job, or educational or career opportunity due to gambling.
- Relies on others for money in financial situations caused by gambling.

ALCOHOL USE DISORDERS (AUDs)

Acute Alcohol Withdrawal

- Symptoms begin within 8 h, peak at 72 h, and resolve within 5–7 d after the last drink of alcohol.
- Symptoms and signs: tremors, agitation, nausea, sweating, vomiting, hallucinations, insomnia, tachycardia, HTN, delirium, seizures.
- Most cases of withdrawal cause only mild symptoms and can be treated safely without medication.
- About 10% of cases have more severe symptoms that are treated with as-needed benzodiazepines (p 80).
- Severity of symptoms dictate whether inpatient or outpatient management is appropriate.
- Assess severity of withdrawal symptoms using a validated instrument (Clinical Institute Withdrawal Assessment for Alcohol Scale-revised [CIWA-Ar] or the Short Alcohol Withdrawal Scale [SAWS]).

Evaluation and Classification of AUDs

Although casual drinking (1 drink/d for women, ≤2 drinks/d for men) has long been felt to have some health benefits, more recent data call that belief into question and suggest that the amount of alcohol consumption that minimizes the risk of death and disability-adjusted life years is zero alcohol.

AUDs are often missed in older adults because of reduced social and occupational functioning; signs more often include poor self-care, malnutrition, and medical illness. Because these disorders occur along a spectrum, it is recommended that all adults are screened for use with validated questionnaires that include the following:

- How many days per week?
- How many drinks on those days?
- Maximal intake on any one day?
- What type (ie, beer, wine, or liquor)?
- What is in "a drink"?

Hazardous or At-Risk Drinking

- Will probably eventually cause harm
- No current alcohol problems
- The National Institute on Alcohol Abuse and Alcoholism (NIAAA) defines at-risk drinking for men as 15 or more drinks/wk or 5 or more on one occasion and for women and anyone aged >65 as >7 drinks/wk or >3 drinks on one occasion.
- A standard drink is 12 oz beer, 5 oz of wine, or 1.5 oz of 80-proof liquor.

***DSM-5* Criteria for AUDs** (see Substance Use Disorders)

Alcohol Misuse Screening: CAGE questionnaire has been validated in the older population.

C Have you ever felt you should **C**ut down?

A Does others' criticism of your drinking **A**nnoy you?

G Have you ever felt **G**uilty about drinking?

E Have you ever had an "**E**ye opener" to steady your nerves or get rid of a hangover?

(Positive response to any suggests problem drinking.)

AUDIT-C

The Alcohol Use Disorders Identification Test Consumption Questions (AUDIT-C) identifies patients along the spectrum of unhealthy alcohol use. It can be self-administered, takes as little as 1–2 min via interview. Scoring (as shown) can also be linked to management (**Table 132**).

Management of Alcohol Use Disorders

First, decide on tx goals: abstinence is the traditional goal, but decreasing alcohol use or eliminating drinking in high-risk situations (eg, before driving, when caring for children) can reduce alcohol-related problems.

Brief Interventions

- *Primary care intervention*—effective for at-risk alcohol use; educate patient on effects of current drinking, point out current AEs, specify safe drinking limits (<7 drinks/wk, <3 on any 1 occasion); for function and longevity, the optimal amount of alcohol is no alcohol. Patients who cannot moderate should abstain.

- Medicare pays for annual screening and up to 4 brief counseling sessions for patients with at-risk drinking who are not yet experiencing adverse effects to their mental or emotional health. No copay or deductible when provided by a primary care provider who accepts assignment.
- The NIAAA provides an online resource: *The Healthcare Professional's Core Resource on Alcohol* (https://www.niaaa.nih.gov/health-professionals-communities/core-resource-on-alcohol)

Table 132. AUDIT-C

	Question	0 points	1 point	2 points	3 points	4 points
Scoring	1. How often did you have a drink containing alcohol in the past year?	Never	Monthly or less	2–4×/mo	2–3×/wk	≥4×/wk
	2. On days in the past year when you drank alcohol how many drinks did you typically drink?	1 or 2	3 or 4	5–6	7–9	10 or more
	3. How often do you have 6 or more drinks on an occasion in the past year?	Never	Less than monthly	Monthly	Weekly	Daily or Almost daily
Management	Total Score =	0–3	4–5	6–7	8–9	10–12
	Health Promotion	✓				
	Brief Intervention		✓	✓		
	Pharmacotherapy			+/–	✓	
	Psychosocial interventions			+/–	+/–	
	Specialty care management				+/–	✓

Psychosocial Interventions

- Have proven benefit for at-risk drinking through the spectrum of AUDs and include:
  - Motivational Interviewing—a counseling technique for eliciting behavior change by exploring and resolving the patient's ambivalence about change
  - CBT
  - Contingency management: creates a system of incentives for sustained abstinence and/or tx adherence

Self-help groups (eg, Alcoholics Anonymous, SMART [Self-Management and Recovery Training])

- Therapeutic communities either inpatient or outpatient

Pharmacotherapy (is underutilized; in the US only 10% of individuals with AUDs receive pharmacotherapy; patients with mild AUD may benefit, but studies are mainly with moderate or severe AUD). See **Table 133** for likely benefits.

- FDA approved
  - Naltrexone 25 mg po × 2 d then 50 mg po 1×/d; Depot naltrexone *(Vivitrol)* 380 mg IM monthly; monitor LFTs, avoid in kidney failure, liver disease and with opioid use. ADRs: ~10% get nausea, headache (L, K). Risk of injection site abscess with depot naltrexone.

- Acamprosate 666 mg q8h po, reduce dosage to 333 mg po q8h if CrCl 30–50 mL/min or weight <132 lb (60 kg); contraindicated if CrCl <30 mL/min; transient dose-related diarrhea is most common ADR (K).
- Addition of counseling to either acamprosate or naltrexone significantly improves abstinence rates (NNT=7.5 and NNT=8.6, respectively).

- Off-Label Alternatives
  - Topiramate 300 mg/d po is effective at reducing relapse; 75–100 mg may be effective. ADRs: cognitive impairment, paresthesia, weight loss, sedation, dizziness, depression
  - Gabapentin (900–1800 mg/d po) ADRs: sedation and edema.

Table 133. Pharmacotherapy for AUD: Expected Outcomes

	Outcomes				
	Abstinence		Reduced		
Drug	Initial	Maintenance	Drinks/d	% Days drinking	% Heavy drinking days
FDA-Approved First-line					
Naltrexone		reduces relapse	×	×	×
Acamprosate	Days increased by 10%	no reduction in relapse			by 11%
Off-Label Alternatives					
Topiramate	×		×	×	×
Gabapentin	only if high withdrawal symptoms in 2 wk before starting	×	×	×	only if high withdrawal symptoms in 2 wk before starting

- The duration of drug tx should be at least 6–12 mo, possibly indefinitely.
- Combining these agents does not improve effectiveness.
- Screen for psychiatric comorbidities; if depression persists after 1 wk of abstinence, tx for depression improves alcohol-related outcomes.
- Disulfiram has limited if any use in older people due to the possible serious (even lethal) consequences when consumed with alcohol.

TOBACCO USE DISORDERS AND SMOKING CESSATION

Smoking is associated with increased mortality, HTN, atherosclerosis, cerebrovascular accidents, increased risk of coronary events and cardiac deaths, decline in pulmonary function, COPD, smoking-related cancers, ED, development of osteoporosis, risk of hip fractures, loss of mobility, and poorer physical functioning.

Approach

First-line tx should include both behavioral tx **and** pharmacotherapy.

Cessation Intervention

Ask about tobacco use at every visit. **Advise** all users to quit; say “the most important thing you can do to improve your health.” **Assess** willingness to quit and when: “if not in the next month, how about in 3 months?” **Assist** the patient with a quit plan by offering both behavioral tx and pharmacotherapy, even if not ready to quit now. Starting tx before quitting improves long-term abstinence.

Offer and Connect to Treatment

- Offer first-line FDA-approved tx varenicline or combined nicotine replacement tx pch + prn gum, inhaler, nasal spray, lozenge (**Table 134**) to control craving.
- If first-line not tolerated or preferred, offer second-line: single nicotine replacement tx or bupropion.
- If second-line insufficient for abstinence offer combination tx:
  - Varenicline + nicotine replacement tx
  - Varenicline + bupropion
  - Bupropion + nicotine replacement tx
- Connect patients to behavioral support:
  - Refer to tobacco tx specialist
  - 1-800-QUIT-NOW for free phone counseling and free sample nicotine replacement tx
  - Smokefree.gov for free counseling by phone, text, or web-based

Pharmacotherapy (Table 134)

- Optimal duration of tx may be 3–6 mo or longer until the patient feels there is no further risk of relapse.
- Nicotine replacement tx is contraindicated with recent MI, uncontrolled high BP, arrhythmias, severe angina, and gastric ulcer.
- Varenicline slightly increases risk of neuropsychiatric disturbance in persons with hx of these disorders.
- E-cigarettes. The safety of e-cigarette and nicotine-vaping products is variable and some are harmful; lung injury and death has occurred related to some products. While there is increasing evidence of effectiveness (recommended for cessation in the UK), these are not recommended in US. If patient is using e-cigarettes with cigarettes, encourage use of only e-cigarettes.

Table 134. Pharmacotherapy for Tobacco Abuse

Drug	Dosage	Comments (Metabolism, Excretion)
Tobacco Abuse		
Bupropion SR	150 mg po q12h × 7–12 wk or longer	Contraindicated with seizure disorders, stroke, brain tumor, brain surgery (L)
Varenicline *(Chantix)*[1]	0.5 mg po × 3 d, 0.5 mg po q12h × 4 d, then 1 mg po q12h × 12–24 wk or longer	Start 7 d before quit date. AEs: nausea, vivid dreams, constipation, depression, small increased risk of cardiovascular events (L, K); reduce dosage if CrCl <30 mL/min

Nicotine Replacement: taper frequency of use and dose over 2–3 mo or longer

Product	Comment
Transdermal patches[1]	Apply to clean, nonhairy skin on upper torso, rotate sites; start 10–15 mg/d with CVD or body weight <100 lb or if smoking <10 cigarettes/d (L)
Polacrilex gum[1]	Chew 1 2-mg piece when urge to smoke; usual 10–12/d, max 30/d; 4 mg if smoking >21 cigarettes/d (L)
Lozenge[1]	Do not exceed 20/d; do not bite or chew; wean over 12 wk
Nasal spray *(Nicotrol NS)*	By prescription: 1 spr each nostril q30–60min; 0.5 mg/spr. Do not exceed 5 applications/h or 40 applications in 24 h; use should not exceed 3 mo
Inhaler *(Nicotrol Inhaler)*	By prescription. 6–16 cartridges/d; 4 mg delivered/cartridge. Max 16 cartridges/d

[1] Partial nicotine agonist that eases withdrawal and blocks effects of nicotine if patients resume smoking.

PRESCRIPTION DRUG USE DISORDERS

Diagnosis of Prescription Medication-Related Use Disorders—see *DSM-5* criteria to classify degree of misuse (p 352); Scope of the problem: prescription benzodiazepine misuse and abuse is highest in the age group 50–64 y; while misuse in those aged >65 is the lowest of all age groups.

Risk factors for prescription misuse/abuse include female sex, social isolation, depression, ADL/IADL disabilities and mental health problems.

Common Prescription Medications Associated with Use Disorders

According to the National Institute on Drug Abuse, the following 3 classes are most common:

- Opioids—usually prescribed to treat pain
- CNS depressants—used to treat anxiety and sleep disorders
- Stimulants—prescribed to treat attention deficit hyperactivity disorder and narcolepsy

Adverse Events

- Benzodiazepines: falls, mobility and ADL disability, cognitive impairment, motor vehicle accidents, pressure ulcers, UI
- Nonbenzodiazepine sedatives: anxiety, depression, nervousness, hallucinations, dizziness, headache, sleep-related behavioral disturbances
- Opioids: falls and fractures
- If a hx or current IV drug abuse, check for hepatitis C infection.

Assessing for Risk of Medication Misuse and Abuse

- Patient education on avoiding misuse is enhanced by a standard patient-prescriber agreement (eg, https://www.exchangecme.com/resourcePDF/btp/resource4.pdf).
- General risk factors include use of a psychoactive drug with abuse potential, use of other substances (alcohol, tobacco, etc), female sex, possibly social isolation, and hx of mental health disorder.
- Persons with a substance abuse hx are more likely to misuse opioids.
- Screen for risk of opioid misuse/abuse with the ORT-OUD, which differentiates low risk from high-risk patients.

Detection of Medication Misuse and Abuse

- Detection relies on clinical judgment; monitor at-risk patients when prescribing benzodiazepines, stimulants, and opioid analgesics.
- Federally mandated prescription drug monitoring programs (PDMPs) track controlled substances prescribed in a state and allow prescribers access to a database to identify other prescribers treating a patient (see Appropriate Prescribing, p 16).
- Observe for behavior that may suggest nonadherence to prescribed medication schedule (eg, early fill request, frequent lost prescriptions).
- Record any suspicious drug-seeking or other aberrant behaviors observed or reported by others, along with actions taken.
- Document evaluation process, rationale for long-term tx, and periodic review of patient status.
- Ask about purchases of medication over the Internet. Controlled substances can readily be purchased through illegitimate Internet-based pharmacies.

Management of Prescription Drug Abuse, Misuse, or Dependence

- Opioids
  - State guidelines require monitoring based on CDC recommendations for use of opioids for chronic pain: https://www.cdc.gov/mmwr/volumes/71/rr/rr7103a1.htm see Pain chapter (p 252).
  - May need to undergo medically supervised detoxification, combined with medications; buprenorphine/naloxone (*Suboxone)* or methadone are first-line tx, naltrexone ER is second-line tx. Behavioral tx might not always be needed.
  - Gradual tapering of opioids (Adjustment of Dosage, p 265) is less successful than pharmacotherapy.
- CNS depressants or stimulants (general rules)
  - Primary provider encouragement to reduce use
  - Behavioral tx is first-line tx.
  - Short-term substitution of other medications (eg, trazodone) or CBT for sleep (see Sleep, p 342)
  - Gradual slow tapering of the drug
- Benzodiazepine dependence
  - Studies show supervised gradual withdrawal to be most effective.
  - An effective program (EMPOWER; see Appropriate Prescribing chapter) uses patient education on adverse effects and very gradual withdrawal guided by symptoms over 4 mo to >1 y (see deprescribing.org; deprescribingresearch.org; or medstopper.com).
  - CBT is directed at the symptom for which the benzodiazepine was originally prescribed, most often insomnia or anxiety; for sleep-specific CBT, see p 343; limited data in older adults.

Medical Marijuana

- Effects of short-term use: impaired short-term memory (learning), impaired coordination (eg, reduced driving skills), altered judgment; in high doses, paranoia and psychosis
- Effects of long-term use: addiction (about 9% of users overall), cognitive impairment, decreased life satisfaction and attainment, chronic bronchitis, and psychosis
- Marijuana (cannabis sativa) contains more than 100 cannabinoids, 2 of which, tetrahydrocannabinol (THC) and cannabidiol (CBD), are considered for medicinal uses. THC is responsible for most AEs. All remain illegal under federal law and are not FDA regulated except for agents specifically approved (nabilone, dronabinol, *Epidiolex),* although most states have legalized some form of medical marijuana.
- **Table 135** summarizes available evidence for conditions studied in RCTs.
- Potential drug interactions: THC is a substrate for CYP2CP and CYP3A4. CBD is a potent inhibitor of CYP3A4, CYP2C19, and CYP2D6.
- For patients who tell you that they are already or plan to start to use CBD or THC, provide guidance (**Table 135**).

Table 135. Medical Reasons Why Adults May Want to Use Cannabis and Evidence for Effectiveness

	Formulation			
	Cannabidiol (low THC)		THC (variable) Cannabis	
Condition	Benefit/SOE	Notes	Benefit/SOE	Notes
Chronic or neuropathic pain	+/ Moderate	Not beneficial in cancer pain NNT=24 NH=6	+/ Substantial	NNT=24 NNH=6
Epilepsy	+/ Moderate	Studies in children; *Epidiolex* is FDA approved	–/ Insufficient	
Antiemetic for CINV		CBD oil is **not** recommended	+/ Substantial	Dronabinol is FDA approved
Insomnia			+/ Moderate	OSA, fibromyalgia, chronic pain, MS
Addiction and withdrawal tx	+/ Limited	Studied in cigarette, THC, heroin, opioid withdrawal		
MS-associated spasticity	+/ Limited		+/ Limited	Synthetic THC (dronabinol, nabiximol) has limited efficacy
Anxiety	+/ Limited	No psychoactive side effects	+/ Limited	
Appetite stimulation			+/ Limited	
Inflammatory bowel disease	+/ Limited	Rectal Sp may be beneficial	–/ Insufficient	
OA/tendinitis	+/ Limited	Topical may be more beneficial		
Dementia symptoms			–/ Limited	Two small studies indicate possible effectiveness
Depression			–/ Limited	Favors ineffective
Glaucoma			–/ Limited	Too short acting to be useful
Huntington disease	–/ Limited	Chorea not improved	–/ Insufficient	
Parkinson disease	+/–/ Limited	Benefits psychiatric but not motor symptoms	–/ Insufficient	

Sources: McDonagh MS et al. *Ann Intern Med* 2022. doi: 10.7326/M21-4520. Pisanti S et al. *Pharmacol Ther* 2017;175:133–150. National Academies of Sciences 2017. Washington DC: The National Academies Press. doi: 10.17226/24625.

CINV, chemotherapy-induced nausea and vomiting; IBS, irritable bowel syndrome; MS, multiple sclerosis; NNH, number needed to harm; NNT, number needed to treat; OSA, obstructive sleep apnea; PD, Parkinson disease; SOE, strength of evidence.

Table 136. Adverse Effects of Cannabis	
Acute	**Chronic**
Cardiovascular: tachycardia, HTN, palpitations, orthostatic hypotension	**Bone health:** reduced BMD
Respiratory: coughing, wheezing, increased sputum	**Respiratory:** chronic bronchitis, impaired alveolar macrophage activity
CNS: disorientation, sedation, dizziness, euphoria, dry mouth, slowed reaction time, impaired coordination, anxiety, psychosis	**CNS:** depression, impaired memory, attention, and decision making **Endocrine**: reduced testosterone **GI**: cannabinoid hyperemesis syndrome

- A 2021 meta-analysis of 46 RCTs (>6200 people aged >50 y [mean 58.6 y ± 7.5 y]) where ADRs were quantified reported that
  - THC-containing cannabinoid medications were associated with side effects of dry mouth, dizziness/lightheadedness, somnolence/drowsiness, disorientation, and impaired mobility, balance, or coordination.
  - THC-CBD combinations might be less acceptable at the dose ranges typically used in RCTs (>2:1 THC:CBD) and their tolerability might be different in people aged >65 and >75.
- A 2022 meta-analysis of 18 placebo-controlled randomized trials and 7 cohort studies (most enrollment for neuropathic pain) reported moderate improvement in pain with products with ≥ 2:1 THC:CBD ratios might be associated with short-term improvements in chronic pain, but increased dizziness and sedation.

COMMON DISORDERS

Breast Cancer

- Screen with mammography q1–2y until age 70–74, perhaps longer in women with life expectancy >10 y.[CW] Continued screening beyond age 75 did not reduce 8-y mortality (Medicare data).

Evaluation of patients over age 65 with newly diagnosed breast cancer should consist of:

- Assess life expectancy (**Table 3**, p 7) and discuss goals of care with the patient.
- The NCCN Clinical Practice Guidelines in Oncology *(NCCN Guidelines®)* recommend that clinicians consider the following 2 questions when evaluating older patients with cancer (breast and other cancers).
  - **Is the patient at moderate or high risk of dying or suffering from cancer considering her overall life expectancy?**
    - If **no**, patients with limited life expectancy and those who are too ill or frail to undergo surgery for the primary tumor, and whose tumors are ER-positive, can be offered tx with an aromatase inhibitor.
    - If **yes**, assess decision-making capacity and identify a surrogate if necessary (Assessment and Approach, **Figure 1**).
  - **Are there any concerns about the patient's ability to tolerate anticancer therapy?**
    - If **no**, screen for fitness using eg, frailty criteria from the Cardiovascular Health Study; (Assessment and Approach, p 14), or the Vulnerable Elders Survey (rand.org/health-care/projects/acove/survey.html), or the Geriatric-8 (siog.org/files/public/g8_english_0.pdf), or other frailty estimator.
      - If unimpaired on screening, may proceed to anticancer tx based on patient preference.
      - If impaired on screening, proceed to Comprehensive Geriatric Assessment (CGA).
    - If **yes**, proceed to CGA.
      - Assess functional status, cognition, social support, psychological status (anxiety/depression), nutrition, and medications (Assessment and Approach, **Table 1**).
      - Address factors identified in CGA before tx or adapt cancer tx plan to accommodate the identified issues.
- If the goal of care is cure or life prolongation, the next steps in evaluation are resection of the tumor and possibly sentinel lymph node (SLN) biopsy.
- Older women with clinically negative axillary exams, small (<2-cm tumors), and who will be treated with adjuvant HT may be managed without axillary surgery. Don't perform axillary lymph node (ALN) dissection for clinical stage I and II without attempting SLN biopsy.[CW]
- If an SLN biopsy is positive, ALN dissection, radiation tx, or both, should be considered depending on whether mastectomy or lumpectomy is planned, the extent of the tumor, and plans for systemic tx.
- Oncology assesses stage of disease and tumor biology to formulate a tx plan.
- Older women are more likely to experience lymphedema after ALN dissection.

Monitoring Women with a History of Breast Cancer

- Hx, physical exam q3–6mo for 3 y, then q6–12 mo for 2 y; pelvic exams as appropriate for age and health status
- Increase surveillance for second primary in breasts, ovaries, colon, and rectum
- Annual mammography

Oral Adjuvant Therapy for Breast Cancer

- Postmenopausal women with ER- or PR-positive tumors at high risk of recurrence (tumors >1 cm, or positive nodes) should be treated with oral adjuvant tx. Tx should be with an aromatase inhibitor (AI) for 5–7 y (**Table 137**).
- Long-term (>5 y) tx is associated with fractures and cardiovascular events.
- For women who wish to discontinue an AI at 5 y to avoid AEs, a switch to tamoxifen is reasonable.
  - Women with higher-risk disease (eg, T3 or lymph node positive), tx with an AI for 7 y is recommended.
  - For smaller node-negative tumors, it is not clear that risk of late recurrence justifies the risks of extended AI tx.
  - Women tolerating endocrine tx and who place a high value on minimizing risk of new breast cancers may choose extended AI tx; those who place a high value on avoiding ADRs may choose to stop after 5 y.
- Obtain BMD before initiating tx with an AI and initiate a bisphosphonate for T score ≤2.5 (Osteoporosis, p 246); encourage all to exercise and take in adequate oral calcium and vitamin D.
- Most patients treated with AIs will experience musculoskeletal side effects. Treat symptomatically (APAP, exercise) or switch to alternate AI or tamoxifen.
- Obtain baseline and sequential lipid profiles.
- Treat dyspareunia with water-soluble lubricants (Sexual Dysfunction, p 328). However, low-dose vaginal estrogens can be used for intractable vaginal symptoms.

Table 137. Oral Agents for Breast Cancer Treatment

Class, Medication	Monitoring	Adverse Events, Interactions (Metabolism)
Antiestrogen Drugs		
Tamoxifen[1]	Annual eye exam; endometrial cancer screening	Avoid fluoxetine, paroxetine, bupropion, duloxetine, and other potent CYPD26 inhibitors that reduce tamoxifen activity; ↑ risk of thrombosis (L)
Toremifene	CBC, Ca, LFTs, BUN, Cr	Drug interactions: CYP3A4–6 inhibitors and inducers; ↑ warfarin effect (L)
Aromatase Inhibitors	*Class AEs*: arthritis, arthralgia, bone pain, carpal tunnel, alteration in lipid profiles, sexual dysfunction, dyspareunia *Other AEs*: fatigue, sleep disorders, self-reported cognitive impairment, depression, asthenia, fracture, MI or ischemia, anemia, leukopenia, pancytopenia, hot flushes, fractures, vaginal bleeding (L)	
Anastrozole	Periodic CBC, lipids, serum chemistry profile, TSH	Inhibits CYP1A2, CYP2C8/9, and CYP3A4
Exemestane		Metabolized by CYP3A4 and aldo-keto reductases; does not inhibit any of the major CYP enzymes
Letrozole		Metabolized by CYP3A4, CYP2A6; strongly inhibits CYP2A6 and moderately inhibits CYP2C19

[1] Reduce dosage if CrCl <10 mL/min.

Adjuvant Chemotherapy: Is used after resection. Reduces risk of recurrence and improves survival, especially when risk of recurrence is >10% at 10 y. Recurrence is reduced by 30–50% with greater benefit in ER-poor or ER-absent breast cancer.

Bisphosphonates:

- Are commonly used in postmenopausal women on other adjuvant tx for breast cancer.
- Among postmenopausal women, bisphosphonate tx reduces bone recurrence, fractures, and breast cancer mortality, and improves overall survival.
- As an adjuvant tx for breast cancer, the recommended dose of zoledronic acid is 4 mg IV q6mo for 3–5 y in women at intermediate and high risk for recurrence.

Therapy for Metastatic Bone Disease: Denosumab monthly or zoledronic acid q3mo reduces time to onset of new skeletal-related events. Denosumab is somewhat more effective.

Cervical Cancer

Prevalence

- More than 20% (US data) or 50% (UK data) of cervical cancers occur in women after age 65.
- In part, the increase is due to a decline in hysterectomy and risk is higher in Black women.

Screening

- Decisions whether to screen should be consistent with life expectancy and goals of care.
- Recommendations by the USPSTF against cervical cancer screening in women age >65 apply only to those who have *had adequate prior screening* (D level recommendation) that includes:
  - 3 consecutive negative cytology ***or***
  - 2 consecutive negative Pap/HPV cotests with the last negative test within 5 y of turning 65
- Some consider screening is less accurate because atrophy affects cytology; however, this does ***not*** apply to HPV testing, which can either be performed in the clinic or using home self-swabbing.

Vulvar Diseases

Nonneoplastic

Patients often do not report symptoms (burning, itching) unless asked.

Table 138. Common Vulvar Dermatoses

Condition	Clinical Presentation and Distribution	Characteristics Used in Diagnosis	Management
Candida vulvovaginitis	Burning, itching, pain involving vulva, vagina, perineum	Classic "satellite" lesions surrounding areas of erythema	Topical antifungal,[1] plus topical steroid speeds relief of symptoms (eg, betamethasone dipropionate 0.05%, clotrimazole 1%); **Table 46**.
Contact dermatitis	Burning, itching over the hair-bearing cutaneous vulva and surrounding skin	Erythema in areas of contact with pads or skincare products, look for superimposed candida	Eliminate offending garment or skincare product

(cont.)

Condition	Clinical Presentation and Distribution	Characteristics Used in Diagnosis	Management
Lichen sclerosis[2]	Burning, itching, or asymptomatic involving the labia minora, majora, clitoral hood; may involve perianus in classic hourglass distribution	Circumscribed pallor, scarring may cause loss of labia minora, stenosis of introitus Biopsy if diagnosis is in doubt, failure to respond to superpotency steroid, or any suspicious areas	Superpotency steroid (**Table 47**) topically q24h for 4 wk, then every other day ×4 wk, then 2–3×/wk for 4 wk and prn
Lichen simplex chronicus	Chronic or intermittent pruritus; often worse in evening or night over the hair-bearing cutaneous vulva	Epidermal thickening, lichenified papules and plaques, ill-demarcated erythema, linear excoriations, erosions	Eliminate all but hypoallergenic skincare products; break scratch-itch cycle with midpotency steroid topically daily for 4 wk (**Table 47**)
Lichen planus	Pain, burning of the labia minora and introitus; most have lesions on either skin, nails, or oral mucosa	Most commonly: bright erythema and erosions, surrounded by white reticulated rim, scarring, vaginal stenosis	Topical superpotency steroids (**Table 47**), but often not sufficient. Often add topical calcineurin inhibitors, oral steroids, etc
Psoriasis	Mild to severe pruritus; pain or burning involving hair-bearing cutaneous vulva, 95% have psoriatic lesions elsewhere	Classic plaque or inverse psoriasis (very red lesions that characteristically appear in body folds)	Topical steroids (**Table 47**), topical vitamin D analogs; topical calcineurin inhibitors; severe disease refer to dermatology.

[1] Severe cases may require oral fluconazole.

[2] Associated with a low risk of SCC; examine the vulva at least yearly, biopsy all suspicious lesions. Ask patients to look at the skin and search for lumps or nonhealing sores monthly.

Neoplastic Vulvar Diseases

- VIN may be asymptomatic or may cause pruritus or dysuria; hypo- or hyperpigmented keratinized plaques most often on the nonhairy areas of the vulva; often multifocal; inspection ± colposcopy of the entire vulva with biopsy of most worrisome lesions; lesions graded on degree of atypia. Tx: surgical or laser ablative tx.
- Vulvar malignancy—Half of cases are in women aged >70; 80% are SCC, with melanoma, sarcoma, basal cell carcinoma, and adenocarcinoma <20%; biopsy any suspicious lesion. Tx: SCC depends on presence of positive nodes and extent of lesion; vulvectomy, radical local excision, or 3-incision surgical techniques.

Postmenopausal Bleeding

Defined as bleeding after 1 y of amenorrhea:

- Exclude malignancy (the cause in 10% of cases), identify source (vagina, cervix, vulva, uterus, bladder, bowel); atrophy of the vagina or endometrium is the most common cause.
- Examine genitalia, perineum, rectum, and obtain cervical cytology.
- If endometrial source, use endometrial biopsy or vaginal probe ultrasound to assess endometrial thickness (<5 mm virtually excludes malignancy).
- D&C when endometrium not otherwise adequately assessed when bleeding reoccurs and when ultrasound shows heterogeneity.

- Evaluation is needed for:
  - Women on combination continual estrogen and progesterone who bleed after 12 mo.
  - Women on cyclic replacement with bleeding at unexpected times (ie, bleeding other than during the second wk of progesterone tx).
  - Women on unopposed estrogen who bleed at any time.

Vaginal Prolapse

- Child-bearing and other causes of increased intra-abdominal pressure weaken connective tissue and muscles supporting the genital organs, leading to prolapse.
- Symptoms include pelvic pressure, back pain, FI, UI, or difficulty evacuating the rectum. Symptoms may be present even with mild prolapse.
- The degree of prolapse and organs involved dictate tx; no tx if asymptomatic.
- Estrogen and pelvic floor muscle training (PFMT) exercises (p 173) may help in mild cases.
- Pessary or surgery indicated with increase in symptoms. Don't exclude pessaries as an option for prolapse.[CW] Surgery needed for fourth-degree symptomatic prolapse.
- Pessaries in addition to PFMT probably improve pelvic organ prolapse symptoms and prolapse-specific quality of life.
- Precise anatomic defect(s) dictates the surgical approach.
- Surgical closure of the vagina (colpocleisis) corrects prolapse as a simple option for frail patients who are not sexually active.
- A common classification (American College of Obstetrics and Gynecology) for degrees of prolapse:
  - First degree—extension to midvagina
  - Second degree—approaching hymenal ring
  - Third degree—at hymenal ring
  - Fourth degree—beyond hymenal ring

HORMONE THERAPY (HT)

Symptoms Associated with the Postmenopausal State

- Hot flushes and night sweats (ie, vasomotor symptoms)
- Sleep disturbances (may affect mood, memory, metabolic syndrome, obesity, and cardiovascular risk)
- Vaginal dryness and dyspareunia (GSM); see Sexuality, p 324
- Depression
- Insufficient evidence exists to link the following commonly reported symptoms to the postmenopausal state: cognitive disturbances, fatigue, sexual dysfunction.

Therapy for Menopausal Symptoms

- Vasomotor and vaginal symptoms respond to estrogen[BC] in a dose-response fashion; start at low dosage (eg, conjugated or esterified estrogen 0.3 mg/d po, which should be combined with medroxyprogesterone or bazedoxifene in women with an intact uterus), titrate to effect.
- Dyspareunia and vaginal dryness respond to either water-soluble moisturizers or lubricants or topical estrogen, ospemifene or prasterone (**Table 127** [see Female Sexual Dysfunction]).
- Conjugated estrogens 0.45 mg/bazedoxifene 20 mg *(Duavee)* po 1×d treats menopausal symptoms without apparent ADRs on the uterus.

- Bioidentical hormone therapy refers to the use of naturally occurring (rather than synthetic or animal-derived) forms of progesterone, estradiol, and estriol. These preparations are compounded by pharmacies and readily available over the Internet but are not FDA approved. Although evidence on their efficacy in controlling symptoms is accumulating, the FDA and the Endocrine Society concur that evidence to evaluate the safety of these agents is insufficient relative to FDA-approved menopausal HT.

Contraindications to Hormone Therapy

- Undiagnosed vaginal bleeding
- Thromboembolic disease
- Breast cancer
- Prior stroke or TIA
- Endometrial cancer more advanced than Stage 1
- Possibly gallbladder disease
- CHD

Risk of Hormone Therapy

- Risks associated with HT use vary based on the length of time between menopause and initiation of HT. For information on the risks and benefits of HT initiated within the first 10 y after menopause (below age 60), see the position statement of the North American Menopause Society (NAMS) at www.menopause.org/docs/default-source/professional/nams-2022-hormone-therapy-position-statement.pdf.
- Overall, HT use in the 50-59 y age group when following the NAMS recommendations is considered safe and may even be beneficial.
- For women taking combined HT, the risk of breast cancer in average-risk women becomes significant at 5 y on tx.
- Beginning HT in women >10 y after menopause or over age 60 is not recommended due to increased risk of MI, DVT, PE, stroke, kidney stones, dementia, and ovarian cancer.
- Women aged ≥60 who started HT at earlier ages should be counselled on the risks and benefits of continuing or withdrawing HT based on individual benefit and harm:
  - Longer durations of tx should be for documented indications (eg, persistent vasomotor symptoms), with shared decision-making and periodic reevaluation.
  - If ongoing vasomotor symptoms and intolerance of other osteoporosis tx, benefits of HT may exceed harm.
  - There is consensus that if HT is continued, it should be at the lowest effective dose and with the safest route, with periodic attempts to trial lower doses or taper and discontinue.
  - Transdermal estrogen is safer for patients who are obese (BMI ≥30), have elevated TG, or have liver disease.
- Older women can get hot flashes if estrogen is discontinued suddenly. Tapering (eg, q48h for 1–2 mo and then q72h for a few months) may be better tolerated.
- The fracture-protective effect from HT is lost rapidly after discontinuation; women at risk of fracture should be evaluated and treated with alternative tx (Osteoporosis, p 246).

Persisting Severe Vasomotor Symptoms After Age 60

- 10% of women continue with vasomotor symptoms 12 y after menopause (on average age >60 y).
- Non–HT tx with safety and effectiveness suggests considering agents in the following sequence:
  - First, antidepressants. SSRIs[BC] and SNRIs[BC] seem to have similar modest beneficial effect: citalopram 10–20 mg/d po; escitalopram 5–20 mg/d po, venlafaxine 75 mg/d po; desvenlafaxine 50–200 mg/d po
  - Avoid paroxetine, sertraline, fluoxetine in patients receiving tamoxifen (**Table 137**); tamoxifen levels will be subtherapeutic; sertraline and fluoxetine do not appear to reduce vasomotor symptoms.

- Second, anticonvulsants: gabapentin[BC] 300 mg po 3×/d or 100–300 mg po hs for primarily nocturnal hot flashes; pregabalin[BC] 75–300 mg/d po.
- Third, α_2-Adrenergic agonists: clonidine 0.1–0.3 mg/d transdermal (Avoid in HTN[BC]); watch for orthostatic hypotension and rebound increase in BP if used intermittently. Common ADRs: dry mouth, constipation, sedation.
- Oxybutynin[BC] 5–10 mg/d po has also shown effectiveness.

CODING IN GERIATRICS 2023

Peter Hollmann, MD, AGSF, 1/3/2023

Geriatricians focus on Medicare, but private payers—including Medicare Advantage plans—may use other valid CPT and HCPCS codes. Every procedure code (CPT or HCPCS) must be accompanied with a diagnosis code (ICD-10). The listed codes are particularly relevant for services performed by geriatrics healthcare professionals, but are not a complete list of all services geriatricians perform. CPT 2023 is an essential reference. A good reference on Medicare rules is the *Medicare Internet-Only Manual for Claims Processing of Physician and Professional Services. Manual 100-4 (Claims Processing),* Chapter 12: https://www.cms.gov/regulations-and-guidance/guidance/manuals/downloads/clm104c12.pdf.

Codes that are new in 2023 are starred (*).

In 2023, all the codes that used history, exam and medical decision making for level selection are now like the Office Visit codes. Medical Decision Making or Total Time on the Date of the Encounter are used for code selection. The AMA has educational materials at ama-assn.org/practice-management/cpt/cpt-evaluation-and-management. Home and ALF codes were merged as were Observation and Hospital Inpatient.

During the Public Health Emergency (PHE), Medicare allows telehealth provided to a patient in their home to be reported as if it was in the office. Telephone codes are allowed. Some services must be audio-video and some may be audio only (eg, the annual wellness visit). https://www.cms.gov/Medicare/Medicare-General-Information/Telehealth/Telehealth-Codes

In 2023 the rules about split (shared) visits are unchanged from 2022 and detailed in the internet manual 100-4, chapter 12 Section 30.6.18.

For a recording on the annual AGS webinar on coding changes, visit geriatricscareonline.org.

All non–face to face services require annual patient consent for payment.

Common Procedure Codes

Procedure Code	Description	Reference/Notes
Evaluation and Management		
99202-99215	Office/Outpatient Visits	Also used for Office/Outpatient (including observation status) Consultations when reporting to Medicare
99221-99223 99231-99233 99234-99236	Hospital Inpatient/Observation	
99242-99245 99252-99255	Consultations	Invalid for Medicare, but may be used by other payers. For Medicare use 99202-99215 for outpatient: 99221-99223, for inpatient: and 99304-99306 for nursing facility. 100-4; 12; 30.6.10
99291-99292	Critical Care	Used in all settings of care, not just the ICU; geriatrician relevant.
99304-99316	Nursing facility Services	See CPT NF code section for a special problem type
99341-99350	Home Services	
99358-99359	Prolonged Services	99358 is for non–face to face services and is no longer allowed by CMS.

(cont.)

99417, 99418* G2211, G0316* G0317*, G0318*		CPT created outpatient (99417) and inpatient (99418) prolonged services codes. CMS disagreed with the start time of prolonged services and created G codes for the same 15 min, but with later start times. They measure time over multiple days for home and NF codes. See page 69614 in the Federal Register: https://www.govinfo.gov/content/pkg/FR-2022-11-18/pdf/2022-23873.pdf
99387, 99397	Comprehensive Preventive Medicine	Non-covered Medicare (see Medicare Preventive Services), may be used by other payers such as Medicare Advantage plans.
99446-99449, 99451, 99452	Interprofessional Telephone/Internet/EHR Consultations	New codes in 2019 and recognized payment for existing codes. Includes "eConsult" and "eReferral."
99483	Cognition Assessment and Care Plan	An assessment for cognition and must include creation of a care plan that is shared with patient and/or caregiver. May not report with other E/M.
99497 99498	Advance Care Planning	If done with IPPE/AWV, use -33 modifier so no patient cost share.

Care Management

cms.gov/Medicare/Medicare-Fee-for-Service-Payment/PhysicianFeeSched/Care-Management.html

99457 99458	Remote physiologic monitoring treatment management	This is similar to CCM, but does not require a care plan, advanced practice, or ≥2 conditions. An example is CHF monitoring management.
99487 99489 99490 99439 99491 99437	Chronic Care Management and Complex CCM	Monthly time-based codes with required services and practice structures (eg, EMR).
99424 99425 99426 99427	Principal Care Management	These are very similar to 99491 (99424 and 99425 for physicians and qualified health care professional time) and 99490 (99426 and 99427 for 30 min of clinical staff time). They are for patients with a single condition of sufficient severity to place the patient at risk of hospitalization or that has been the cause of a recent hospitalization. The practice must have the attributes of a CCM practice, but the care plan is disease specific. There is a limit of 2 units for 99427
99495 99496	Transitional Care Management Services	For 30 d postdischarge hospital/obs or SNF. In 2020, CMS removed almost all exclusions for other services in the same 30 d.
99484 G0323*	Care management for behavioral health conditions	This is the BH equivalent of 99490, except that there does not need to be either a comprehensive care plan or practice requirements, such as EMR G0323 is when the time is spent by a psychologist or licensed social worker.

(cont.)

G0506	Comprehensive assessment of and care planning for patients requiring chronic care management services (list separately in addition to primary monthly care management service) (Add-on)	This is for assessment and care management initiation that is beyond the reported E/M initiating visit. It is added to the E/M or Medicare IPPE/AWV code.
Digital Services and Telephone Services		
99091	Collection and interpretation of physiologic data, 30 mins, each 30 d	May use for 30 min of physician time in 30 d when no more specific code exists. Can use with Care Management codes.
G2010	Image evaluation	HCPCS code for the interpretation of an image sent by the patient with report back to the patient
G2012 G2252	Remote check-in	A check-in with patient to avoid a face-to-face visit. During the PHE these codes are less useful than 99441-99443.
99421-99423 98970-98972	Online digital E/M	CPT created a set of time-based codes for professionals who can report E/M (99421-99423) and those who cannot (98970-98972). CPT outlines extensive rules.
99441-99443	Telephone Services	During the PHE these are covered and pay at the level of 99212-99214.
	Medicare Preventive Services	
G0008, G0009	Flu and Pneumonia Vaccine Administration	Use CPT and Q codes for vaccine supply
G0402	IPPE "Welcome to Medicare" Preventive Exam	If necessary and performed, E/M may be reported same date with modifier -25.
G0438 G0439	Annual Wellness Visits	If necessary and performed, E/M may be reported same date with modifier -25.
G0442 G0444	Alcohol misuse Screening Depression Screening	Medicare relabeled these as 5-15 minutes in 2023. (5 is a minimum).

(cont.)

Other Important Procedure Codes		
93793	Warfarin Management	Use for each INR reviewed with follow-up instructions to patient.
G0179, G0180	Home Care Certification	These services are for time spent with professionals on patients who are receiving covered home care or hospice.
G0181, G0182	Home/Hospice Care Plan Oversight	Manuals: 100-2 Chapters 7 and 9; 100-1 Chapter 4 https://www.cms.gov/Regulations-and-Guidance/Guidance/Manuals/Downloads/ge101c04.pdf https://www.cms.gov/Regulations-and-Guidance/Guidance/Manuals/Downloads/bp102c07.pdf https://www.cms.gov/Regulations-and-Guidance/Guidance/Manuals/Downloads/bp102c09.pdf
HCPCS "J" codes	Codes for drugs administered (eg, steroids)	

Many other codes are relevant to practice (eg, EKG), but for brevity are not listed. Psychiatric Collaborative Care Management, Mental Health, and Neuropsychological Testing codes are not listed. RHCs and FQHCs use different codes for Care Management.

Index

Page references followed by *t* and *f* indicate tables and figures, respectively.

Trade names are in *italics*.

D

E

G

H

J

K

M

S

V

X

Y

Z